Atlas of Cardiovascular Emergencies

NOTICE

Medicine is an ever-changing science. As new research and clinical experience broaden our knowledge, changes in treatment and drug therapy are required. The authors and the publisher of this work have checked with sources believed to be reliable in their efforts to provide information that is complete and generally in accord with the standards accepted at the time of publication. However, in view of the possibility of human error or changes in medical sciences, neither the authors nor the publisher nor any other party who has been involved in the preparation or publication of this work warrants that the information contained herein is in every respect accurate or complete, and they disclaim all responsibility for any errors or omissions or for the results obtained from use of the information contained in this work. Readers are encouraged to confirm the information contained herein with other sources. For example and in particular, readers are advised to check the product information sheet included in the package of each drug they plan to administer to be certain that the information contained in this work is accurate and that changes have not been made in the recommended dose or in the contraindications for administration. This recommendation is of particular importance in connection with new or infrequently used drugs.

Atlas of Cardiovascular Emergencies

Editors

Cedric Lefebvre, MD
Assistant Professor
Department of Emergency Medicine
Wake Forest School of Medicine
Winston-Salem, North Carolina

James C. O'Neill, MD
Assistant Professor
Department of Emergency Medicine
Wake Forest School of Medicine
Winston-Salem, North Carolina

David M. Cline, MD
Professor
Department of Emergency Medicine
Wake Forest School of Medicine
Winston-Salem, North Carolina

New York   Chicago   San Francisco   Athens   London   Madrid
Mexico City   Milan   Singapore   Sydney   Toronto

Atlas of Cardiovascular Emergencies

Copyright © 2015 by McGraw-Hill Education. All rights reserved. Printed in China. Except as permitted under the United States Copyright Act of 1976, no part of this publication may be reproduced or distributed in any form or by any means, or stored in a database or retrieval system, without the prior written permission of the publisher.

1 2 3 4 5 6 7 8 9 0   CTP/CTP   19 18 17 16 15

ISBN 978-0-07-179394-0
MHID 0-07-179394-1

This book was set in Minion Pro Regular by MPS Limited.
The editors were Anne M. Sydor, Brian Belval, and Peter J. Boyle.
The production supervisor was Catherine H. Saggese.
Project management was provided by Vipra Fauzdar, MPS Limited.
The cover designer was Thomas De Pierro.
China Translation & Printing Services, Ltd., was printer and binder.

This book was printed on acid-free paper.

Cataloging-in-publication data for this book is on file at the Library of Congress.

McGraw-Hill Education books are available at special quantity discounts to use as premiums and sales promotions, or for use in corporate training programs. To contact a representative please visit the Contact Us pages at www.mhprofessional.com.

To my wife, Jen, and my daughters, Ava and Alexis, for their love and encouragement; to my parents and Isabella for their steadfast support; to my residents and faculty colleagues for their collaboration on this project; and to Frank, Maggie, and José, for inspiring me to explore the world of medical science.

Cedric Lefebvre

To my wife, Spence, my boys, Frank and Steven, my parents, Frank and Patricia, for all their enduring support and love, and to the residents and fellows who have inspired and challenged me.

James C. O'Neill

To my family for their continued support, to my fellow faculty who contributed to this project, to the residents and students who inspired me to take on this project by asking questions I could not answer without images to illustrate my point.

David M. Cline

Contributors ix
Preface xv
Acknowledgments xvii

Chapter 1
ANATOMY 1

NORMAL CORONARY ARTERY ANATOMY 2
NORMAL CHAMBERS 4
NORMAL VALVES 6
PROSTHETIC VALVES 8
ANOMALOUS LEFT CORONARY ARTERY 10
DEXTROCARDIA 12

Chapter 2
ELECTROCARDIOGRAPHY: NORMAL HEART, ACUTE ISCHEMIA, AND CHRONIC DISEASE 13

Normal Heart 14
NORMAL CARDIAC CONDUCTION 14
NORMAL RESTING ELECTROCARDIOGRAM (ECG) 16

Acute Ischemia and Chronic Disease 18
SUPPLEMENTAL ECG LEADS 18
ST-ELEVATION MYOCARDIAL INFARCTION (BY ANATOMIC REGION, INCLUDES SGARBOSSA CRITERIA) 23
T-WAVE INVERSION 28
HYPERACUTE T-WAVES 29
ST SEGMENT DEPRESSION 30
Q WAVES 32
WELLENS' SYNDROME 33

Chapter 3
PRINCIPLES OF CARDIOVASCULAR IMAGING 35

CHEST RADIOGRAPHS 36
BEDSIDE ULTRASOUND/ECHOCARDIOGRAPHY 39
TRANSTHORACIC ECHOCARDIOGRAPHY 43
TRANSESOPHAGEAL ECHOCARDIOGRAPHY 46
BEDSIDE ULTRASOUND: EVALUATION FOR DEEP VEIN THROMBOSIS 51
CARDIAC COMPUTED TOMOGRAPHY 56
CARDIAC MAGNETIC RESONANCE IMAGING 59
CT ANGIOGRAM FOR PULMONARY EMBOLISM 62
VENTILATION/PERFUSION SCAN (V/Q SCAN) 64
DOPPLER ULTRASOUND OF PERIPHERAL VENOUS SYSTEM 66
DOPPLER ULTRASOUND OF PERIPHERAL ARTERIAL SYSTEM 70
ULTRASOUND GUIDED VASCULAR ACCESS 72

Chapter 4
DEVICES 77

TRANSCUTANEOUS PACEMAKER 78
TRANSVENOUS PACEMAKER 81
COMPLICATIONS OF IMPLANTED PACEMAKERS 84
IMPLANTED CARDIOVERTER-DEFIBRILLATOR: COMPLICATIONS 88
LVAD: LEFT VENTRICULAR ASSIST DEVICE 90
AUTOMATED CPR DEVICE 92
EXTERNAL RHYTHM RECORDER: HOLTER MONITOR AND KING OF HEARTS 94
EXTRACORPOREAL MEMBRANE OXYGENATION 96

Chapter 5
ARRHYTHMIAS 99

Sinus Arrhythmias 100
SINUS BRADYCARDIA/TACHYCARDIA INCLUDING RESPIRATORY VARIABLITY 100

Atrial Arrhythmias 103
PREMATURE ATRIAL CONTRACTIONS (PAC) 103
WANDERING ATRIAL PACEMAKER 105
CLASSIFICATION AND MECHANISMS OF SUPRAVENTRICULAR TACHYCARDIA 107

Atrioventricular Tachycardias 111
AV NODAL REENTRY TACHYCARDIA SLOW-FAST CONDUCTION, FAST-SLOW CONDUCTION 111
AV RECIPROCATING TACHYCARDIA, ORTHODROMIC AVRT, ANTIDROMIC AVRT 113
WOLFF–PARKINSON–WHITE SYNDROME AND PRE-EXCITATION SYNDROMES 116
LOWN–GANONG–LEVINE SYNDROME 119

Atrial Tachycardias 120
MULTIFOCAL ATRIAL TACHYCARDIA 120
ECTOPIC (UNIFOCAL) ATRIAL TACHYCARDIA 122
ATRIAL FLUTTER 124

ATRIAL FIBRILLATION WITH/WITHOUT
RVR, WITH ABERRANCY 126

Aberrant Atrial Conduction 128
ASHMAN PHENOMENA, ATRIAL FIBRILLATION WITH
PREMATURE SUPRAVENTRICULAR
ABERRANT BEATS 128

Junctional Rhythms 129
JUNCTIONAL ESCAPE RHYTHM 129
JUNCTIONAL TACHYCARDIA 131

Ventricular Arrhythmias 133
PREMATURE VENTRICULAR CONTRACTIONS 133
ACCELERATED IDIOVENTRICULAR RHYTHM 135
VENTRICULAR TACHYCARDIA INCLUDING
POLYMORPHIC, MONOMORPHIC 137
TORSADES DE POINTES 139
VENTRICULAR FIBRILLATION 141
BRUGADA SYNDROME 144

Conduction Disorders 146
FIRST-DEGREE ATRIOVENTRICULAR BLOCK 146
SECOND-DEGREE-ATRIOVENTRICULAR BLOCK,
MOBITZ TYPE I 149
SECOND-DEGREE-ATRIOVENTRICULAR BLOCK,
MOBITZ TYPE II 151
THIRD-DEGREE ATRIOVENTRICULAR BLOCK 153
BIFASCICULAR BLOCK 155
LEFT ANTERIOR FASCICULAR BLOCK 157
RIGHT BUNDLE BRANCH BLOCK 159
LEFT BUNDLE BRANCH BLOCK 161
LONG QT SYNDROME 162

Pacemaker Rhythms 164
ECG INTERPRETATION OF PACED RHYTHM 164

Chapter 6
VASCULAR DISEASE 169

ABDOMINAL AORTIC ANEURYSM 170
AORTIC DISSECTION 172
ACUTE ARTERIAL OCCLUSION 174
DVT: UPPER/LOWER, PHLEGMASIA ALBA DOLENS,
PHLEGMASIA CERULEA DOLENS 176
PULMONARY EMBOLISM 178
SYSTEMIC AND PULMONARY HYPERTENSION 181
LEFT VENTRICULAR ANEUYRSM 185

Chapter 7
CARDIOMYOPATHIES 187

DILATED CARDIOMYOPATHY 188
RESTRICTIVE CARDIOMYOPATHIES 190
HYPERTROPHIC CARDIOMYOPATHY 193
AORTIC STENOSIS 196
MITRAL STENOSIS 199
ACUTE AORTIC INSUFFICIENCY 201
MITRAL REGURGITATION AND ACUTE MITRAL INSUFFICIENCY 203

Chapter 8
PEDIATRIC CARDIOLOGY 207

Pediatric Electrocardiogram Norms 208
NORMAL ECG AT AGE INTERVALS (NEWBORN,
1MO, 3MO, 12MO, 3Y, 5Y, 8Y, 13Y) 208

Congenital Heart Disease 214
NEONATAL CONGENITAL HEART DISEASE 214
INFANTILE CONGENITAL HEART DISEASE 217
PEDIATRIC CONGENITAL HEART DISEASE 221

Inflamatory and Infectious Disorders 225
MYOCARDITIS AND PERICARDITIS 225
KAWASAKI DISEASE 230
RHEUMATIC HEART DISEASE 232

Obstructive Shock 234
CARDIAC TAMPONADE 234

Cardiac Rhythm Disorders 237
SUPRAVENTRICULAR TACHYCARDIA IN CHILDREN 237
HEART BLOCK IN CHILDREN 241
WOLFF–PARKINSON–WHITE IN CHILDREN 245
LONG QT SYNDROME IN CHILDREN 248

Chapter 9
PROCEDURES 251

RADIOFREQUENCY ABLATION 252
ANKLE BRACHIAL INDEX 254
CARDIAC CATHETERIZATION 256
PERICARDIOCENTESIS 261
PERICARDIAL WINDOW 263
CARDIOVERSION/EXTERNAL DEFIBRILLATION 265

INDEX 267

CONTRIBUTORS

William Alley, MD, RDMS
Assistant Professor
Department of Emergency Medicine
Wake Forest School of Medicine
Winston-Salem, North Carolina
Chapter 3

Kim Askew, MD
Assistant Professor
Department of Emergency Medicine
Wake Forest School of Medicine
Winston-Salem, North Carolina
Chapter 5

Shad Baab, MD, FAAP
Assistant Professor
Department of Emergency Medicine
Wake Forest School of Medicine
Winston-Salem, North Carolina
Chapter 8

P. Matthew Belford, MD, FACC
Assistant Professor
Department of Medicine
Section on Cardiology
Wake Forest School of Medicine
Winston-Salem, North Carolina
Chapter 9

Erin Boyd, DO
Clinical Instructor
Department of Emergency Medicine
Wake Forest School of Medicine
Winston-Salem, North Carolina
Chapter 5

Glenn M. Brammer, MD
Assistant Professor
Department of Medicine
Section on Cardiology
Wake Forest School of Medicine
Winston-Salem, North Carolina
Chapters 4 and 5

Joshua S. Broder, MD
Associate Professor
Department of Surgery,
Division of Emergency Medicine
Duke University School of Medicine
Durham, North Carolina
Chapters 1 and 6

Ron Buchheit, MD
Instructor
Department of Emergency Medicine
University of Tennessee College of Medicine Chattanooga
Chattanooga, Tennessee
Chapter 5

Joseph Hayes Calvert, DO
Clinical Instructor
Department of Emergency Medicine
Wake Forest School of Medicine
Winston-Salem, North Carolina
Chapter 5

Cheryl Cammock, MD
Assistant Professor
Department of Pediatrics
Section of Cardiology
Wake Forest School of Medicine
Winston-Salem, North Carolina
Chapter 8

Alan T. Chiem, MD, MPH
Assistant Clinical Professor
Department of Emergency Medicine
Olive View-UCLA Medical Center
Geffen School of Medicine at UCLA
Los Angeles, California
Chapters 2 and 8

Jason W. Christie, MD
Fellow in Vascular Surgery
Department of Vascular and Endovascular Surgery
Wake Forest School of Medicine
Winston-Salem, North Carolina
Chapter 3

David M. Cline, MD
Professor
Department of Emergency Medicine
Wake Forest School of Medicine
Winston-Salem, North Carolina
Chapters 5 and 6

Kristi Colbenson, MD
Fellow in Sports Medicine
Department of Orthopedics
Vanderbilt University
Nashville, Tennessee
Chapter 7

Sean Collins, MD, MSc
Associate Professor
Department of Emergency Medicine
Vanderbilt University
Nashville, Tennessee
Chapter 7

Thomas D. Conlee, MD
Fellow in Vascular Surgery
Department of Vascular and Endovascular Surgery
Wake Forest School of Medicine
Winston-Salem, North Carolina
Chapter 3

CONTRIBUTORS

Casey Jae Davis, MD
Resident in Emergency Medicine
Department of Emergency Medicine
Wake Forest School of Medicine
Winston-Salem, North Carolina
Chapter 9

Deborah Diercks, MD, MSc
Professor
Department of Emergency Medicine
University of California, Davis
Sacramento, California
Chapter 2

Daniel Entrikin, MD
Associate Professor
Department of Radiology
Wake Forest School of Medicine
Winston-Salem, North Carolina
Chapter 3

Sanjay K. Gandhi, MD
Associate Professor
Department of Medicine
Section on Cardiology
Wake Forest School of Medicine
Winston-Salem, North Carolina
Chapter 9

Casey Glass, MD
Assistant Professor
Department of Emergency Medicine
Wake Forest School of Medicine
Winston-Salem, North Carolina
Chapter 3

Scott Goldston, MD
Clinical Instructor
Department of Emergency Medicine
Wake Forest School of Medicine
Winston-Salem, North Carolina
Chapter 5

Heather Heaton, MD
Instructor
Department of Emergency Medicine
Mayo Clinic
Rochester, Minnesota
Chapter 4

Jackson Henley, MD
Resident in Emergency Medicine
Department of Emergency Medicine
Wake Forest School of Medicine
Winston-Salem, North Carolina
Chapter 5

Jeffrey W. Hinshaw, MS, PA-C, NREMT-P
Assistant Professor
Department of Emergency Medicine/Physician
  Assistant Studies
Wake Forest School of Medicine
Winston-Salem, North Carolina
Chapters 4 and 9

Judd E. Hollander, MD, FACEP
Professor
Department of Emergency Medicine
University of Pennsylvania
Philadelphia, Pennsylvania
Chapter 2

Kathleen Hosmer, MD
Assistant Professor
Department of Emergency Medicine
Wake Forest School of Medicine
Winston-Salem, North Carolina
Chapter 5

Justin B. Hurie, MD
Assistant Professor
Department of Vascular and Endovascular
  Surgery
Wake Forest School of Medicine
Winston-Salem, North Carolina
Chapter 3

Joshua T. James, MD
Resident in Emergency Medicine
Department of Emergency Medicine
Wake Forest School of Medicine
Winston-Salem, North Carolina
Chapter 4

Justin B. Joines, DO
Clinical Instructor
Department of Emergency Medicine
Wake Forest School of Medicine
Winston-Salem, North Carolina
Chapters 3 and 9

Jason N. Katz, MD, MHS
Assistant Professor
Department of Medicine
University of North Carolina School of Medicine
Chapel Hill, North Carolina
Chapter 4

Erica Kellenbeck, MD
Resident in Emergency Medicine
Department of Emergency Medicine
University of California, Davis School of Medicine
Sacramento, California
Chapter 2

Jieun Kim, MD
Resident
Department of Internal Medicine
Singapore General Hospital
Singapore
Chapter 7

Nicholas E. Kman, MD, FACEP
Assistant Professor
Department of Emergency Medicine
The Ohio State University College of Medicine
Columbus, Ohio
Chapter 2

Cedric Lefebvre, MD, FACEP
Assistant Professor
Department of Emergency Medicine
Wake Forest School of Medicine
Winston-Salem, North Carolina
Chapters 1, 2, 3, 5, and 9

Chad McCalla, MD
Assistant Professor
Department of Emergency Medicine
Wake Forest School of Medicine
Winston-Salem, North Carolina
Chapter 8

Chadwick D. Miller, MD, MS
Associate Professor
Department of Emergency Medicine
Wake Forest School of Medicine
Winston-Salem, North Carolina
Chapter 3

Michael S. Mitchell, MD
Assistant Professor
Department of Emergency Medicine
Wake Forest School of Medicine
Winston-Salem, North Carolina
Chapter 8

Jennifer Mitzman, MD
Fellow in Pediatric Emergency Medicine
Department of Emergency Medicine
Wake Forest School of Medicine
Winston-Salem, North Carolina
Chapter 5

James C. O'Neill, MD
Assistant Professor
Department of Emergency Medicine
Wake Forest School of Medicine
Winston-Salem, North Carolina
Chapters 6, 7, and 8

Manoj Pariyadath, MD
Assistant Professor
Department of Emergency Medicine
Wake Forest School of Medicine
Winston-Salem, North Carolina
Chapter 3

W. Frank Peacock, MD, FACEP
Professor, Emergency Medicine
Research Director
Department of Emergency Medicine
Baylor College of Medicine
Houston, Texas
Chapter 7

Nicholas R. Phillips, MD
Chief Resident in Emergency Medicine
Department of Emergency Medicine
Wake Forest School of Medicine
Winston-Salem, North Carolina
Chapter 7

Min Pu, MD, PhD
Professor
Department of Internal Medicine
Section of Cardiology
Wake Forest School of Medicine
Winston-Salem, North Carolina
Chapter 3

Michael D. Quartermain, MD
Assistant Professor
Department of Pediatrics
Wake Forest School of Medicine
Winston-Salem, North Carolina
Chapter 8

Daniel Renner, MD
Resident in Emergency Medicine
Department of Emergency Medicine
University of North Carolina
Chapel Hill, North Carolina
Chapter 4

Kevin Rooney, BA
MD MS Candidate
Department of Emergency Medicine
University of California, Irvine School of Medicine
Irvine, California
Chapter 8

Bryon E. Rubery, MD
Assistant Professor
Department of Medicine
Section of Cardiology
Wake Forest School of Medicine
Winston-Salem, North Carolina
Chapters 4 and 5

xii CONTRIBUTORS

Michael Schinlever, MD
Fellow in Critical Care
Department of Medicine
Wake Forest School of Medicine
Winston-Salem, North Carolina
Chapters 3 and 9

Jon W. Schrock, MD, FAHA, FACEP
Associate Professor
Department of Emergency Medicine
Case Western Reserve University School of Medicine
Metro Health Medical Center
Cleveland, Ohio
Chapter 3

Ahren Shubin, DO
Resident in Emergency Medicine
Department of Emergency Medicine
Wake Forest School of Medicine
Winston-Salem, North Carolina
Chapter 5

Benjamin C. Smith III, MD
Attending Physician
Department of Emergency Medicine
University of Tennessee
Chattanooga, Tennessee
Chapters 4 and 5

Dina M. Sparano, MD
Fellow in Cardiology
Section of Cardiology
The University of Chicago Medicine
Chicago, Illinois
Chapter 2

J. Stephan Stapczynski, MD
Executive Chair and Professor
Department of Emergency Medicine
University of Arizona College of Medicine – Phoenix
Phoenix, Arizona
Chapter 5

Sherrill Stockton, MD, PhD
Resident in Emergency Medicine
Department of Emergency Medicine
Wake Forest School of Medicine
Winston-Salem, North Carolina
Chapter 1

David James Story, MD
Assistant Professor
Department of Emergency Medicine
Wake Forest School of Medicine
Winston-Salem, North Carolina
Chapter 6

Joshua Thomas, MD
Resident in Emergency Medicine
Department of Emergency Medicine
Wake Forest School of Medicine
Winston-Salem, North Carolina
Chapter 1

Wiley D. Thuet, MD
Resident in Emergency Medicine
Department of Emergency Medicine
Wake Forest School of Medicine
Winston-Salem, North Carolina
Chapter 7

Elizabeth Turner, MD
Director of the Medical Intensive Care Unit
Department of Medicine University of California
Irvine, California
Chapter 8

Samuel Turnipseed, MD
Professor
Department of Emergency Medicine
University of California Davis Medical Center
Sacramento, California
Chapter 2

Bharathi Upadhya, MD
Assistant Professor
Department of Medicine
Section of Cardiology
Wake Forest School of Medicine
Winston-Salem, North Carolina
Chapter 3

Michael J. Walsh, MD
Assistant Professor
Department of Pediatrics
Section of Pediatric Cardiology
Wake Forest School of Medicine
Winston-Salem, North Carolina
Chapter 8

Sidney Larken Ware, MD
Resident in Emergency Medicine
Department of Emergency Medicine
Wake Forest School of Medicine
Winston-Salem, North Carolina
Chapters 4 and 8

Christopher Watkins, DO
Assistant Professor
Department of Emergency Medicine
Wake Forest School of Medicine
Winston-Salem, North Carolina
Chapter 8

Jeremy Webb, MD
Resident in Emergency Medicine
Department of Emergency Medicine
Wake Forest School of Medicine
Winston-Salem, North Carolina
Chapter 1

Derick M. Wenning, MD
Fellow in Pediatric Emergency Medicine
Department of Emergency Medicine
Wake Forest School of Medicine
Winston-Salem, North Carolina
Chapters 6 and 8

Mary A. Wittler, MD
Assistant Professor
Department of Emergency Medicine
Wake Forest School of Medicine
Winston-Salem, North Carolina
Chapter 5

John D. Wofford, MD
Resident in Emergency Medicine
Department of Emergency Medicine
Wake Forest School of Medicine
Winston-Salem, North Carolina
Chapters 2 and 5

Joseph Yeboah, MD, MS
Assistant Professor
Center for Cardiovascular Medicine
Wake Forest School of Medicine
Winston-Salem, North Carolina
Chapter 3

Laura Yoder, MD
Resident in Emergency Medicine
Department of Emergency Medicine
Wake Forest School of Medicine
Winston-Salem, North Carolina
Chapter 5

Daniel Zelinski, MD, PhD
Associate Professor
Department of Emergency Medicine
The Ohio State University
Columbus, Ohio
Chapter 2

Stacie Zelman, MD
Assistant Professor
Department of Emergency Medicine
Wake Forest School of Medicine
Winston-Salem, North Carolina
Chapter 5

PREFACE

"Use a picture, it's worth a thousand words," wrote influential newspaper editor Arthur Brisbane in 1911. However, a medical image may be worth very little to the untrained observer. Even experienced clinicians may find they lack the specific skills to read complex diagnostic images. This atlas is designed to empower the reader to correctly interpret cardiovascular medical images, and, in particular, time critical images for emergency management.

It has been 119 years since the very first non-artist rendered image representing heart function was published by Willem Einthoven in 1895.[1] This was a very simple one-lead electrocardiogram, which gave us the designations for the now familiar wave forms: Q, R, S, and T. At approximately the same time, Conrad Roentgen discovered X-rays,[2] but it would be decades before these devices would be used to manage patients with emergencies. Indeed at this point in history, emergency care was provided by general practitioners making house calls, and diagnoses were made on the basis of history and physical exam alone. Critically ill patients rarely survived long enough to be tested. Much has changed in the past 100 to 120 years. Now pattern recognition of findings on electrocardiograms, plain radiographs, ultrasound images, computed tomography images, magnetic resonance images, and other sophisticated cardiovascular images is essential to making real-time diagnoses in the emergency department.

This atlas was written as a concise guide to acute care cardiovascular image interpretation for the diagnosis and management of emergency conditions. Just as the management of these patients requires the input from a number of specialists, including emergency physicians, cardiologists, radiologists, and cardiovascular surgeons, this book has drawn on the expertise of these specialists to write chapters, review materials, critique content, or provide classic images. We the editorial team are deeply grateful to all the contributors who made this atlas a possibility.

Cedric Lefebvre, MD
James C. O'Neill, MD
David M. Cline, MD

---

1. *Einthoven W.* "Ueber die Form des menschlichen Electrocardiogramms." *Arch f d Ges Physiol.* 1895;60:101-123.
2. Stanton A. Wilhelm Conrad Röntgen On a New Kind of Rays: translation of a paper read before the Würzburg Physical and Medical Society, 1895. *Nature.* 1896;53(1369):274–276.

ACKNOWLEDGMENTS

We the medical editors, gratefully acknowledge the work of our Project Manager, Sarah M. Granlund; the Senior Editors at McGraw-Hill, Anne Sydor and Brian Belval; our Project Development Editor, Peter Boyle; our Senior Project Manager at MPS Limited, Vipra Fauzdar; the copy editors; the staff of the Heart Station at Wake Forest Baptist Health (especially Simone Holmes); and all the technical experts who helped us produce this book.

Chapter 1

ANATOMY

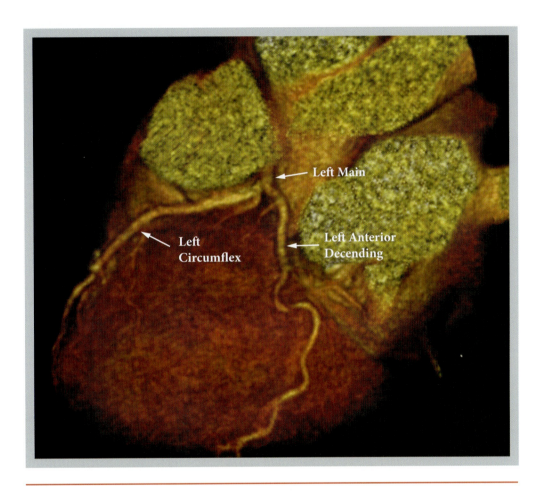

NORMAL CORONARY ARTERY ANATOMY

Joshua Thomas
Jeremy Webb

Clinical Highlights

The coronary arteries provide oxygenated blood to the myocardium and originate from the proximal aorta. There are two main branches: the left coronary artery (LCA) and the right coronary artery (RCA). The LCA branches into the left circumflex, the left marginal, and the left anterior descending arteries. The RCA branches into the right marginal artery and commonly the posterior descending artery (PDA).

Heart "dominance" is determined by which of the initial coronary arteries supplies the PDA which, in turn, supplies the AV node. The heart is right dominant (85%) if the PDA is supplied by the RCA. The heart is left dominant (7.5%) if

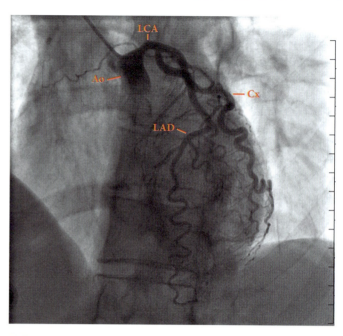

FIGURE 1.2 ■ Cardiac catheterization demonstrating healthy left coronary arterial vasculature in a right dominant heart. (Ao, aorta; Cx, circumflex artery; LAD, left anterior descending artery; LCA, left coronary artery.)

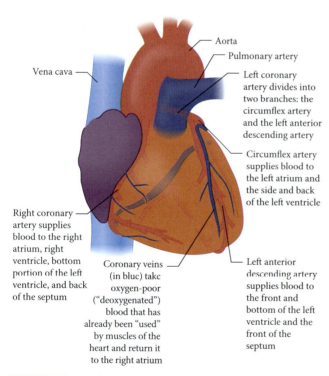

FIGURE 1.1 ■ Left coronary artery (left main), circumflex artery, left anterior descending artery, and the right coronary artery are detailed in the figure. Reproduced, with permission, from Piktel JS. Cardiac rhythm disturbances. In: Tintinalli JE, Stapczynski J, Ma O, Cline DM, Cydulka RK, Meckler GD. eds. *Tintinalli's Emergency Medicine: A Comprehensive Study Guide.* 7th ed. New York, NY: McGraw-Hill; 2011.

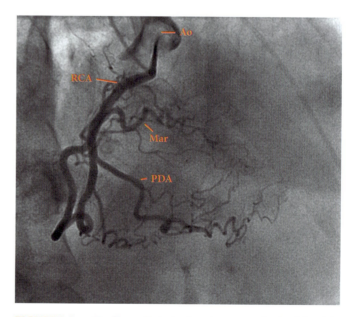

FIGURE 1.3 ■ Cardiac catheterization demonstrating healthy right coronary arterial vasculature in a right dominant heart. (Ao, aorta; Mar, marginal artery; PDA, posterior descending artery; RCA, right coronary artery.)

the PDA is supplied by the circumflex branch of the LCA. If the PDA is supplied by parts of the right and left circulation, then the heart is codominant (7.5%). In a right dominant heart, the right ventricle is supplied by the right marginal branch. In a left dominant heart, the right ventricle is supplied by the circumflex artery. The left ventricle, which contains the majority of the heart's myocardium, is supplied by both right and left circulation. Coronary arteries are considered end arteries, meaning that there is little collateralization and if blockages develop, ischemia will occur in dependent cardiac tissue.

The coronary veins remove deoxygenated blood from the myocardium. The precise venous anatomy varies from patient to patient but commonly mirrors the arterial supply. The coronary veins drain into the coronary sinus, which empties directly into the right atrium. Below figures show the origins of the left and right coronary arteries on cardiac computed tomography (CT) scanning.

ED Care and Disposition

Although coronary structures are rarely imaged directly in the emergency department, it is important for the astute emergency physician to understand the basic coronary anatomy. Knowledge of cardiac structures can be helpful in the emergency department when taking care of patients experiencing myocardial ischemia. Determining the location of ischemia, particularly right versus left ventricular infarction, allows the emergency physician to better manage resuscitation of the patient.

Pearls and Pitfalls

- Variations of normal coronary anatomy are very common.
- Heart dominance is determined by which coronary artery supplies the AV node via the PDA.

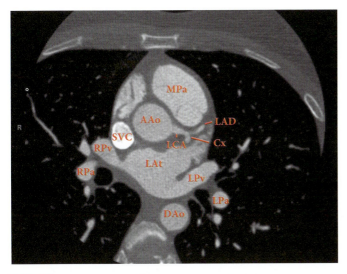

FIGURE 1.4 ■ Cardiac CT demonstrating the left coronary artery arising from its source at the ascending aorta. (AAo, ascending aorta; Cx, circumflex artery; DAo, descending aorta; LAD, left anterior descending artery; LAt, left atrium; LCA, left coronary artery; LPa, left pulmonary artery; LPv, left pulmonary vein; MPa, main pulmonary artery; RPa, right pulmonary artery; RPv, right pulmonary vein; SVC, superior vena cava.)

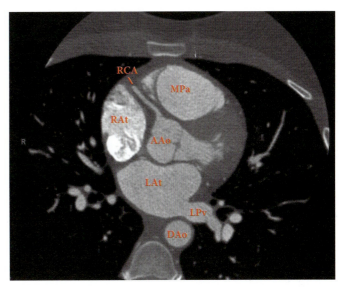

FIGURE 1.5 ■ Cardiac CT demonstrating the right coronary artery arising from its source at the ascending aorta. (AAo, ascending aorta; DAo, descending aorta; LAt, left atrium; LPv, left pulmonary vein; MPa, main pulmonary artery; RAt, right atrium; RCA, right coronary artery.)

NORMAL CHAMBERS

Jeremy Webb
Cedric Lefebvre

Anatomical Region

The heart is a four-chambered muscular organ, consisting of two atria and two ventricles, with an internal fibrous skeleton. It maintains a right anterior position in the left chest. The atria and ventricles are separated from their contralateral equivalents by septa and from each other by cardiac valves. Deoxygenated blood enters the heart from the superior vena cava, inferior vena cava, and coronary sinus at the right atrium (RA). The RA is composed of a smooth sinus venarum at these connections and a muscular wall consisting of pectinate muscles. The border between these structures is the crista terminalis. The right ventricle (RV) is a trabeculated structure that makes up most of the sternocostal surface of the heart and receives blood from the RA via the tricuspid valve. A distinguishing feature of this chamber is the moderator band, which encases the right bundle of the AV conducting system. The RV propels blood through the pulmonary valve into the pulmonary trunk, which bifurcates into right and left main branches of the pulmonary artery. Blood then continues into the lungs to acquire oxygenation.

Oxygenated blood reenters the heart via pulmonary veins into the posteriorly positioned left atrium (LA). Posterior structures in contact with the LA include the coronary sinus, esophagus, and descending aorta. The LA is connected to the left ventricle (LV) via the mitral valve. The LV has three times the wall diameter of the RV which assists in pumping against systemic pressures. It comprises most of the diaphragmatic surface of the heart.

Clinical Highlights

The heart chambers can be easily viewed with multiple radiologic modalities including chest radiograph, computerized tomography (CT), magnetic resonance imaging (MRI), and bedside cardiac ultrasound. For example, bedside ultrasound can be used to identify an enlarged right ventricle and septal bowing in the setting of massive pulmonary embolism. Understanding the orientation of these chambers and how they are affected by varying disease processes can guide emergency decision making.

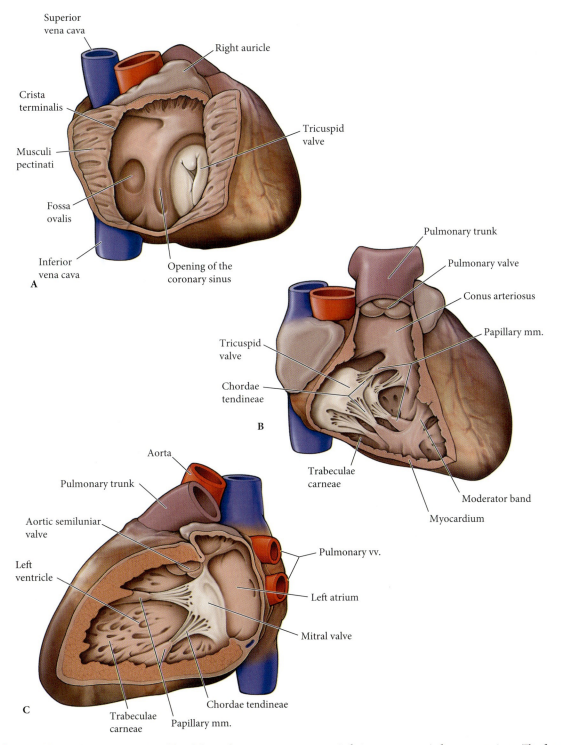

FIGURE 1.6 ■ (A) The right atrium receives blood from the superior vena cava, inferior vena cava and coronary sinus. The fossa ovalis, an oval depression in the septal wall of the right atrium, is a remnant relating to the foramen ovale during development. Congenital defects in this area can result in a patent foramen ovale. (B) The right ventricle consists of trabeculae carneae, which are muscular columns originating from the inner surfaces of the ventricle. Papillary muscles (mm) from the ventricular wall connect to the leaflets of the tricuspid valve via chordae tendineae. (C) The left cardiac chambers are characterized by a thin-walled left atrium and a muscular, thick-walled left ventricle. Pulmonary veins (vv) return oxygenated blood from the pulmonary circulation to the left atrium. Chordae tendineae and papillary muscles (mm) attach to the cusps of the mitral valve to prevent prolapse during ventricular systole. Blood is propelled into the aorta and systemic circulation by the left ventricle via the aortic valve. Reproduced, with permission, from Morton DA, Foreman K, Albertine KH. eds. *The Big Picture: Gross Anatomy*. New York, NY: McGraw-Hill; 2011.

NORMAL VALVES

Jeremy Webb

Clinical Highlights

There are four cardiac valves. The valves open to allow forward blood flow, then close to prevent backward blood flow, thereby allowing blood flow in only one direction when valvular function is normal.

The tricuspid and mitral valves are atrioventricular valves that lie between the right and left atria and ventricles, respectively. They consist of five distinct components: annulus, leaflets, commissures, chordae tendineae, and papillary muscles. The tricuspid valve typically has three leaflets that are connected to right ventricular papillary muscles by chordae tendineae, which prevent leaflet prolapse into the atrium. The mitral valve is a bicuspid valve, whose leaflets are connected to left ventricular papillary muscles by their own chordae tendineae.

During diastole, these valves are closed to allow for atrial filling. As atrial pressure exceeds ventricular pressure, the valves open to allow passive filling of the ventricles, and remain open through the end of diastole for atrial contraction to complete ventricular filling. They close during systole as ventricular pressure exceeds atrial pressure.

The pulmonary and aortic valves are referred to as the semilunar valves, and separate the right and left ventricular outflow tracts from the pulmonary artery and aorta, respectively. They only consist of three components: annulus, cusps, and commissures. The pulmonary and aortic valves typically have three cusps that open during ventricular systole to deliver deoxygenated blood to the lungs, and oxygenated blood to the remainder of the body.

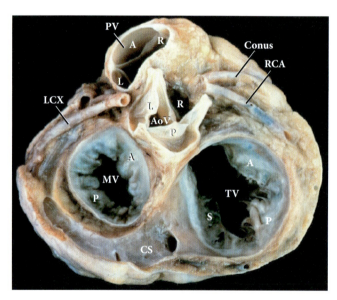

FIGURE 1.7 ■ Gross cadaveric dissection of the heart revealing the cardiac valves. (A, anterior; AoV, aortic valve; AV, atrioventricular; CS, coronary sinus; IV, interventricular; L, left; LCX, left circumflex coronary artery; MV, mitral valve; P, posterior; PV, pulmonary valve; R, right; RCA, right coronary artery; S, septal; TV, tricuspid valve.) Reprinted, with permission, from Fuster V, Walsh RA, Harrington RA. *Hurst's The Heart*. 13th ed. New York, NY McGraw-Hill; 2011.

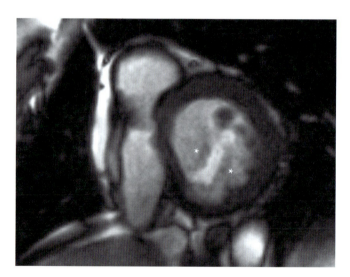

FIGURE 1.8 ■ Cross-sectional magnetic resonance imaging of the mitral valve during diastole as the valve begins to open. Note the bicuspid anatomy (cusps are denoted by asterisks).

ED Care and Disposition

The cardiac valves and their associated components can be afflicted by a variety of pathology including infection, ischemia, and congenital abnormality. Presentation of these entities can range from benign murmurs to advanced cardiac failure accompanied by poor perfusion and pulmonary congestion.

Pearls and Pitfalls

- The emergency provider should be familiar with the cardiac cycle and the corresponding normal heart sounds associated with normal and abnormal valve closure.
- Functional anatomy and physiology of the cardiac valves is best appreciated with ultrasound, which can also help grade the severity of dysfunction.

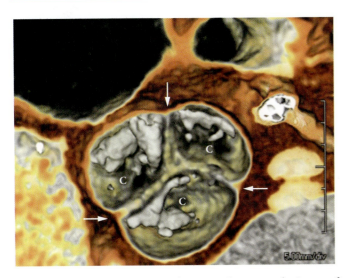

FIGURE 1.9 ■ This reconstructed computed tomography image of the aortic valve demonstrates the tricuspid (C) appearance of semilunar valves as well as the valve commissures (arrows).

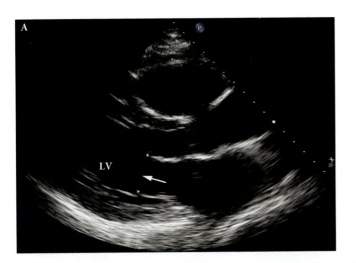 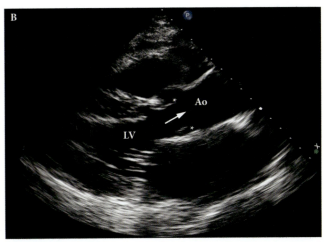

FIGURE 1.10 ■ (A) Echocardiogram showing open mitral valve with left ventricular filling. Arrow denotes the path of blood flow through open valve into left ventricle (LV); asterisks show valve leaflets. (B) Echocardiogram showing subsequent opening of the aortic valve during left ventricular (LV) contraction. Arrow denotes the path of blood flow from left ventricle (LV) through open aortic valve into the aorta (Ao); asterisks show valve leaflets.

PROSTHETIC VALVES

Jeremy Webb

Clinical Highlights

As a result of infection, ischemia, or congenital abnormalities, the heart valves may obstruct flow due to critical narrowing (stenosis) or failure to halt retrograde flow (regurgitation). Prosthetic valves were designed to correct this pathology.

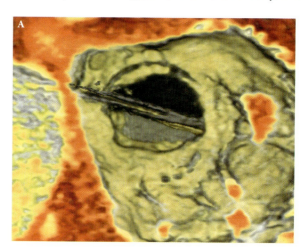

Two types of prosthetic heart valves exist: mechanical valves and bioprosthetic valves. Mechanical valves are of several designs. The first were caged-ball designs. Modern valves consist mainly of the *tilting disc* and the newer *bileaflet valve*

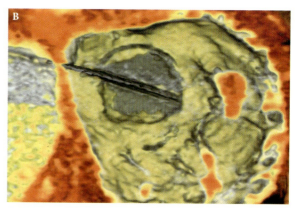

FIGURE 1.11 ■ Three mechanical valve types. The three types of mechanical valve implants from left to right: ball-valve, tilting disc, and bileaflet valve designs. Panel **A** reveals the route of blood flow around these valves, while panel **B** illustrates each valve type's profile in situ. Reproduced, with permission, from Fuster V, Walsh RA, Harrington RA. *Hurst's The Heart*. 13th ed. New York, NY: McGraw-Hill; 2011. Figure 80-3.

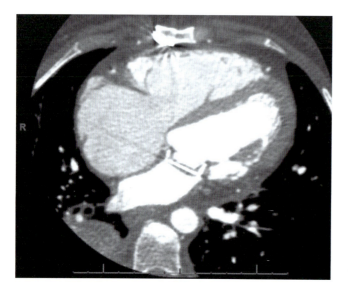

FIGURE 1.12 ■ Computed tomography of a mechanical valve. A mechanical mitral valve (thin disc on-side orientation) as viewed on classic chest computed tomography imaging.

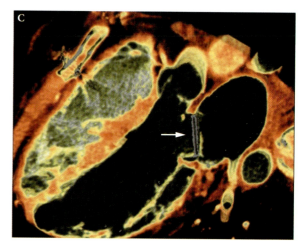

FIGURE 1.13 ■ Mechanical valve on reconstructed computed tomography images. These reconstructed computed tomography images reveal the structure of a mechanical bileaflet valve in open (**A**) and closed (**B**) condition as viewed from the left ventricle. Its location (arrow) at the left atrioventricular junction is seen on a sagittal cut (**C**).

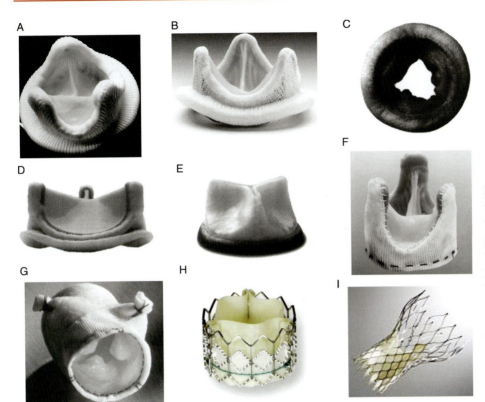

FIGURE 1.14 ■ Examples of bioprosthetic valves. (**A**) Carpentier-Edwards porcine valve. (**B**) Hancock Modified Orifice II porcine valve. (**C**) Mosaic stented porcine valve. (**D**) Carpentier-Edwards Magna pericardial valve. (**E**) Mitroflow pericardial valve. (**F**) Toronto Stentless porcine valve. (**G**) Medtronic Freestyle stentless valve. (**H**) Cribier-Edwards transcatheter pericardial valve. (**I**) CoreValve transcatheter pericardial valve. Reproduced, with permission, from Fuster V, Walsh RA, Harrington RA. *Hurst's The Heart*. 13th ed. New York, NY: McGraw-Hill; 2011. Figure 80-4.

designs. Their circular ring frames are made of combinations of nickel or titanium alloys covered in Dacron or Teflon to permit suturing. They are increasingly manufactured to be MRI safe but are only slightly radiopaque. The frame of the tilting disc valves has two supports that hold a single door that opens and closes to function as a valve. The bileaflet valves consist of two semicircular carbon leaflets. These valves are less likely to cause mechanical hemolysis than their predecessors.

All mechanical valves require the use of anticoagulation, to prevent clot formation. Bioprosthetic valves, on the other hand, consist of either porcine aortic valves or pericardium from bovine, porcine, or equine origin. They may or may not be mounted on stents for implant.

ED Care and Disposition

Prosthetic heart valves are durable but can play a role in various emergent presentations. Mechanical valve failure is sometimes encountered, and the symptoms are likely to be those of acute heart failure. Urgent cardiology and/or cardiothoracic surgery consultations should be strongly considered. Bioprosthetic heart valves tend to present with subacute degeneration and symptoms of slowly progressive heart failure. The immediate temporizing treatment of prosthetic valvular dysfunction is the same as for the valve's native counterpart. Functional assessment of the valve is made with echocardiography. Mechanical assessment is often possible with advanced MRI or gated multidetector computed tomography (MDCT) studies.

Thromboembolic events should be considered in these patients and coagulation parameters should be checked. Infectious symptoms should raise suspicion for infective endocarditis. Anemia, from mechanical destruction of red cells, can also present emergently.

Pearls and Pitfalls

- Mechanical valves are often difficult to appreciate on plain film chest radiography.
- Consider heart failure, thromboembolic events, infective endocarditis, and anemia in patients with prosthetic heart valves.
- Functional anatomy and physiology of the prosthetic valve is best appreciated with ultrasound, which can also help grade the severity of dysfunction. CT or MRI may be necessary as well.

ANOMALOUS LEFT CORONARY ARTERY

Joshua S. Broder

Clinical Highlights

The normal left coronary artery originates at the left sinus of Valsalva of the aorta and follows the left atrioventricular groove and anterior interventricular groove. The vessel is normally epicardial (superficial to the myocardium) until near its termination at the myocardial capillaries. An anomalous coronary artery is present when the origin or path of the coronary artery differs from this anatomic norm. Myocardial bridging occurs when a coronary artery prematurely enters the myocardium before resuming an epicardial location. Intramyocardial course of a coronary artery occurs when the artery enters the myocardium and remains intramyocardial for the remainder of its course.

An anomalous path can result in abnormal compression of the artery during cardiac contraction. For example, a coronary artery that passes between the aorta and the main pulmonary artery can be dynamically compressed during high cardiac output states, resulting in cardiac ischemia, chest pain or dysrhythmia, sometimes presenting with syncope or sudden cardiac death. Similarly, intramyocardial course

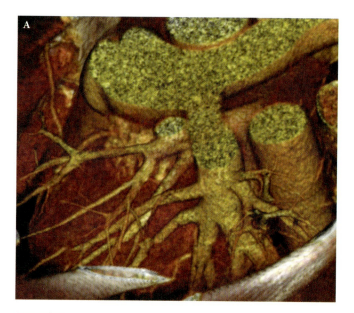

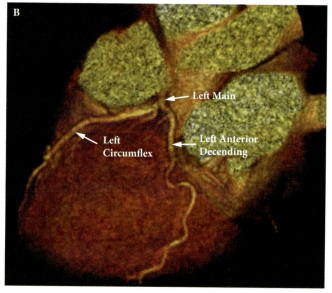

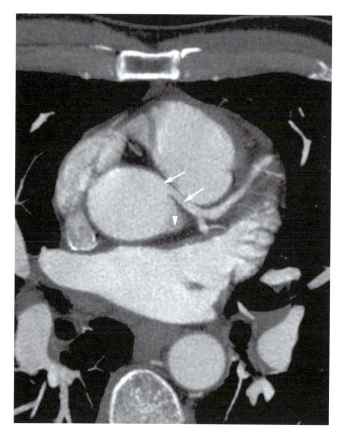

FIGURE 1.15 ■ CT coronary angiogram, axial image. The left main coronary artery originates anomalously from the right sinus of Valsalva (arrows) immediately adjacent to the left sinus (arrowhead marks the expected site of origin of the left main). This patient had been incidentally noted to have an anomalous coronary artery on a previous CT, prompting this more detailed evaluation.

FIGURE 1.16 ■ Three-dimensional CT reconstruction of the heart generated from the same CT dataset as the previous figure. (A) Multiple structures overlie the surface of the heart, obstructing the view of the left coronary artery. (B) Overlying structures have been digitally subtracted, revealing the left coronary artery and its main divisions labeled.

of a coronary artery can result in systolic compression of the artery, diminished coronary artery blood flow, and cardiac ischemia during exercise. Patients with anomalous coronary arteries may have a normal resting electrocardiogram (ECG), as no ischemia is present at rest. During stress testing, ischemia is reproduced as described earlier, resulting in a positive stress test. If standard left heart catheterization is performed (done at rest), the anomalous vessel may not be recognized. In the absence of atherosclerotic disease, true ischemia revealed by stress testing may be dismissed as a "false positive" result in light of the apparently "normal" cardiac catheterization. Myocardial bridging or intramyocardial course may not be appreciated. Additionally, in a traditional coronary angiogram performed for evaluation of coronary artery disease, the left heart is catheterized but the right heart is not, leaving right heart structures invisible. Consequently, the path of the left coronary artery relative to right heart structures such as the pulmonary artery may not be evident.

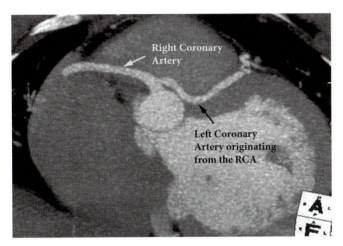

FIGURE 1.17 ■ Anomalous left coronary artery. In a different patient, the left coronary artery (black arrow) arises as a proximal branch of the right coronary artery (white arrow).

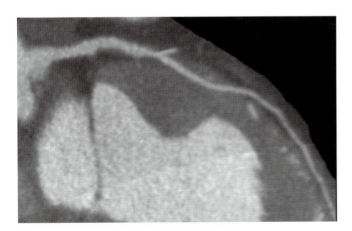

FIGURE 1.18 ■ Myocardial bridging. The left coronary artery normally is epicardial through most of its course. Here, the artery traverses the ventricular myocardium (notice the arterial compression during myocardial contraction), a process called myocardial bridging.

ED Care and Disposition

When an anomalous coronary artery is suspected, CT coronary angiography (CTCA) can reveal the diagnosis. CTCA has advantages over traditional catheter angiography: it simultaneously reveals the left and right heart and associated structures, and it visualizes the myocardium as well as coronary artery lumen. Treatment options include reimplantation to alter the origin or path, restoring perfusion, and eliminating dynamic compression. Coronary artery bypass grafting for symptomatic myocardial bridges has also been described. When an anomalous coronary artery is discovered, restrict exercise or other activities that could lead to dynamic compression until the patient is evaluated by a cardiologist.

Pearls and Pitfalls

- Suspect anomalous left coronary artery in young patients without CAD risk factors, presenting with exertional chest pain or syncope.
- Recognize the potential for anomalous coronary artery when stress testing is positive but coronary angiography shows no occlusive coronary artery disease.
- Use CTCA to depict the course of coronary arteries when anomaly is suspected.

DEXTROCARDIA

Sherrill Stockton

Clinical Highlights

Dextrocardia is a cardiac positional variant in which the heart lies in the right hemithorax and maintains a mirror image of the normal base-to-apex axis of the heart. There are different types of dextrocardia, each with different embryological and developmental etiologies, and some exhibit tendencies to coexist with different defects of the heart, great vessels, and abdominal organs. When all of the major visceral organs are transposed, the condition is called *situs inversus with dextrocardia* or *situs inversus totalis*.

These individuals often live normal healthy lives. However, when only the heart assumes an anomalous position in the right chest—a condition called *dextrocardia without situs inversus*—defects of the heart and other organs predominate. Similarly, transposition of the visceral organs that maintains the normal position of the heart—*situs inversus with levocardia*—is also associated with myriad important defects of the heart, great vessels, and other organs.

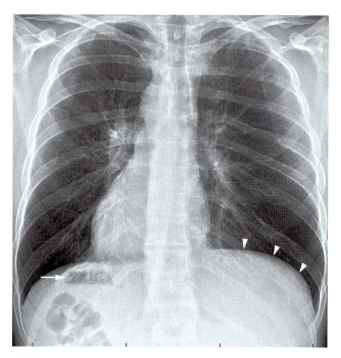

FIGURE 1.19 ■ *Situs inversus totalis* on AP chest radiograph. The heart is in the right hemithorax. Importantly, the stomach and liver are transposed as well, indicated by the air fluid level in the right abdomen (stomach, see arrow) and the elevated diaphragm (see arrowheads) above the liver in the left abdomen.

ED Care and Disposition

Positional irregularities of the heart, great vessels, or major visceral organs may be noted on chest radiograph, CT studies, MRI studies, or ultrasound studies. These positional abnormalities may inform treatment and disposition decisions in the emergency department. In emergent presentations, for example, ECG lead and defibrillation pad/paddle placement and pericardiocentesis approach must necessarily be adjusted to the corresponding anatomy in the right hemithorax. Less emergent presentations are also possible in patients with chronic complaints that have not been imaged previously or diagnosed with an anatomical or functional abnormality. Patients with these irregularities, especially dextrocardia without situs inversus and situs inversus with levocardia, should be dispositioned with great care given the propensity for structural defects of the great organs. Abdominal complaints in this population may result from malpositioned or dysfunctional great organs. Infectious symptoms are to be taken seriously as many patients with this spectrum of disease possess poor or absent splenic function, putting them at risk for infection by encapsulated organisms. In the pediatric population, unstable patients with dextrocardia without situs inversus and situs inversus with levocardia should raise a concern for structural heart defects and prostaglandin therapy should be considered. In short, disposition decisions should be made carefully in this population. Conversely, stable healthy patients with complaints not likely related to major organ systems, especially those with suspected *situs inversus totalis*, are candidates for close outpatient follow-up.

Pearls and Pitfalls

- Suspected or newly diagnosed dextrocardia can represent a healthy patient with normal life expectancy or may suggest serious underlying disease.
- Suspected cardiac and great organ positional defects such as *situs inversus with levocardia* and *dextrocardia without situs inversus*, portend serious underlying defects that may have acute ramifications for treatment and stabilization in the emergency department.
- Acute management of patients with dextrocardia requires the reversal of ECG leads, defibrillation pads/paddles, and approaches to various procedures including pericardiocentesis and lateral thoracotomy.

Chapter 2

ELECTROCARDIOGRAPHY: NORMAL HEART, ACUTE ISCHEMIA, AND CHRONIC DISEASE

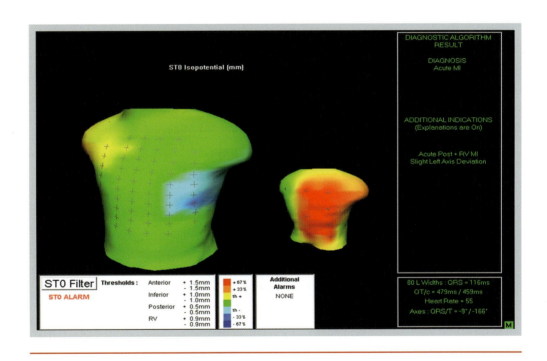

Normal Heart
NORMAL CARDIAC CONDUCTION

John D. Wofford
Cedric Lefebvre

Normal cardiac conduction follows a precisely coordinated pattern from the initiation of an electrical impulse to myocardial repolarization after ventricular contraction. Under normal conditions, the electrical cardiac cycle begins at the sinoatrial (SA) node—a collection of pacemaker cells located at the junction of the superior vena cava and the right atrium. These cells possess an intrinsic ability to initiate electrical impulses spontaneously. This is achieved by the depolarization of a polarized cell membrane, primarily from the flow of ions (Na^+, K^+, and Ca^{2+}) through ion channels embedded in the membrane. The term "action potential" is used to describe the depolarization–repolarization cycle of a cell.

The SA node is the dominant pacemaker of the cardiac cycle and typically fires at a rate of 60–100 action potentials per minute. The rate is influenced by sympathetic and vagal stimulation. The action potential of one cell triggers the action potentials in adjacent cells. Thus, the impulse initiated by the SA node is propagated through nearby cells. This causes both contraction of the atrial myocardium (atrial systole) and further electrical impulse propagation through the cardiac conduction system. Specialized conducting cells are responsible for delivering this electrical signal to the remainder of the myocardium. Long, thin, and efficient in relaying electrical impulses, these cells are similar to wires carrying electricity. Once an electrical impulse reaches a myocardial cell, calcium ions are released within the cell causing contraction. This contraction, known as excitation–contraction coupling, is achieved through the coupling of actin and myosin molecules, which are abundant within the myocardial cell.

Starting at the SA node, an electrical impulse travels through internodal atrial pathways to the atrioventricular (AV) node. The AV node acts as a relay site by connecting atrial electrical impulses with the ventricular conducting system. Conduction through the AV node, which is located at the base of the atrial septum, is slowed momentarily, allowing for ventricular filling of blood prior to ventricular systole. Signal conduction is then accelerated rapidly through the bundle of His and its right and left bundle branches. The right bundle branch continues toward the apex of the right ventricle (RV), whereas the left bundle branch splits into left anterior superior and left posterior inferior fascicles. Electrical impulses progress through the fibers of the Purkinje system and are ultimately delivered to the ventricular myocardium that causes ventricular contraction (ventricular systole).

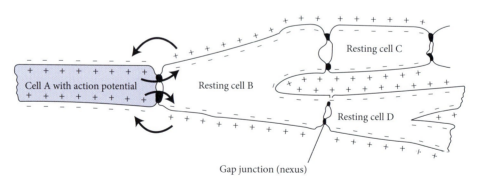

FIGURE 2.1 ■ Action potentials in cardiac myocytes produce local currents that depolarize the membranes of adjacent cells and propagate electrical signals. Cell-to-cell conduction is also achieved by end-to-end connections called gap junctions. Reproduced, with permission, from Chapter 2. Characteristics of cardiac muscle cells. In: Mohrman DE, Heller LJ. eds. *Cardiovascular Physiology*. 7th ed. New York, NY: McGraw-Hill; 2010.

NORMAL CARDIAC CONDUCTION (CONTINUED)

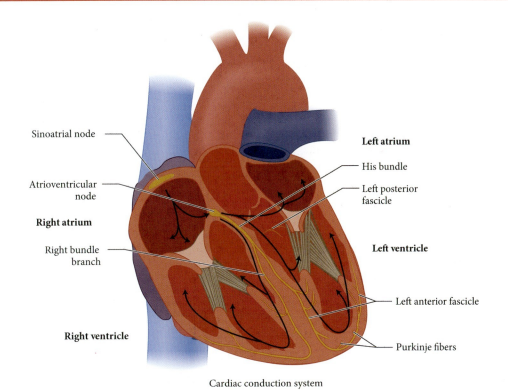

FIGURE 2.2 ■ The cardiac conduction system propagates electrical signals that originate from the SA node (under normal conditions) to myocytes in the atria and ventricles to stimulate sequential contraction of these chambers. Reproduced, with permission, from Fauci AS, Kasper DL, Braunwald E, et al. *Harrison's Principles of Internal Medicine.* 17th ed. New York, NY: McGraw-Hill; 2008.

Clinical Highlights

Through the coordinated propagation of electrical impulses throughout the entirety of the myocardium, the heart is able to provide a coordinated contraction that is necessary to pump blood throughout the pulmonary and systemic circulation. Electrolyte disturbances, myocardial ischemia, medications, structural abnormalities, and other factors can result in alterations of electrical conduction. Disruption of this highly coordinated system can lead to various electrocardiac pathologies and is the basis of several cardiovascular emergencies.

NORMAL RESTING ELECTROCARDIOGRAM (ECG)

Nicholas E. Kman
Daniel P. Zelinski

Technology/Technique

An electrocardiogram (ECG) is a graphic representation of the electrical events of the cardiac cycle. The normal ECG waveform results from an electrical current that originates in the SA node in the right atrium and is propagated through healthy myocardial tissue. The electrical current is transmitted from the atria to the ventricles via the AV node where it spreads throughout the ventricular myocardium.

A standard ECG records the heart's electrical cycle across 12 channels simultaneously. Waveforms are printed on a special grid depicting amplitude and duration of electrical events. Electrical data are collected from electrodes applied to 12 distinct anatomical locations on the human torso and limbs. Abnormalities in ECG waveform morphology can indicate several clinical conditions including arrhythmias, myocardial ischemia/infarction, peridarditis/myocarditis, chamber hypertrophy, electrolyte disturbances, and drug toxicity.

Interpretation

Normal sinus rhythm depicts a normal electrical cardiac cycle. It is characterized by regular P waves followed by normal QRS complexes at a rate of 60 to 100 beats per minute. *P waves* represent atrial depolarization. Inverted or larger amplitude P waves can indicate atrial enlargement. The *PR interval* is measured from the beginning of the P wave to the start of the QRS complex. The *QRS complex* represents ventricular depolarization. Widening of the QRS complex is caused by a delay in intraventicular conduction. Immediately following the

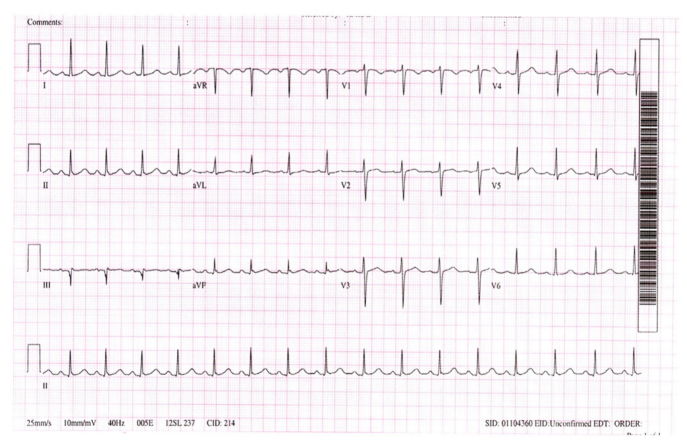

FIGURE 2.3 ■ Normal resting ECG. The ECG is recorded on graph paper divided into 1 mm × 1 mm squares. With a paper speed of 25 mm/s, each square represents 40-millisecond duration along the horizontal axis and 0.1 mV amplitude along the vertical axis. Darker lines mark 5 mm × 5 mm squares, or 0.2 seconds and 0.5 mV.

NORMAL RESTING ELECTROCARDIOGRAM (ECG) (CONTINUED)

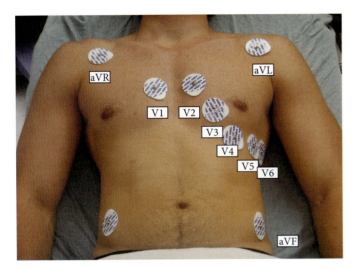

FIGURE 2.4 ■ ECG 12 lead placement. Four extremity electrodes are applied to the skin: left arm (aVL), right arm (aVR), neutral to the right leg, and left foot (aVF) to the left leg. Six electrodes are applied to the precordial region (V1–V6). Photograph courtesy of Dan Zelinski.

TABLE 2.1 ■ NORMAL ECG WAVEFORM AND INTERVAL MEASUREMENTS

	Amplitude (mV)	Duration (s)
P wave	<0.25	<0.12
PR interval	—	0.12–0.20
Q wave	<¼ R wave, usually ≤0.1	<0.04
QRS complex	Variable	<0.1
QT interval	—	<½ R–R interval
QTc interval	—	≤0.44*
T wave	Variable	0.04–0.08
U wave	≤0.1	—

*There are various methods for calculating the QTc and there are several definitions for a "normal," "abnormal," and "borderline" QTc. These values may also vary with gender.

P wave, any downward deflection is a *Q wave*, and any upward deflection is an *R wave*. Small Q waves can be seen in leads I, aVL, V5, and V6 and represent septal activation. Pathological Q waves (>¼ R-wave amplitude, >0.04 seconds) can signal old myocardial infarction (MI) or septal hypertrophy. An increase in *R-wave* amplitude from lead V1 to its maximum amplitude in V5 is considered normal *R-wave progression*. The *S wave* represents late ventricular depolarization. The *ST segment*, or interval, begins at the end of the QRS complex. Depression or elevation of the ST segment can represent myocardial ischemia or infarction. The *T wave* represents ventricular repolarization. Normally, T waves are upright in every lead except aVR and V1. Inverted or broad T waves can indicate myocardial ischemia or infarction. Peaked T waves can signal hyperkalemia. The *QT interval* is primarily a measure of ventricular repolarization. The QT interval varies with heart rate and its measurement can be adjusted accordingly using the *corrected QT interval* (QTc). A prolonged QTc interval can be a marker for ventricular arrhythmia and a risk factor for sudden cardiac death. *U waves* are small waves following T waves and may be normal in some leads, especially the precordial leads V2 to V4. U waves can also signal hypokalemia and other metabolic conditions. See Table 2.1 for normal ECG waveform and interval measurements.

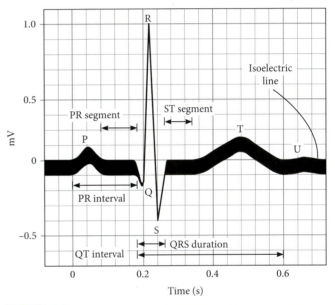

FIGURE 2.5 ■ ECG waves are labeled alphabetically and begin with the P wave. Normal waveform and interval measurements are included in Table 2.1. Reprinted, with permission, from Chapter 29. Origin of the heartbeat & the electrical activity of the heart. In: Barrett KE, Boitano S, Barman SM, Brooks HL. eds. *Ganong's Review of Medical Physiology*. 24th ed. New York, NY: McGraw-Hill; 2012.

Pearls and Pitfalls

- Electrodes should be placed flat against the skin. When lead wires are attached, ensure lead wires are not pulling on the skin.
- When interpreting an ECG, use a systematic approach to evaluate the rate, rhythm, axis, and waveforms.

Acute Ischemia and Chronic Disease
SUPPLEMENTAL ECG LEADS

Cedric Lefebvre

Technology/Technique

A key component of acute MI (AMI) management includes rapid acquisition of ECG on patients presenting with anginal symptoms and early reperfusion therapy for patients in whom ST-segment elevation is noted. Identifying ST-segment elevation on ECG in certain cases can be challenging. The use of ECG leads beyond the conventional 12-lead anatomic territory can supplement electrocardiographic evaluation for ST-elevation MI (STEMI).

Posterior Myocardial Infarction

Occlusion of the left circumflex artery causes infarction of the posterobasal wall of the left ventricle (LV), resulting in posterior AMI. Because conventional ECG leads are placed on the anterior chest wall, posterior AMI may escape detection by ECG. Although the true incidence of ST-segment elevation posterior AMI is unknown, studies have shown a 3.3% incidence of isolated posterior wall infarction among all cases of AMI and an incidence of 15% to 21% of posterior AMI associated with inferior and/or lateral AMI. Patients with posterior wall involvement during inferior or lateral AMI have a greater incidence of LV dysfunction and death.

Right Ventricular Infarction

In right dominant coronary circulations (most common), the inferior wall and RV receive vascular supply from branches of the right coronary artery (RCA). Occlusion of the right coronary circulation may cause inferior wall AMI with or without RV infarction. Although isolated RV infarctions are relatively rare, up to 30% to 40% of inferior wall infarctions are associated with RV infarction. Inferior AMI with RV involvement confers unique hemodynamic sequelae, has a relatively high rate of mortality, and requires a specific therapeutic approach. As RV infarction progresses, cardiac output decreases and cardiogenic shock may ensue. The clinical manifestations of RV infarction are elevated neck veins and hypotension. Although RV infarction may be suspected when these clinical findings are present or when ST-segment elevation is noted in the inferior leads, RV infarction can be missed because conventional 12-lead ECG is not sensitive for injury patterns in this region of the heart.

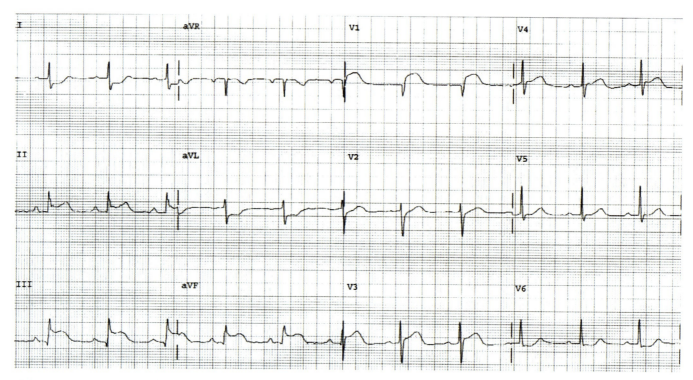

FIGURE 2.6 ■ ST-segment elevation is noted in the inferior leads II, III, and aVF.

Interpretation

Posterior Leads (V7–V9)

Indirect ECG changes associated with posterior AMI such as ST-segment depression and prominent R waves in the anterior precordial leads (V1–V3) may be evident on 12-lead ECG. If posterior AMI is suspected, the American College of Cardiology/American Heart Association (ACC/AHA) practice guidelines advise the use of posterior leads (V7–V9) to investigate the presence of this phenomenon (class IIa recommendation). Posterior leads are placed on the left posterior chest wall, just below the scapula. ST-segment elevation of ≥1 mm in leads V7–V9 is highly suggestive of posterior AMI. If such ECG changes are noted, AMI treatment should be expedited and immediate cardiology consultation should be obtained for consideration of reperfusion therapies.

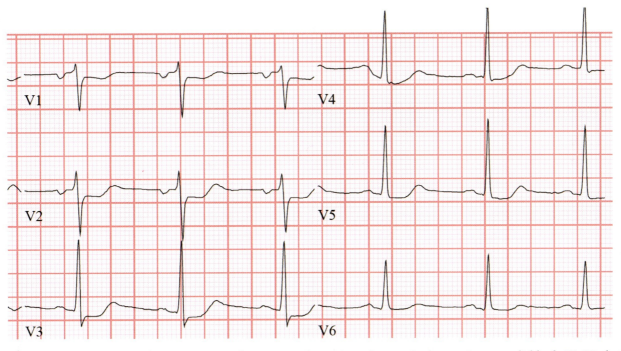

FIGURE 2.7 ■ This ECG tracing shows ST-segment depression and prominent R waves in the anterior precordial leads V1–V3 that may represent posterior AMI.

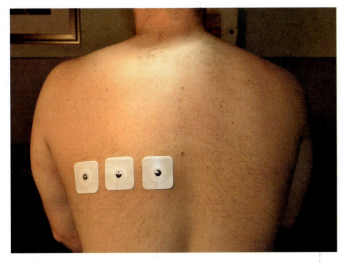

FIGURE 2.8 ■ To investigate a posterior STEMI, leads are placed on the left posterior chest wall, just below the scapula.

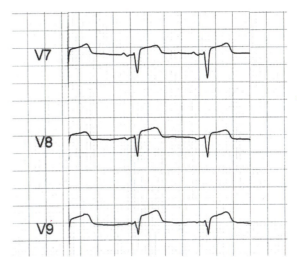

FIGURE 2.9 ■ ST-segment elevation of ≥1 mm in posterior leads V7–V9 is highly suggestive of posterior AMI.

Right-Sided Leads (V1R–V6R)

The clinician should investigate the presence of RV infarction in cases of inferior AMI. A class I recommendation of the ACC/AHA practice guidelines on the management of STEMI is the use of right-sided ECG leads to screen for RV involvement in cases of inferior AMI. The addition of right-sided chest leads may improve the sensitivity of 12-lead ECG for the detection of RV infarction by up to 9%. Leads V1R–V6R are placed to the right of the sternum as a mirror image of the locations for V1–V6 on the left. ST-segment elevation in these leads, particularly V4R (mid-clavicular line, fifth intercostal space), is highly suggestive of RV infarction. If RV infarction is detected, therapy should include preload optimization, RV afterload reduction, inotropic support if necessary, and consideration of early reperfusion therapy. Nitrates, diuretics, morphine, and other agents that decrease preload should be avoided. Emergent cardiology consultation should be obtained and/or transfer to a medical center capable of percutaneous coronary intervention (PCI) should be arranged.

Body Surface Mapping

Body surface mapping (BSM) is an extension of the ECG extra-lead concept. Using multiple (up to 80) individual leads to measure electrocardiographic potentials on the human torso, surface mapping collects and analyzes data from a broader thoracic area, permitting greater spatial sampling of the myocardium. Some BSM software can display information as ECG tracings or a topographic color map. It includes the RV, posterior, and high left lateral regions of the heart

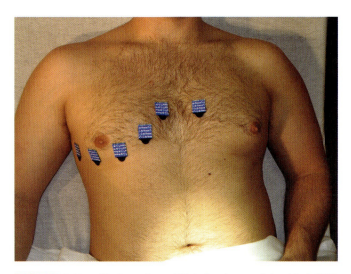

FIGURE 2.10 ■ To investigate RV infarction, a right-sided ECG is obtained by placing leads V1R–V6R as a mirror image of the locations for V1–V6 on the left.

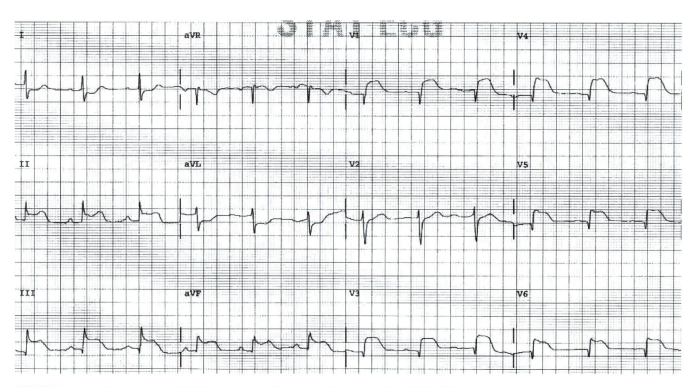

FIGURE 2.11 ■ This right-sided ECG demonstrates ST-segment elevation in leads V1R–V6R.

allowing the clinician to detect injury patterns in these areas. BSM has shown up to 9% greater sensitivity for AMI than 12-lead ECG and has shown potential for detecting AMI in the setting of bundle branch block (BBB) and other conduction abnormalities. With the emergence of more user-friendly computer hardware/software and electrode application, BSM is becoming feasible in clinical practice for the evaluation of patients with chest pain.

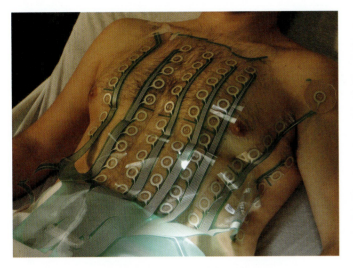

FIGURE 2.12 ■ Multiple leads aligned in self-adhesive strips are placed on the anterior chest wall to perform BSM.

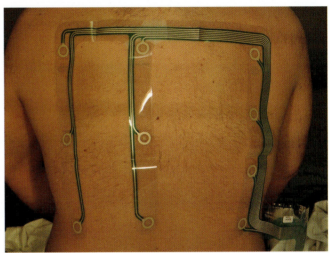

FIGURE 2.13 ■ Multiple leads are applied to the posterior torso for BSM evaluation.

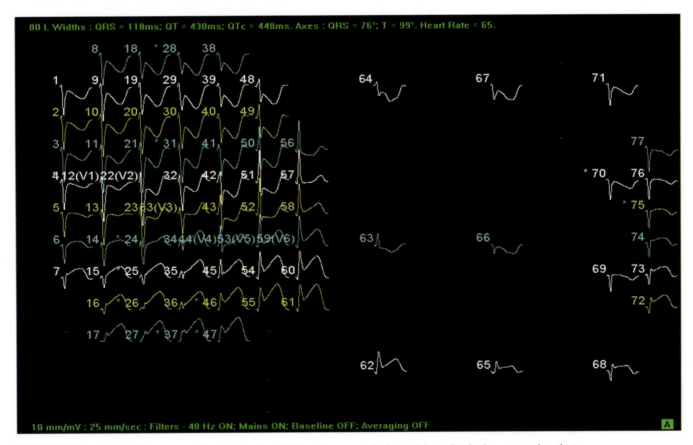

FIGURE 2.14 ■ BSM information can be displayed as ECG tracings at each channel for individual or regional analysis.

22 ■ SUPPLEMENTAL ECG LEADS (CONTINUED)

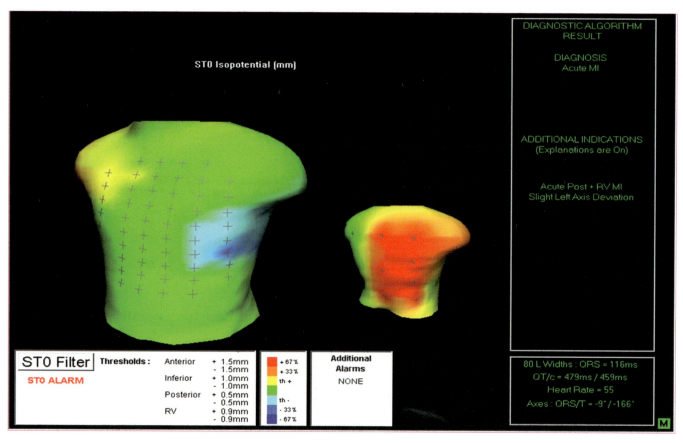

FIGURE 2.15 ■ This BSM torso color display portrays ST-segment elevation in red, ST-segment depression in blue, and isoelectric signals in green. The color distributions noted here are consistent with posterior and RV infarctions.

Pearls and Pitfalls

- Posterior leads should be utilized when ST-depression is noted on the anterior leads of a 12-lead ECG to investigate the presence of posterior AMI.
- Failure to identify ST-segment elevation in a patient with posterior AMI may lead to delays in diagnosis, underutilization of aggressive treatment strategies, and poor outcomes.
- Consider a right-sided ECG to investigate RV involvement in patients who present with inferior ST-segment elevation AMI.
- Failure to recognize RV involvement during an inferior AMI can lead to inappropriate therapy that may result in cardiovascular collapse.

ST-ELEVATION MYOCARDIAL INFARCTION (BY ANATOMIC REGION, INCLUDES SGARBOSSA CRITERIA)

Erica Kellenbeck
Samuel Turnipseed
Deborah Diercks

Clinical Highlights

MI is diagnosed by ECG, cardiac biomarkers, and/or imaging modalities that detect new loss of viable myocardium or new regional wall motion abnormality. In a patient with symptoms suggestive of acute coronary syndrome (ACS; eg, chest pain, dyspnea, diaphoresis, nausea, and vomiting), ST-segment elevation on ECG indicates complete occlusion of a coronary artery resulting in transmural infarction, or STEMI. Such electrocardiographic changes are dependent upon the location of infarction and the degree of coronary artery occlusion.

Clinically significant ST-segment elevation is considered to be present if greater than 1 mm (0.1 mV) in at least two anatomically contiguous leads or 2 mm (0.2 mV) in two contiguous precordial leads.

Left Coronary Artery Occlusion

The left coronary artery begins as the left main coronary artery (LMCA) and branches into the left anterior descending (LAD) artery and the circumflex artery. The LAD travels along the anterior interventricular groove to the apex, supplying blood to the anterior septum and anterior LV. Occlusion of the LAD causes anterior myocardial ischemia with ST elevation in the anterior leads, V1–V5. Elevation in lead aVR greater than elevation in V1 is predictive of LMCA occlusion. Occlusion of a diagonal branch of the LAD can lead to ST elevation in the lateral leads, I, aVL, V5, and V6.

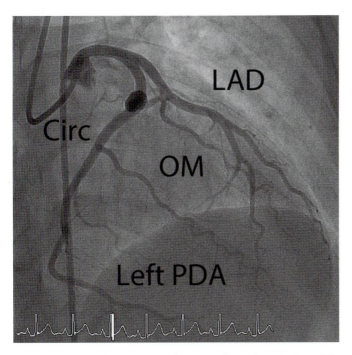

FIGURE 2.16 ■ This is an image from a cardiac catheterization while contrast material is injected into the LMCA. The LAD is running anteriorly toward the apex of the heart. The circumflex is running away from the viewer along the left AV sulcus. OM, obtuse marginal.

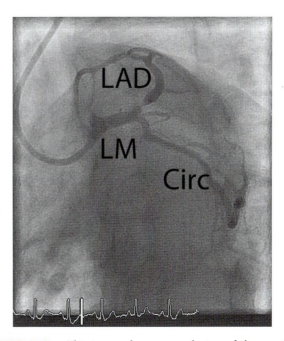

FIGURE 2.17 ■ This image shows an occlusion of the proximal LAD. It is not a total occlusion because contrast material reaches the artery distal to the occlusion. The image is shot looking from the apex toward the aortic root with the LAD anterior and the circumflex again in the left AV sulcus.

24 ST-ELEVATION MYOCARDIAL INFARCTION (CONTINUED)

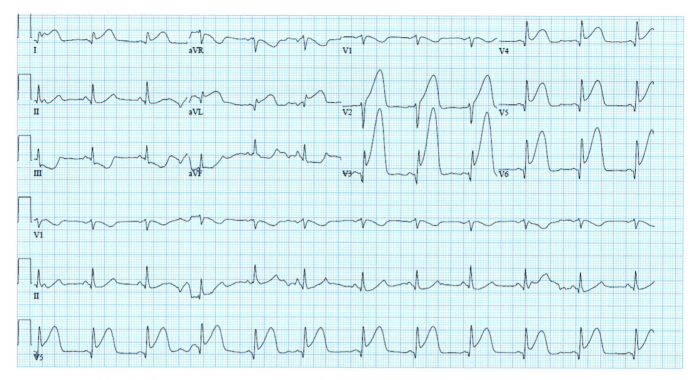

FIGURE 2.18 ■ This ECG shows an anterior STEMI due to occlusion of a mid-LAD lesion.

Circumflex Occlusion

After branching off the LMCA, the circumflex artery runs along the left AV sulcus, supplying blood to the lateral LV through the obtuse marginal branches. Occlusion of the circumflex artery leads to lateral MI with ST elevation in high lateral leads I and aVL. In left dominant systems, described later, inferolateral or inferoposterior MI can be seen with elevation in the corresponding leads.

Right Coronary Artery Occlusion

The RCA runs along the right AV groove to the inferior sinus, supplying blood to the right side of the heart and the inferoposterior heart. The right marginal artery is a branch of the RCA, which runs along the anterior RV, supplying blood to this area. Occlusion of the RCA results in an inferior MI with ST elevation in leads II, III, and aVF. Posterior MI or inferoposterior MI can be seen in right dominant systems, described later. Posterior MI is suggested by depression in V1–V4, which is an electrical mirror image of elevation in leads V7–V9 placed on the patient's back (see Supplemental ECG Leads). Elevation in lead III greater than in lead II is

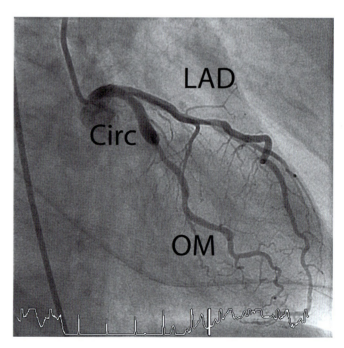

FIGURE 2.19 ■ This image shows a completely occluded circumflex artery just distal to the off-take of the obtuse marginal. The LAD is anterior, apex is to the bottom left, and the circumflex artery is heading away from the viewer.

ST-ELEVATION MYOCARDIAL INFARCTION (CONTINUED)

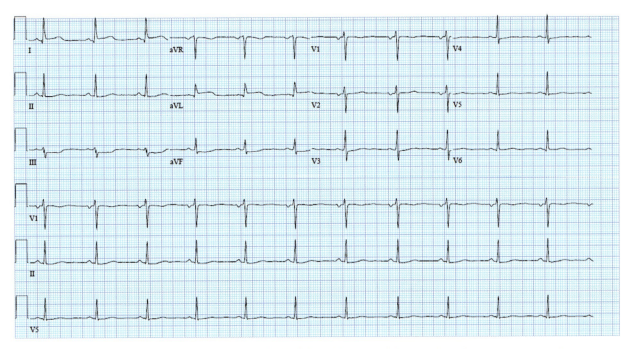

FIGURE 2.20 ■ This ECG shows ST-segment elevation in the high lateral leads (I, aVL); a result of circumflex artery occlusion.

suggestive of a RV infarct and should be investigated with right-sided leads to look for ST elevation in V3R–V6R. STEMI due to RCA occlusion is more frequently associated with conduction abnormalities because the RCA often supplies the SA node, AV node, and bundle of His.

Posterior Descending Artery Occlusion

The posterior descending artery (PDA) supplies the inferior and posterior wall of the LV and the inferior portion of the septum. In a majority of people, the PDA arises as a branch from the RCA, known as a right dominant system. In a minority,

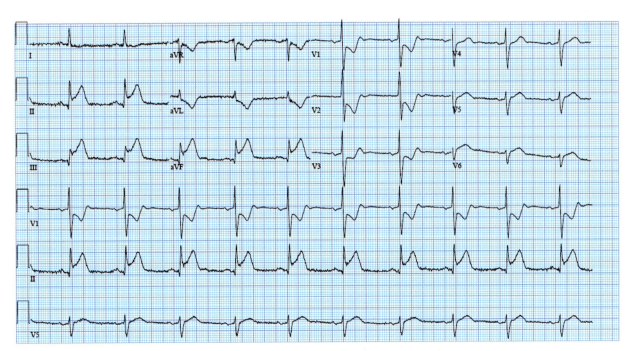

FIGURE 2.21 ■ This ECG reveals ST-segment elevation in the inferior leads (II, III, and aVF) with reciprocal changes in the anterior leads resulting from RCA occlusion.

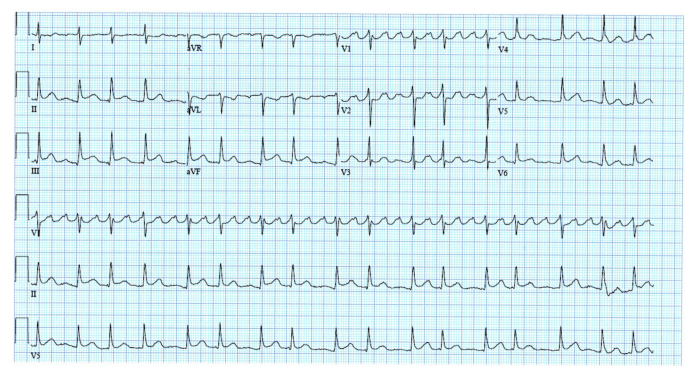

FIGURE 2.22 ■ This ECG shows ST-segment elevation in the inferior leads (II, III, and aVF) and subtle ST-segment depression in lead V2 after PDA occlusion.

less than 10% in most studies, the PDA arises from the circumflex, constituting a left dominant system. A codominant system in which circulation is supplied by branches of both the circumflex and the RCA is also possible. Occlusion of the PDA often leads to inferior MI with ST-segment elevation in the inferior leads (II, III, and aVF), ST-segment depression in leads V1–V4, and elevation in posterior leads V7–V9 (if obtained).

Sgarbossa Criteria

A left BBB (LBBB) is present in roughly 7% of MI and may be associated with total occlusion of a coronary artery. The sequence of repolarization is altered when a LBBB is present, which may make ST-segment changes difficult to discern. The Sgarbossa criteria were developed to help diagnose AMI in patients with LBBB. They include (1) ST-segment elevation of 1 mm or more that is concordant with (in the same direction as) the QRS complex, (2) ST-segment depression of 1 mm or more in lead V1, V2, or V3, and (3) ST-segment elevation of 5 mm or more that is disconcordant with (in the opposite direction from) the QRS complex. The presence of these findings has been shown to have a positive likelihood ratio of 9.5, 6.5, and 3.6.

ED Care and Disposition

The overall therapeutic goal in patients with STEMI is to restore myocardial perfusion as soon as possible. PCI and fibrinolysis are available reperfusion strategies. PCI is associated with increased survival rates, decreased intracranial hemorrhage, and repeated MI. It is recommended for any patient with an acute STEMI who can undergo the procedure within 90 minutes of first medical contact. Fibrinolytic therapy, administered within 30 minutes of first medical contact, is recommended in patients presenting within 12 hours

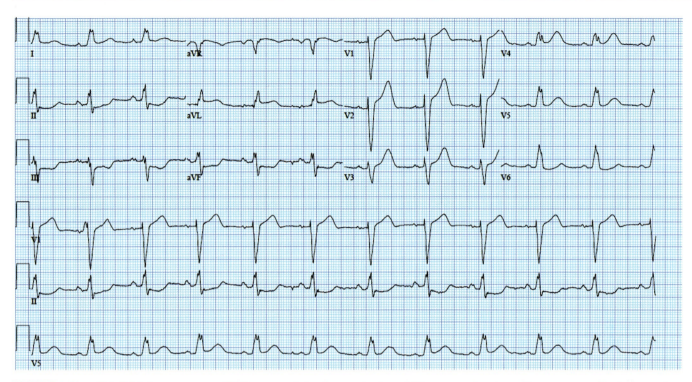

FIGURE 2.23 ■ This ECG demonstrates a LBBB pattern. A Sgarbossa criterion of ST-segment elevation of 1 mm or more that is concordant with the QRS complex (in leads I and AVL) is met.

of symptom onset if PCI is not available within 90 minutes. Recent studies suggest that even patients initially treated with fibrinolysis should be rapidly transferred to a PCI center.

Adjunctive therapy such as oxygen, nitrates, antiplatelet agents, and anticoagulants may also be initiated. Aspirin should be given to all patients with ACS to prevent further thrombosis. In addition, a thienopyridine may be administered. Treatment of ischemic pain, hypertension, and tachycardia can mitigate increased myocardial oxygen demand. Oral or parenteral nitroglycerin can be administered to achieve vasodilation, but should be avoided in patients with hypotension, suspected RV infarct, bradycardia, tachycardia, or those who have taken a phosphodiesterase inhibitor within 24 hours. Anticoagulants may also be administered in the acute setting. The selection of antiplatelet and anticoagulant agents and the timing of their administration may be dependent on the reperfusion strategy selected.

Pearls and Pitfalls

- Older patients, diabetics, and women with ACS are more likely to present with symptoms such as dyspnea, weakness, nausea, vomiting, palpitations, and syncope than with classic symptoms such as chest discomfort.
- ST-segment elevation on ECG should prompt rapid initiation of reperfusion therapy.
- The utilization of adjunctive therapy should not delay the initiation of the appropriate reperfusion strategy.
- LBBB on ECG can make the diagnosis of STEMI difficult. The Sgarbossa criteria can aid in the diagnosis.

T-WAVE INVERSION

Judd E. Hollander
Dina M. Sparano

Clinical Highlights

T-wave inversions can be evidence of cardiac ischemia, follow a tachycardia, be associated with intrinsic heart disease (myocarditis, pericarditis, and ventricular hypertrophy), be a normal variant (persistent juvenile pattern), or be associated with noncardiac conditions, such as intracranial injury or pulmonary embolism. When evaluating a patient with chest pain or other anginal symptoms, T-wave inversions are concerning for cardiac ischemia. When these T-wave inversions are >1 mm, are symmetrically inverted in a pointed fashion, and/or are either concordant with the QRS complex or biphasic, they can be a marker of severe coronary artery stenosis. Concomitant subtle doming of the ST segment is an additional worrisome feature. T-wave inversions can appear when ischemia is transient (ie, unstable angina) and may recover when the patients symptoms resolve; commonly referred to as dynamic T-wave changes. When cardiac ischemia progresses to transmural infarction, T-wave inversions are likely to persist and eventually be accompanied by the other electrocardiographic changes of MI in evolution. In patients whose baseline ECG shows T-wave inversions, ischemic conditions can cause the T waves to flip upright and appear normal, a term called pseudo-normalization.

ED Care and Disposition

New T-wave inversions in symptomatic patients likely indicate unstable angina. Cardiac biomarkers may or may not be elevated initially, because the ECG reveals changes during acute ischemia while biomarkers can take several hours to become elevated. Patients with new T-wave inversions in a setting of concerning symptoms and historical features should be admitted and treated according to the ACC/AHA guidelines for ACS.

Pearls and Pitfalls

- T-wave inversions that appear in the setting of anginal symptoms are highly suggestive of severe coronary stenosis and ischemia.
- A comparison should be made to the patient's baseline ECG when possible. New T-wave inversions or pseudo-normalization of baseline T-wave inversions should raise concern for ACS.
- ED patients with potential ACS who have T-wave inversions are at increased risk of adverse outcomes relative to those who do not have T-wave inversions.

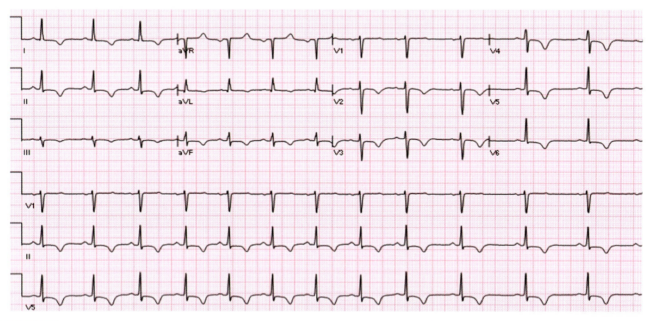

FIGURE 2.24 ■ This tracing shows concordant T-wave inversions in the anterolateral (V2–V6, as well as I and AVL) and inferior (II, III, and AVF) leads. In addition, the subtle doming of the ST segment in the anterior leads is worrisome in the right clinical context.

HYPERACUTE T-WAVES

Judd E. Hollander
Dina M. Sparano

Clinical Highlights

In the very early stages of a MI, the T waves corresponding to the affected myocardial territory will peak, becoming tall and narrow. This typically occurs within 15 minutes from the onset of transmural ischemia and is very transient, thus infrequently captured on ECG. This is particularly true because most patients delay, up to 2 hours on average, activating emergency medical response services or seeking medical attention once their chest discomfort begins. Thus, capturing hyperacute T waves on an ECG would likely necessitate the patient already being in the hospital/emergency department when their symptoms begin or shortly thereafter.

ED Care and Disposition

In patients with symptoms suggestive of myocardial ischemia, the presence of hyperacute, or peaked, T waves on ECG should prompt immediate concern for MI. After a brief period of persistent transmural ischemia, these T-wave changes may evolve into ST-segment elevations. Tall or peaked T waves can also be seen in healthy patients as a normal variant, typically in the precordial leads. The presence of tall, peaked T waves is also an electrocardiographic finding associated with hyperkalemia. As such, hyperacute T waves in a dialysis patient should prompt consideration of hyperkalemia in the appropriate clinical setting. Tall T waves can also be seen in LV hypertrophy, LBBB, and intracranial bleeding.

Pearls and Pitfalls

- Hyperacute T waves are infrequently captured on ECG because they typically appear within minutes after the onset of symptoms, long before most patients present to the emergency department.
- This abnormality is transient, lasting briefly before evolving into ST-segment elevations, which can last for hours. Therefore, the absence of hyperacute T waves should not discourage the diagnosis of AMI.
- In the appropriate clinical setting, hyperacute T waves can be caused by an entirely different life-threatening condition: hyperkalemia. This electrolyte abnormality requires rapid stabilization and treatment.

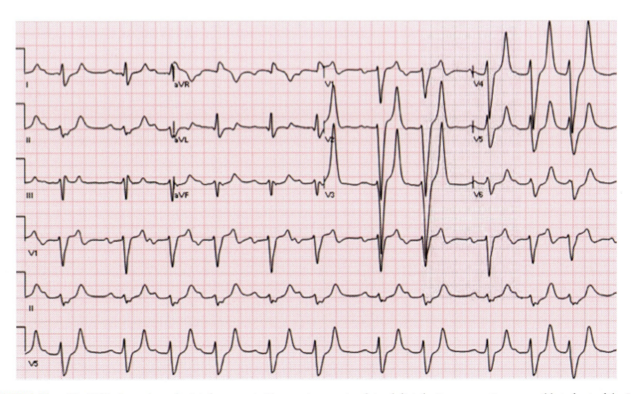

FIGURE 2.25 ■ The ECG shown here depicts hyperacute T waves in an anterolateral distribution, suggesting a possible infarct of the LAD artery and an associated diagonal branch.

ST SEGMENT DEPRESSION

Judd E. Hollander
Dina M. Sparano

Clinical Highlights

ST-segment depressions on an ECG can be electrocardiographic evidence of cardiac ischemia. In healthy patients, the ST segment is isoelectric as all myocytes maintain similar potential during early repolarization. Deviation from this is an electrocardiographic surrogate for myocardial ischemia. While transmural ischemia classically results in ST-segment elevation in the corresponding leads, subendocardial ischemia typically results in the overall ST-segment vector pointing toward the inner ventricular layer and appears as ST-segment depression.

Depression of the ST segment is a repolarization abnormality suggestive of myocardial ischemia. Horizontal or downsloping depression >1 mm and up-sloping depression >2 mm is considered positive. ST-segment depressions can occur with or without T-wave inversion. The magnitude of ST-segment depression correlates with the severity of ischemic burden.

The presence and characteristics of ST-segment depression are a key factor in risk-stratifying patients with non-ST-segment elevation myocardial infarction (NSTEMI)/unstable angina (UA). Patients with ACS and ST-segment depressions fare worse than those with T-wave inversions or the absence of ECG changes. These patients demonstrate increased mortality and are more likely to have MI.

Magnitude and location of ST-segment depression lend diagnostic and prognostic information. Mortality is higher for patients with ST-segment depression >2 mm. However, ST-segment depression of <1 mm showed an increased mortality relative to those who remain isoelectric. A focal distribution, while it may correlate to territorial groups of leads (eg, II, III, AVF for inferior or V1–V4 for anterior, etc.), does not necessarily match the area of ischemia on stress imaging or coronary angiography because ST-segment depressions may be reciprocal to contralateral ST-segment elevations. The number of leads with ST-segment depression as well as a higher sum of ST-segment depression in all leads is associated with a worse outcome.

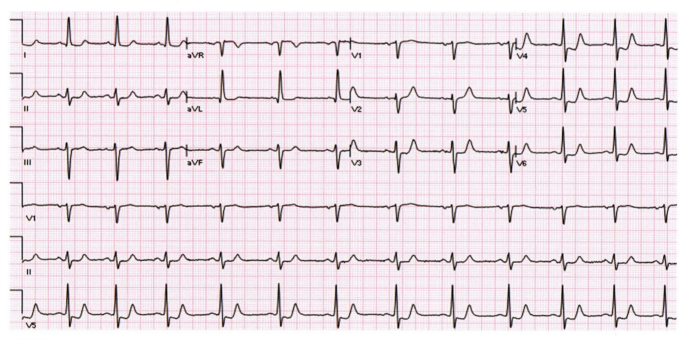

FIGURE 2.26 ■ ST-segment depression (seen here in leads V3–V6) with simultaneous ST-segment elevation in lead AVR is an ominous finding in the setting of anginal symptoms. This abnormality, particularly in conjunction with ST-segment elevation in AVL, is 75% predictive of severe stenosis in the LMCA or three-vessel disease.

ST SEGMENT DEPRESSION (CONTINUED)

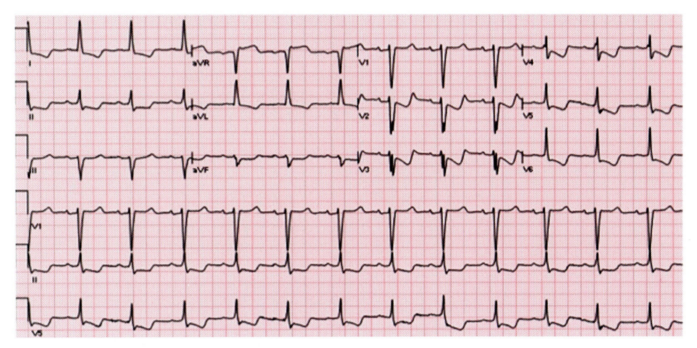

FIGURE 2.27 ■ This ECG shows isolated ST-segment elevation in AVR with deep ST-segment depression and T-wave inversion in nearly all other leads except V1. In the right clinical context, this ECG is worrisome for either left main or proximal (to the first diagonal branch) LAD occlusion.

ED Care and Disposition

During stress, ST-segment changes are measured from the isoelectric baseline of the ECG, determined by the PR interval. If the ST segments are elevated at baseline, ST-segment depressions are still measured from the isoelectric baseline. If, however, the ST segments are depressed at baseline, further ST-segment depression with stress is measured from the resting ST segment. Significant ST-segment depression, particularly if it can be confirmed that it constitutes a change from baseline, in patients presenting with angina or equivalent symptoms should raise concern for subendocardial ischemia. ST-segment depressions can occur unrelated to ischemia. They can be seen in patients with LV and RV hypertrophy, electrolyte abnormalities (hypokalemia), and digitalis toxicity. Patients should be treated according to the ACC/AHA guidelines for NSTEMI/UA and considered for early revascularization strategies when appropriate.

Pearls and Pitfalls

- While ST-segment elevations are a result of transmural infarctions, subendocardial ischemia results in ST-segment depression.
- ST-segment depressions in the setting of ACS (ie, NSTEMI/UA) are an ominous finding as they portend a worse prognosis.
- Magnitude of ST-segment depression and number of leads involved have been shown to aid in risk stratification of patients presenting with NSTEMI and guide revascularization strategies.

Q WAVES

Judd E. Hollander
Dina M. Sparano

Clinical Highlights

When MI occurs, ensuing myocyte necrosis leads to a reduction or absence of electrical forces in the affected area. This is represented on the ECG as decreased R-wave amplitude or the appearance of Q waves. Pathologic Q waves are defined as >0.04 s or more than 25% of the R-wave amplitude. Q waves, along with other ECG changes of AMI, may persist or resolve. Persistence of Q waves and ST-segment elevations for several days to weeks after infarction is associated with wall motion abnormalities in the affected territory and/or the development of a ventricular aneurysm.

Q waves may also appear in the absence of MI. They may be physiologic, particularly in leads V1, V2, III, and AVF. They may appear with ventricular hypertrophy or conduction disturbances as well. Rarely, they can be seen in chronic myocardial diseases, such as amyloidosis or myocarditis, and in certain electrolyte disturbances.

ED Care and Disposition

When patients present with symptoms of angina and ECG changes suggestive of acute myocardial ischemia, the presence of Q waves suggests myocardial necrosis has occurred. Despite the fact that this may represent a MI that began hours to days before the patient presents, cardiology consultation should be obtained as early as possible and the patient should be treated according to the ACC/AHA guidelines for ACS. There still may be ongoing ischemia for which the patient may benefit from early reperfusion strategies.

Pearls and Pitfalls

- Pathologic Q waves are typically defined as being >0.04 s (one small box) or at least 25% of the R-wave amplitude on ECG.
- While they appear later in the sequence of ECG changes that occur with AMI, the presence of Q waves does not exclude the use of reperfusion strategies if a patient has ST-segment elevation and is within the treatment window.
- The persistence of Q waves and ST-segment elevation on ECG suggests the development of ventricular wall akinesis or dyskinesis that is suggestive of aneurysm formation.

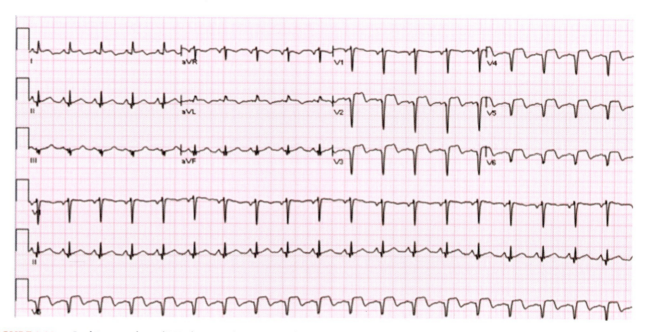

FIGURE 2.28 ■ In this anterolateral MI, there are dramatic ST elevations in leads V2–V6 as well as in lead I, suggesting involvement of either the proximal LAD before it gives rise to diagonal branch(es) that supply the lateral wall, or a left main artery occlusion that involves both the LAD and left circumflex systems. Q waves are already apparent in the precordium, suggesting the patient is at least several hours to days into the event. In the setting of symptoms, however, there is presumably ongoing ischemia as well.

WELLENS' SYNDROME

Alan T. Chiem

Clinical Highlights

Wellens syndrome is characterized by T-wave changes in the anterior ECG leads and is a warning sign of impending MI. The characteristic ECG findings of Wellens syndrome are biphasic or deep, inverted symmetric T waves in the anterior precordial leads. Such electrocardiographic changes signal critical stenosis of the proximal LAD coronary artery. Patients with Wellens syndrome are at imminent risk of developing significant MI, ventricular arrhythmia, and death.

Wellens syndrome was first described by the Dutch cardiologist Hein Wellens and his colleagues in 1982. In early studies by Wellens et al., all study subjects with these characteristic ECG changes demonstrated obstructive LAD disease on coronary angiography. The LAD coronary artery supplies the septal wall, anterior wall, and apex of the LV. Due to the high risk of congestive heart failure, ventricular arrhythmias, and death associated with an acute occlusion of the LAD coronary artery, it is sometimes referred to as a "widow maker" lesion.

In a majority of patients, the ECG abnormalities associated with Wellens syndrome occur only when the patient is pain-free. During a bout of anginal pain, these ECG changes can disappear, pseudonormalize or progress to ST-segment elevation. Furthermore, cardiac biomarkers are often normal or minimally elevated in patients with Wellens syndrome. Therefore, findings on ECG may be the only warning signal of imminent MI and must be recognized by the provider.

The ECG abnormalities associated with Wellens syndrome consist of deep, symmetrically inverted T waves (most

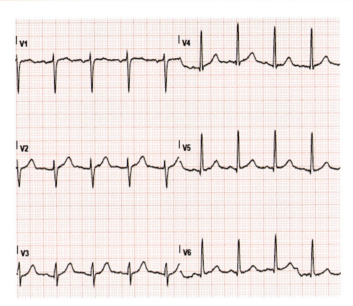

FIGURE 2.30 ■ This ECG was acquired upon presentation to emergency department, when the patient still had moderate chest pain. There is no Wellens-type abnormality.

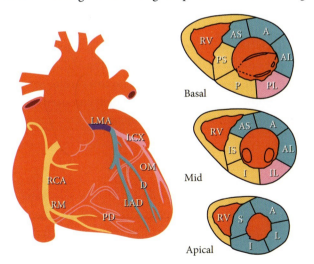

FIGURE 2.29 ■ Coronary distribution using a 16-segment model. LCX, left circumflex artery; D, diagonal branch of the LAD; OM, obtuse marginal branch of the LCX; and RM, right marginal branch of the RCA. Notice that the LAD and its branches supply the septal, anterior, and lateral walls of the LV at the base and mid portion, while supplying the entire apex. Reprinted, with permission, from Malouf JF, Edwards WD, Tajik A, Seward JB. Chapter 4. Functional anatomy of the heart. In: Fuster V, Walsh RA, Harrington RA. eds. *Hurst's The Heart*. 13th ed. New York, NY: McGraw-Hill; 2011.

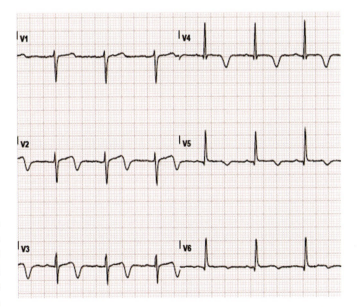

FIGURE 2.31 ■ This ECG was obtained after the patient's chest pain had resolved, demonstrating biphasic T waves in V2–V3 and inverted T waves in V4–V5.

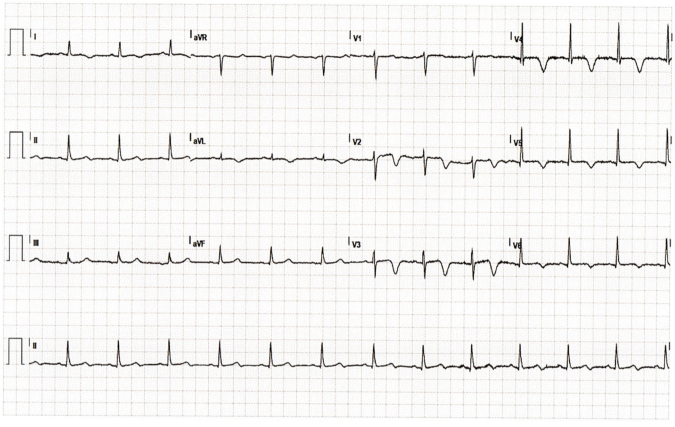

FIGURE 2.32 ■ This is an example of deep, symmetrically inverted T waves in leads V2–V4; an ECG pattern associated with Wellens syndrome.

common) in leads V2 and V3 (sometimes in V1, V4-6) or biphasic T waves (less common) in leads V2 and V3.

The ST segment is typically isoelectric but elevations are sometimes present with either convex or concave morphology. Recent cardiac MRI studies suggest that the ECG changes may be related to myocardial edema. Because T-wave inversions can result from a number of other clinical conditions, the combination of either T-wave abnormality described earlier plus the following criteria can help distinguish between Wellens pathology and other clinical syndromes: (1) a history of angina but the absence of ongoing anginal pain, (2) the absence of precordial Q waves, (3) normal or mildly elevated cardiac biomarkers, and (4) the presence of isoelectric or minimally elevated ST segments.

ED Care and Disposition

Patients with suspected Wellens syndrome, as with any other high-risk ACS, should not undergo stress testing. Patients with Wellens syndrome are at high risk for total occlusion of the proximal LAD coronary artery and resultant infarction of the inferior, anterior, and septal walls. Medical therapy should be optimized in accordance with the ACC/AHA guidelines for high-risk ACS and admission to a cardiology service should be obtained. Subsequent inpatient coronary angiography with reperfusion strategy is indicated.

Pearls and Pitfalls

- The ECG changes associated with Wellens syndrome often occur when anginal symptoms have resolved. Therefore, a recent *history* of anginal pain in addition to these characteristic ECG findings should alert the provider to the presence of Wellens syndrome and the potential for significant adverse cardiac events.
- The natural historical course of Wellens syndrome is progression to significant MI. Therefore, patients with these characteristic ECG findings should undergo inpatient monitoring as well as aggressive diagnostic and therapeutic strategies.
- A stress test is contraindicated in Wellens syndrome due to the risk of precipitating MI.

Chapter 3
PRINCIPLES OF CARDIOVASCULAR IMAGING

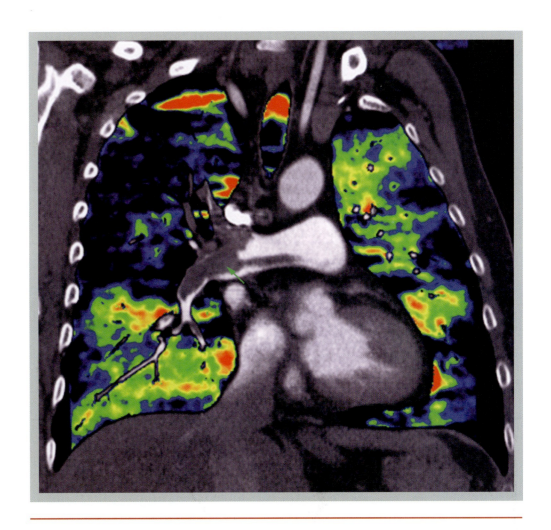

CHEST RADIOGRAPHS

Justin B. Joines
Cedric Lefebvre

Technology/Technique

Chest radiographs are the most commonly performed diagnostic radiographs in emergency departments. A chest radiograph can help identify cardiovascular emergencies and other medical problems such as pneumothorax, pulmonary edema, aortic dissection, pneumonia, perforation of the gastrointestinal tract, fractures, masses, and foreign bodies (Table 3.1).

A radiograph, or "x-ray," is customarily performed by a trained radiologic technician. The x-ray apparatus typically consists of x-ray film or a special plate that digitally records the picture and an x-ray tube. The x-ray film is positioned next to the patient while the x-ray tube is located at a distance of about 6 feet from the patient. Two views are taken for a conventional chest radiograph: a posterior–anterior (PA) view, in which the x-ray beam passes through the chest from the back, and a lateral view such that x-rays pass through the chest from one side to the other. When the clinical scenario mandates a portable radiograph at the bedside, an anterior–posterior (AP) view can be obtained with the patient in a seated position. The technician may use a lead apron to protect certain parts of the patient's body (eg, reproductive organs) from radiation. The amount of radiation used in a chest radiograph is relatively small and confers approximately 0.1 milli-severts (1/10,000 Sv) to the patient.

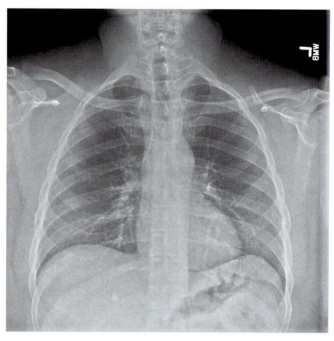

FIGURE 3.1 ■ The conventional PA view of a chest radiograph provides an image of the lungs, heart, great vessels, mediastinum, ribs, clavicles, trachea, esophagus, spine, and diaphragms.

TABLE 3.1 ■ MEDICAL CONDITIONS AND ASSOCIATED FINDINGS ON CHEST RADIOGRAPH

Diagnosis	Important Finding
Pulmonary edema	Vascular congestion, increased cephalization of vascular flow
Pneumothorax	Absence of lung markings, deep sulcus sign, mediastinal deviation
Aortic dissection/aneurysm	Abnormal mediastinum, aortic knob or cardiac contour; pleural effusions, displaced intimal calcification, tracheal deviation
Pneumonia	Focal or lobar consolidation, localized infiltration, patchy opacifications
Cardiac tamponade	Possible presence of enlarged cardiac silhouette
Pulmonary embolus	Westermark sign, Hamptons hump, atelectasis
Esophageal rupture	Widened mediastinum, free air

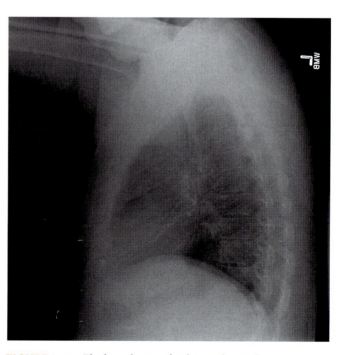

FIGURE 3.2 ■ The lateral view of a chest radiograph.

CHEST RADIOGRAPHS (CONTINUED)

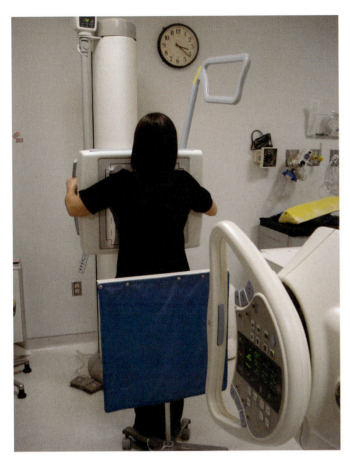

FIGURE 3.3 ■ For a PA view, the patient is positioned so that the chest rests against the image plate.

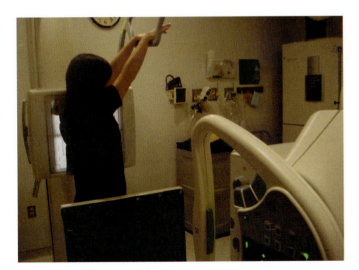

FIGURE 3.4 ■ For a lateral view, the patient is turned with one side against the image plate and arms raised above the head.

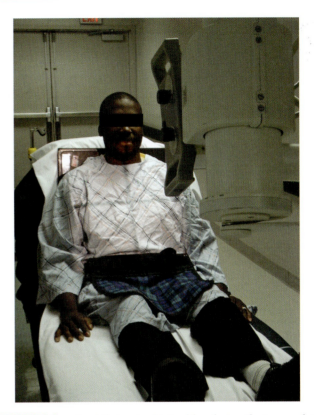

FIGURE 3.5 ■ An AP view is obtained by placing the image plate behind a patient sitting upright.

Interpretation

Most chest radiographs today are viewed and stored in a digital format. Chest radiographs use the ionizing radiation of x-rays to produce images of the structures within the human torso. Visual contrast is achieved by the different degrees to which various tissue types absorb radiation. Lungs are air-filled structures that appear dark, whereas bony structures are dense and appear white. The interpretation of a chest radiograph should be approached in a consistent and stepwise fashion. Consider the following format: review identifying patient information, observe the trachea for midline position and caliber, view the lungs and pleura for abnormal appearance, screen the pulmonary vasculature for enlargement or cephalization of flow, and investigate the hila for masses or lymphadenopathy. Next, examine the heart-to-thorax ratio and mediastinal contour, identify bony lesions or fractures, inspect soft tissues for swelling or air, and confirm supporting medical apparatus when applicable (eg, tubes and intravenous [IV] lines).

38 ■ CHEST RADIOGRAPHS (CONTINUED)

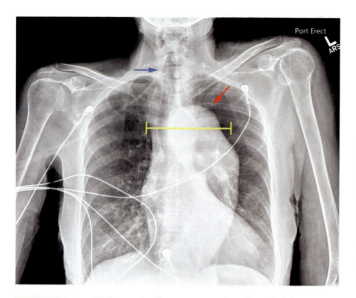

FIGURE 3.6 ■ This aortic dissection can be identified by a widened mediastinum (yellow bracket), tracheal deviation (blue arrow), abnormal cardiac contour and a distorted aortic knob (red arrow).

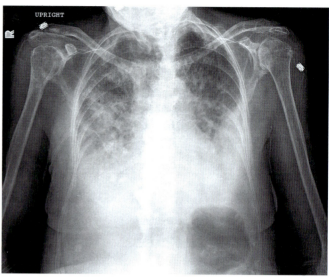

FIGURE 3.7 ■ The interstitial prominence and pleural effusions seen here are evidence of pulmonary edema in this patient with congestive heart failure.

Pearls and Pitfalls

- The patient must take a deep breath and hold it for an adequate image. The diaphragm should be found at about the level of the eighth to tenth posterior rib or fifth to sixth anterior rib.
- The AP view will magnify the size of the cardiac silhouette.
- Adequate penetration is required for a good study. For a point of reference, the thoracic spine disc spaces should be barely visible through the heart on a PA film.
- Rotation of the patient may cause the mediastinum to look abnormal. Ensure that the clavicular heads are at equal distances from the spine.

BEDSIDE ULTRASOUND/ECHOCARDIOGRAPHY

Casey Glass

Video in this chapter is available at http://mhprofessional.com/sites/lefebvre

Technology/Technique

Bedside echocardiography can assist the emergency physician in narrowing the differential diagnosis and improving treatment decisions for a number of clinical scenarios. Common Emergency Department (ED) applications include assessment of global left ventricular (LV) function, investigation of acute right-sided heart failure or symptomatic pericardial effusion, and evaluation of volume status through measurement of the inferior vena cava (IVC). The measurement of ejection fraction, the assessment of diastolic dysfunction, and Doppler evaluation of valvular function can also be obtained using bedside echocardiography.

The quality of images obtained is greatly dependent on the quality of the ultrasound equipment and the skill of the operator. Generally, point-of-care machines produce images inferior to their dedicated echocardiography counterparts. Ideally, a phased array probe will be used for cardiac ultrasound. However, images can be obtained with a curved linear array probe as well. The ultrasound probe is oriented to produce images of the same screen appearance as formal echocardiography studies. Typically a bedside echocardiogram will include a four-chamber subcostal view, a long axis view of the vena cava, parasternal long and short axis views, and an apical four-chamber view.

Interpretation

The subcostal view is obtained by placing the ultrasound probe in the subxiphoid space with the indexed side of the probe to the patient's right and the beam aimed at the left shoulder. This view visualizes all four chambers of the heart as well as the anterior and posterior pericardium. A pericardial effusion appears as a dark stripe around the heart. Portions of the chambers may be out of plane and chamber size may be distorted. Caution should be exercised when deciding if there is abnormal chamber size.

The probe is then rotated 90° clockwise so that the indexed side of the probe is oriented toward the patient's head. The right upper quadrant (RUQ) is swept from midline to the right flank to locate the vena cava, which appears as an anechoic tube connecting to the right atrium. In this position, an M-mode tracing can be performed approximately 2 cm caudal to the diaphragm to evaluate for respiratory movement of the

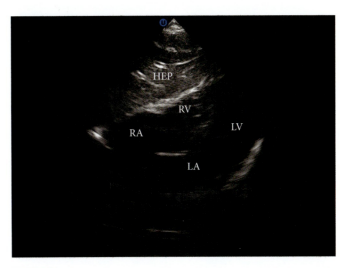

FIGURE 3.8 ■ In the subcostal four-chamber view of the heart, the base of the heart is toward screen left and the apex toward screen right. The right ventricle (RV), right atrium (RA), LV, and left atrium (LA) are imaged using the liver (HEP) as a window.

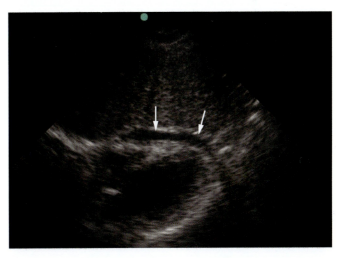

FIGURE 3.9 ■ A pericardial effusion (arrows) as seen from a subcostal view. Effusion fluid may be anechoic as in the case of a transudate or mixed-echogenicity as in pericardial abscess or hemorrhage. The fluid should follow the outer contour of the heart.

 VIDEO 3.1 ■ A subcostal view of the heart. This view is the most familiar view among emergency physicians and is well suited for assessment of pericardial effusion and global function. The operator should increase the depth of the image as needed to visualize the posterior pericardium.

IVC and IVC diameter. The ratio of the inspiratory and expiratory diameter of the IVC (the caval index) correlates with central venous pressure (CVP). A diameter greater than 1.5 to 2 cm with little change during respiration correlates with

an elevated CVP (>20 cm H$_2$O), and a small or collapsed IVC <1 cm with more than 50% collapse with respiration correlates with a low CVP (<10 cm H$_2$O).

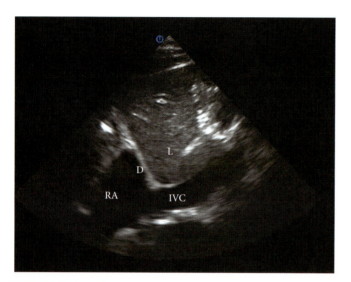

FIGURE 3.10 ■ The IVC is imaged in the long axis as it enters the right atrium (RA). The liver (L) provides a window for imaging the IVC. IVC diameter is measured caudal to the diaphragm (D).

 VIDEO 3.2 ■ Respiratory variation of the vena cava. The vena cava collapses as the negative intrathoracic pressure associated with inspiration draws blood from the abdomen into the chest. These dynamic changes are reduced or eliminated by congestive heart failure, extrinsic pressure on the heart as in tamponade or tension pneumothorax, or with positive pressure ventilation.

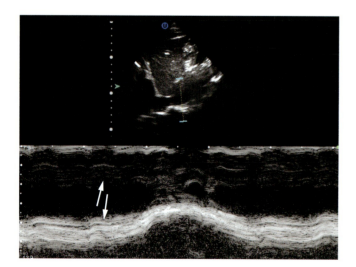

FIGURE 3.11 ■ For m-mode measurement of vena cava size, the vena cava diameter is measured at end expiration (large arrows) and again during inspiration when it reaches its least diameter (arrowheads).

Parasternal views are obtained when the probe is placed in the third or fourth intercostal space along the left side of the sternum. The probe is first oriented with the indexed side to the lower left costal margin producing an image of the heart in the long axis. The parasternal long axis view visualizes the LV and left atrium as well as the aortic outflow tract. The RV is only partially imaged and the right atrium is excluded. This view is helpful for assessing volume status and global cardiac function as well as aortic root diameter.

The parasternal short axis view is obtained by rotating the probe 90° clockwise until it is oriented toward the lower right costal margin producing an image of the LV in the short axis. The probe should be angled or moved laterally to image the LV at the level of the papillary muscles. In cases of acute pulmonary hypertension, the septum may deviate toward the LV producing a "D-shaped" ventricle. The short axis view is also useful for assessing global LV function.

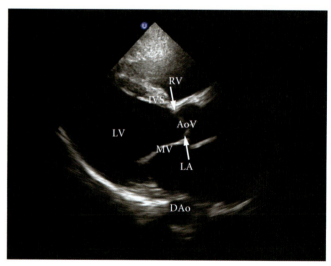

FIGURE 3.12 ■ The parasternal long axis view gives a good representation of the LV, left atrium (LA), interventricular septum (IVS), and aortic outflow tract (AO). The mitral (MV) and aortic (AoV) valves are seen. Aortic root measurements are performed at the level of the aortic valve (arrows). The descending aorta is also imaged posterior to the heart (DAo).

 VIDEO 3.3 ■ The parasternal view is useful for estimating cardiac function and ejection fraction. The degree of anterior mitral valve excursion is one surrogate for ejection fraction. In most individuals, it should approach the septum at the start of diastole as blood rushes in from the left atrium to fill the ventricle.

BEDSIDE ULTRASOUND/ECHOCARDIOGRAPHY (CONTINUED) ■ 41

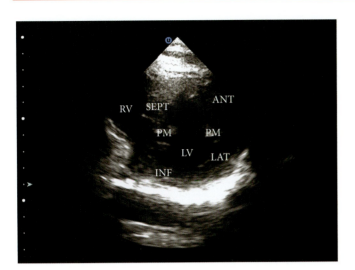

FIGURE 3.13 ■ The parasternal short axis view allows assessment of the anterior (ANT), septal (SEPT), lateral (LAT), and inferior (INF) LV walls. The RV usually extends out of the screen. Ideally, we would like to image at the level of the papillary muscles (PM).

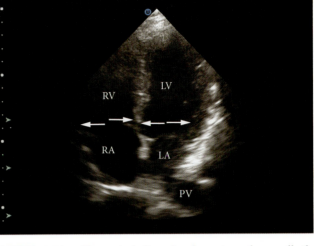

FIGURE 3.14 ■ The apical four-chamber view shows all the chambers in their anatomic size when the probe is on plane with the heart. The ventricle diameters are measured from the outside wall to the septum (arrows). Pulmonary veins (PV) can sometimes be seen posterior to the left atrium.

VIDEO 3.4 ■ The parasternal short axis view is useful for assessing wall motion abnormalities and global function.

VIDEO 3.6 ■ The apical four-chamber view is useful for investigating an effusion and for evaluating global function and RV enlargement.

VIDEO 3.5 ■ Deviation of the septum toward the LV is an indicator of acute severe pulmonary hypertension as in the setting of massive PE. In the short axis, the LV has a rounded "O" appearance. In the setting of right heart strain the septum moves toward the LV making it appear as a "D."

The apical four-chamber view is obtained when the probe is placed over the point of maximal impulse with the indexed side of the probe aimed anteriorly and toward the patient's right. The beam is aimed at the right shoulder producing a four-chamber image of the heart. This view is helpful for assessing RV size, global function, and the presence of effusion. To measure ventricle size, the ventricles are measured at the level of the tricuspid or mitral valve from the outer wall to the middle of the septum at end diastole.

Clinical scenarios where bedside echocardiography is often employed include evaluation of unexplained hypotension, possible aortic dissection, and for estimation of ejection fraction.

Advanced skills include evaluation for systolic dysfunction by evaluating the degree of E-point septal separation and measured ejection fraction, evaluation for diastolic dysfunction

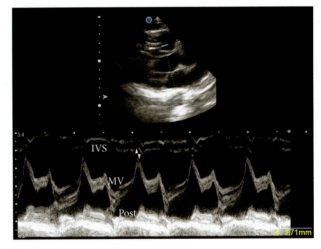

FIGURE 3.15 ■ E-point septal separation is a useful surrogate for impaired ejection fraction due to systolic dysfunction, valvular dysfunction, or ventricular septal defect. The probe must be perpendicular to the heart to ensure an axis view. The maximal excursion of the anterior mitral leaflet is measured with reference to the interventricular septum (arrowheads). A normal measurement is less than 4 mm.

through measurement of the E to A ratio and E wave duration, and measurement of cardiac output. These studies require significant additional ultrasound skill and an understanding of their limitations.

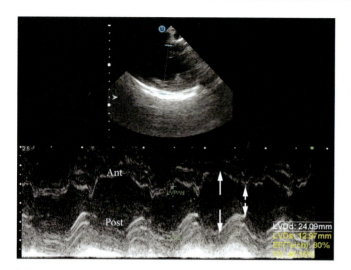 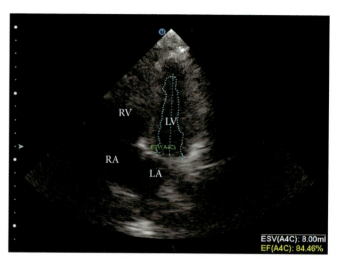

FIGURE 3.16 ■ When patients have known systolic dysfunction without significant regional wall motion abnormalities, ejection fraction can be estimated by comparing the systolic (small arrows) and diastolic (large arrows) diameters of the LV. This measurement is usually obtained in the parasternal short axis view at the level of the papillary muscles.

FIGURE 3.17 ■ Simpson's method of disks is a more accurate estimation of ejection fraction, is appropriate for all patients and is necessary for those with significant regional wall motion abnormalities. The ventricle is imaged in the apical four- or two-chamber view and the endocardium is traced at end diastole and end systole.

Pearls and Pitfalls

- The left lateral decubitus position is helpful for improving the parasternal and apical views.
- Positive pressure ventilation can reduce or eliminate the normal respiratory variation in IVC size.
- Cardiac views may be improved by having the patient hold their breath at end expiration.
- Pleural and peritoneal fluid can be mistaken for a pericardial effusion if several views of the heart are not assessed.

TRANSTHORACIC ECHOCARDIOGRAPHY

Joseph Yeboah
Bharathi Upadhya

Technology/Technique

Transthoracic echocardiography (TTE) has evolved into a diagnostic cornerstone in cardiovascular emergency management. It is safe, noninvasive, highly accurate, and offers a quick assessment of the heart and a portion of the aorta. A crystal-containing TTE probe projects ultrasound waves at the organ of interest and these waves are reflected back to the probe. The reflected waves are processed and reconstituted into images. TTE imaging includes M-mode, in which the ultrasound beam is aimed manually at selected cardiac structures, as well as color and Doppler imaging by which the direction and velocities of moving objects can be measured. More recently, strain/speckle tracking imaging has been developed for non-invasive assessment of myocardial deformation. Standardized imaging protocols have been established for TTE of the heart and thoracic aorta. These standardized views include parasternal long and short axes, apical long and short axes, subcostal and suprasternal notch views.

The scope of the diagnostic capabilities of TTE includes evaluating the cause of chest pain, investigating the etiology of hypotension/shock, and exploring the source of dyspnea. In the setting of chest pain, TTE can help differentiate between myocardial ischemia/infarct during which wall motion abnormalities may be noted, and acute pericarditis during which wall motion is normal but a small amount of pericardial effusion may be seen. Stress-induced cardiomyopathy, or Takotsubo cardiomyopathy, is another cause of chest pain that can be investigated by TTE. In Takotsubo cardiomyopathy, characteristic apical ballooning and hyperdynamic movement of the base of the LV is noted. Thoracic aortic dissection is another etiology of chest pain that can be found on TTE.

When investigating the cause of severe hypotension/shock, TTE can accurately identify cardiac emergencies contributing to hemodynamic instability. In cases of cardiogenic shock due to massive myocardial infarction (MI), TTE will often reveal reduced LV ejection fraction with wall motion abnormalities. In cases of cardiac tamponade, an accumulation of fluid in the pericardial sac with evidence of hemodynamic compromise can be observed with TTE. TTE can also detect hypovolemia as the cause of hypotension by identifying underfilling of the cardiac chambers.

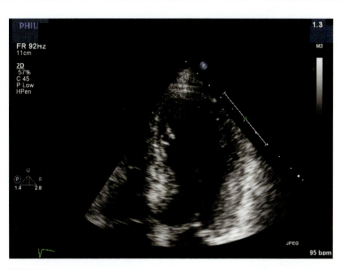

FIGURE 3.18 ■ Apical ballooning, seen here on TTE, imparts the characteristic shape of the LV during ventricular systole in Takotsubo cardiomyopathy. Takotsubo means "octopus trap" in Japanese.

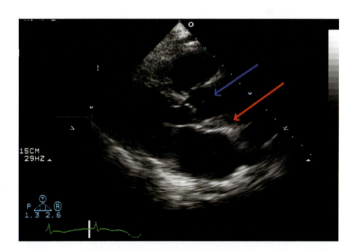

FIGURE 3.19 ■ This parasternal long axis view of a patient with chest pain reveals a dissection of the aortic root and ascending aorta. The true (blue arrow) and false lumens (red arrow) of the ascending thoracic aorta are indicated.

When evaluating a patient with acute shortness of breath, TTE can help identify causes such as massive pulmonary embolism (PE), congestive heart failure, and chronic obstructive pulmonary disease (COPD) exacerbation. It is the ideal tool for identifying complications such as free wall rupture, ventricular septal defects, and papillary muscle rupture. Identification of cardiac masses, such as tumors and thrombi, can be achieved with TTE as well. TTE can be used as an adjunct to therapy during cardiovascular emergencies such as pericardiocentesis.

FIGURE 3.20 ■ This parasternal short axis view of a patient with massive PE in ventricular systole shows dilation and severe hypokinesis of the base and midwall of the RV with a hyperkinetic apex (McCullen's sign).

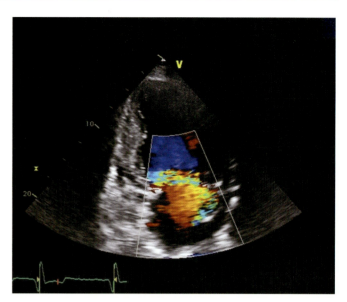

FIGURE 3.22 ■ This apical two-chamber view with color Doppler of a patient with acute MI shows papillary muscle rupture and severe mitral regurgitation.

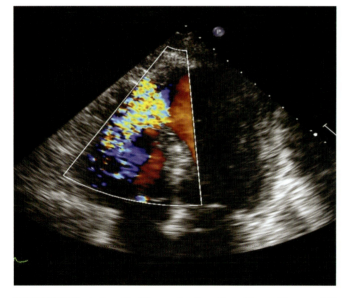

FIGURE 3.21 ■ An apical long axis view of a patient with acute MI complicated by a ventricular septal defect is demonstrated by color Doppler showing a left to right shunt.

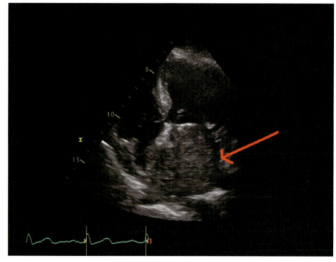

FIGURE 3.23 ■ In a patient who presented with syncopal episodes, an apical long axis view of the heart revealed a large tumor obstructing flow (atrial myxoma).

Interpretation

TTE during cardiovascular emergencies should be performed by a qualified echocardiography technician or physician. Images from TTE should be interpreted by a qualified physician. A systematic review of the TTE images (overall anatomy, chamber sizes and function, and valve morphology), evaluation of color and Doppler flow velocities (pressure gradients), and careful consideration of patient's history and hemodynamic status are always recommended. In many cardiovascular emergencies, however, time is restricted and only a focused exam is feasible. Therefore, interpretation of TTE

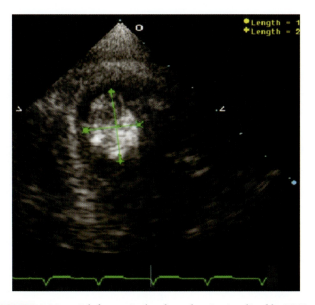

FIGURE 3.24 ■ A left ventricular thrombus is visualized by TTE.

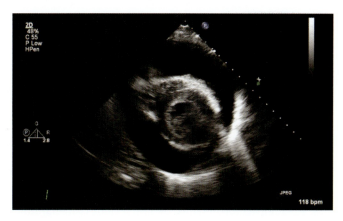

FIGURE 3.25 ■ This parasternal short axis view on TTE reveals a large pericardial effusion compressing the right heart and causing tamponade.

must be made with limited information at times. Limitations of TTE imaging include inadequate resolution of images and poor echocardiographic windows. These can occur in patients on mechanical ventilation and in obese patients. Assistance from other providers may be necessary to help position the patient for adequate imaging. Misinterpretation of TTE images can lead to the misdiagnosis of critical cardiovascular emergencies and a delay to therapeutic measures.

Pearls and Pitfalls

- In patients with chest pain not relieved by nitroglycerin and with no obvious ST-segment elevation on electrocardiogram (ECG), be certain to visualize the aorta (root, arch, and descending). The patient may have an aortic dissection.
- Beware of image artifact. If image artifact is suspected, check to see whether a structure is visible in multiple views. If it is not, artifact is likely and should not be included in the interpretation of the TTE.
- A large pericardial effusion does not *always* result in cardiac tamponade. Cardiac tamponade is a clinical diagnosis that can be assisted by findings on TTE. If a patient with a pericardial effusion is hemodynamically unstable, one should investigate TTE evidence of tamponade such as RV collapse in early diastole, right atrial inversion in late diastole, and respiratory variation of mitral/tricuspid inflow velocity.

TRANSESOPHAGEAL ECHOCARDIOGRAPHY

Min Pu

Technology/Technique

Transesophageal echocardiography (TEE) is a semi-invasive procedure that provides real-time imaging of the heart. To overcome the shortcomings of TTE, TEE was developed after miniaturization of the echocardiographic probe. Indications for TEE include the need for real-time data about cardiac function that will help guide clinical and therapeutic strategies. The information obtained by TEE includes valvular function, pericardial conditions, aortic anatomy, and heart wall motion. Severe esophageal disease (cancer or obstruction) is an absolute contraindication to performing TEE.

Moderate sedation of the patient is required to perform TEE. Clinical practice guidelines for safe and effective conscious sedation should be followed. Benzocaine spray and/or gargled lidocaine preparations may be used for local anesthesia. The patient is positioned in the lateral decubitus position and a bite guard is used. The TEE probe is introduced into the mouth and down the esophagus. The probe is manipulated to acquire images and to optimize picture quality. With the probe in the mid-esophagus, multiple mid-transesophageal views can be obtained. In order to acquire transgastric images, the probe is advanced into the stomach, flexed anteriorly, and slowly withdrawn while monitoring the images. With biplane views, short and long axis images of the LV and RV can be simultaneously obtained. The descending aorta can be imaged by rotation of the probe to near 180° facing the back of the patient. Slow withdrawal and rotation of the probe enables visualization of the thoracic aorta.

A complete or targeted TEE examination can be performed depending on the clinical question and the patient's condition. Although serious complications are rare, the risks of TEE include injury to laryngeal structures and rupture of the esophagus. The potential side effects and risks associated with sedation must also be considered and disclosed to the patient or consenting party. Postprocedural management includes monitoring of vital signs for at least 30 minutes and until the patent returns to baseline. Patients should not eat or drink for at least 2 hours after the procedure or until oral sensation and swallowing function return to normal. General postprocedural sedation precautions should be observed.

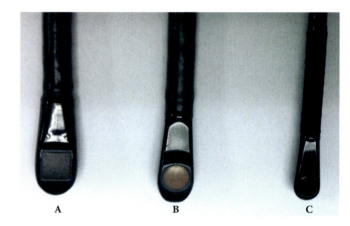

FIGURE 3.26 ■ A series of TEE probes are pictured here. From the left to right: (**A**) adult real-time 3D probe; (**B**) adult multiplane probe; and (**C**) pediatric probe.

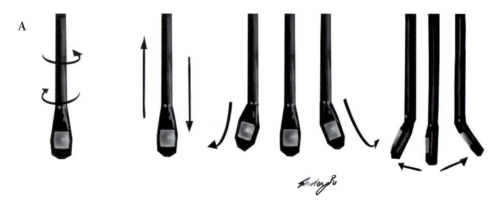

FIGURE 3.27 ■ (**A**) The TEE probe can be flexed anteriorly, posteriorly, and laterally via manipulation of the control knob. (**B**) Short and long axis views of the LV are demonstrated here. (**C**) TEE images of the descending aorta and aortic arch are displayed.

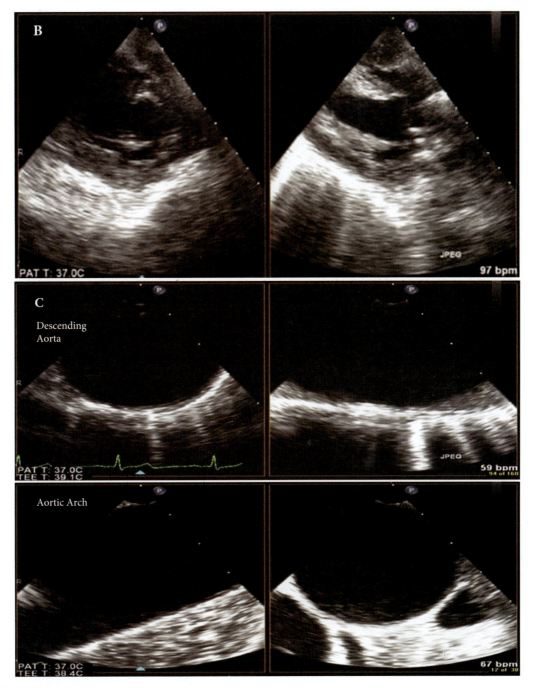

FIGURE 3.27 ■ *(Continued)*

Interpretation

Interpretation of TEE requires a thorough understanding of echocardiography and a familiarity with the basic principles of ultrasound. Special training for the implementation and interpretation of TEE is recommended by the American Society of Echocardiography. Imaging of cardiovascular anatomy and the Doppler study of hemodynamics and blood flow are essential for transesophageal examination. A complete TEE should be obtained in a systematic fashion when the patient's condition allows.

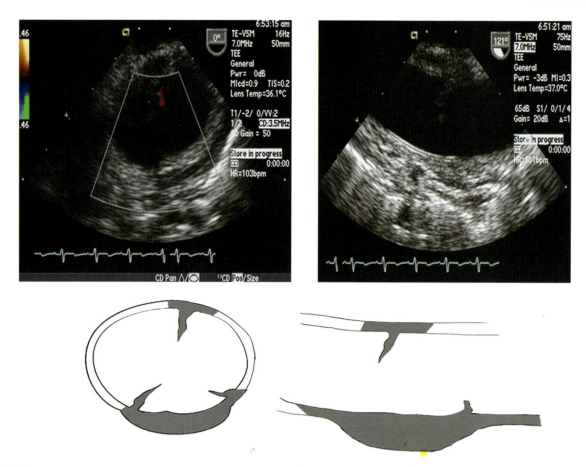

FIGURE 3.28 ■ This image series of aortic transection reveals the flap of aortic transection in the lumen with concomitant hematoma around the vessel.

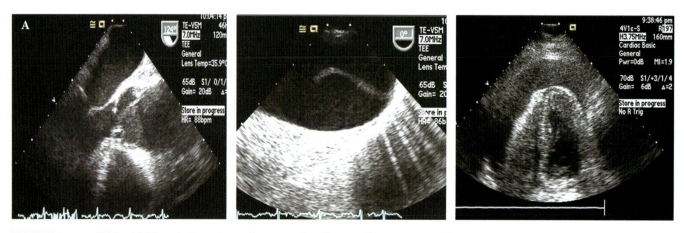

FIGURE 3.29 ■ (A) In this Type A dissection, a flap is noted in the ascending aorta. TEE demonstrated a large pericardial effusion caused by the rupture of the dissected ascending aorta into the pericardium. (B) The flap of dissected intima may prolapse into the LV outflow tract (pictured here) through the aortic valve during diastole and cause severe aortic regurgitation. It is important to differentiate whether the aortic regurgitation is caused by a tear of the aortic sinus/aortic valve or by the prolapsed flap. Patients with intact valves only require aortic root repair with sparing of the native aortic valve. Patients with torn aortic valves and sinus may require aortic valve replacement along with aortic root repair.

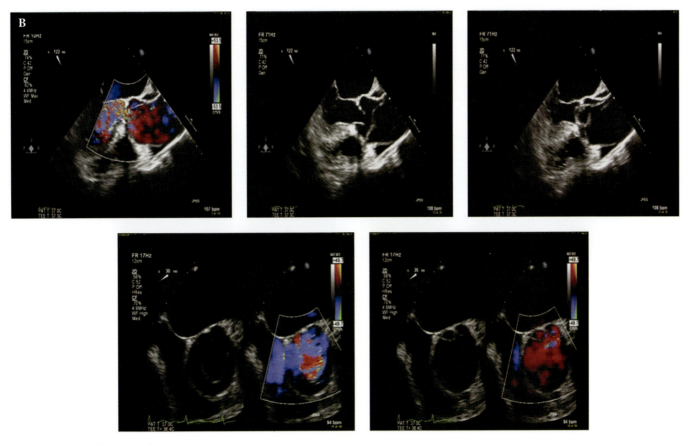

FIGURE 3.29 ■ (Continued)

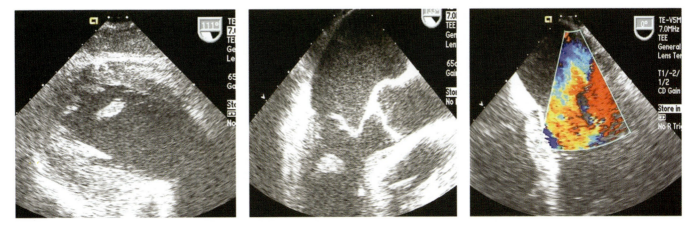

FIGURE 3.30 ■ This patient with MI presented with cardiogenic shock and pulmonary edema due to posteromedial papillary muscle rupture. Transgastric view (left) shows the mobile head of the papillary muscle. The mid-transesophageal view (middle) shows the flailed mitral anterior leaflet and ruptured papillary muscle. Color Doppler imaging (right) shows severe mitral regurgitation.

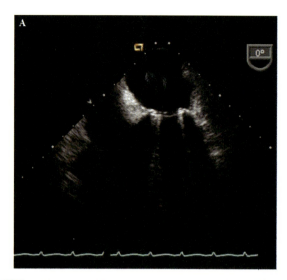 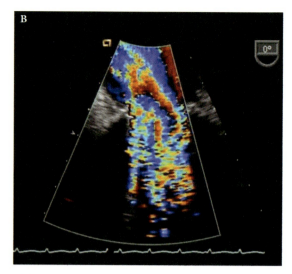

FIGURE 3.31 ■ Severe mitral regurgitation was caused by malfunction of this mechanical prosthetic valve (Bjork–Shiley). The strut fracture of the prosthetic valve led to dislodgment of the occluding disc leaving the mitral valve wide open (**A**) associated with severe mitral regurgitation illustrated by color Doppler study (**B**).

Pearls and Pitfalls

- TEE can be performed at the bedside, and it provides simultaneous anatomical and hemodynamic assessment. It does not interfere with patient monitoring or treatment, making it extremely suitable for unstable patients and for use in the intensive care unit, emergency room and operating room.
- TEE may not fully display the aortic arch and descending aorta.
- Recent development of real-time 3D TEE significantly enhances its application.

BEDSIDE ULTRASOUND: EVALUATION FOR DEEP VEIN THROMBOSIS

William Alley

Technology/Technique

For patients with a swollen or painful lower extremity, with or without erythema, deep vein thrombosis (DVT) should be considered as a possible cause. Generally, the evaluation for DVT requires lower extremity duplex ultrasonography. This study has some distinct benefits over other studies including lack of ionizing radiation and relatively low cost. Unfortunately, it also has limitations. First, many institutions cannot provide duplex ultrasonography at all times of the day and/or every day of the week. Second, formal duplex ultrasonography can take up to 45 minutes to perform, and it may require sending a patient to another location. This may not be feasible for a clinically unstable patient.

An alternative to formal duplex ultrasonography is physician-performed bedside ultrasound of the lower extremity. In contrast to duplex ultrasonography, limited bedside venous ultrasound focuses on the compressibility of the common femoral and popliteal veins. This test is based on the premises that clots distal to the popliteal vein are less likely to embolize and that isolated DVTs between the common femoral and popliteal veins are uncommon.

A high-frequency linear probe is used throughout the procedure. If greater image depth is needed, a lower-frequency probe can be used at the expense of image resolution. The patient should be positioned with leg slightly externally rotated with knee slightly flexed. Placing the patient in reverse Trendelenburg or a semi-sitting position will help distend the veins.

Begin by finding a transverse view of the common femoral vein just distal to the inguinal ligament. At this level, the vein is usually medial to the artery. If identification of the vein is uncertain, remember that it is generally larger, thinner walled, and more ovoid than the artery. It is also more compressible, though the presence of a DVT can affect compressibility. Doppler can also be used to detect arterial versus venous waveform.

Interpretation

Once the common femoral vein is identified, the physician should apply pressure using the ultrasound probe to compress

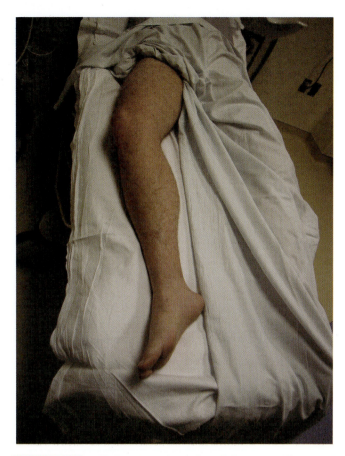

FIGURE 3.32 ■ The leg is positioned with hip externally rotated and knee slightly flexed.

the vessel about every centimeter, proceeding distally until the bifurcation into the superficial femoral and deep femoral veins. The sonographer should also pay special attention to the branching-in point of the greater saphenous vein just proximal to the superficial femoral vein.

Next, attention turns to the popliteal vein. The vein is visualized from about 12 cm proximal to the popliteal crease to the trifurcation of the calf vessels or 10vcm distal to the crease, whichever occurs more proximally. The probe is placed on the posterior aspect of the leg and pressure is applied to the vessel every centimeter along the course of the vein. The vein should appear superficial to the artery.

Once both the femoral and popliteal veins have been imaged and compressibility is confirmed, the study is finished. If the vein is not completely compressible, the diagnosis of DVT is made. The test usually takes less than 5 minutes for a skilled operator to complete.

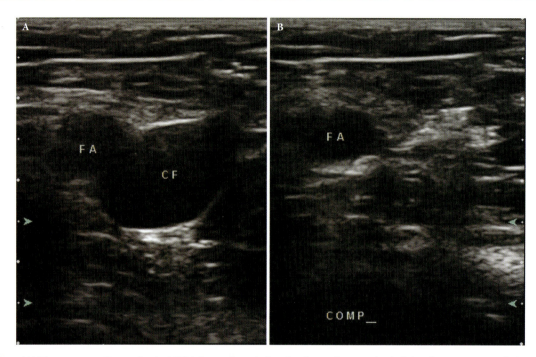

FIGURE 3.33 ■ (A) The common femoral vein (CF) is located medial to the femoral artery (FA). (B) When compressed, the normal CF vein is completely collapsed.

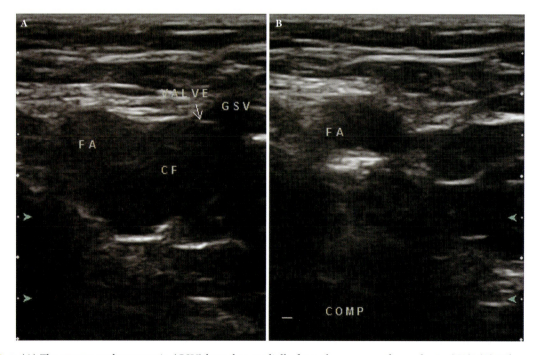

FIGURE 3.34 ■ (A) The greater saphenous vein (GSV) branches medially from the common femoral vein (CF). (B) When compressed, all of the veins are completely collapsed.

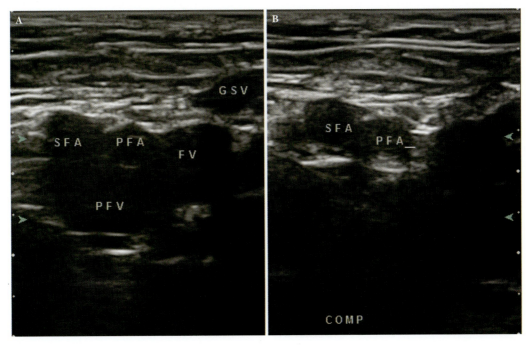

FIGURE 3.35 ■ (A) The femoral artery bifurcates into superficial and deep femoral arteries (SFA and PFA, respectively). Near the arterial bifurcation, the vein bifurcates into superficial and deep femoral vein (FV and PFV, respectively). (B) All venous structures compress easily.

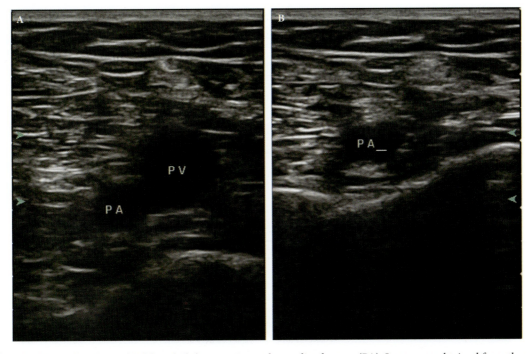

FIGURE 3.36 ■ (A) The popliteal vein (PV) lies slightly posterior to the popliteal artery (PA). Images are obtained from the posterior aspect of the leg, so the vein is viewed superficial to the artery. (B) The normal popliteal vein is easily compressed.

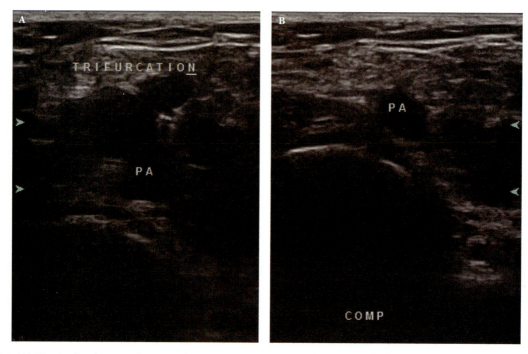

FIGURE 3.37 ■ (A) The popliteal vein trifurcation located anterior to the popliteal artery (PA). Anatomy varies, so all three branches may not be visible. (B) The normal venous structures compress easily.

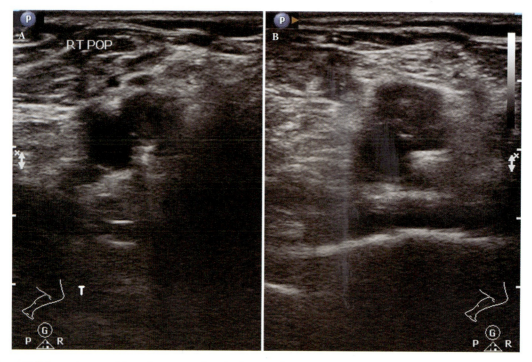

FIGURE 3.38 ■ (A) Echogenic material can be seen within the lumen of this popliteal vein. (B) When compressed, the popliteal vein does not collapse.

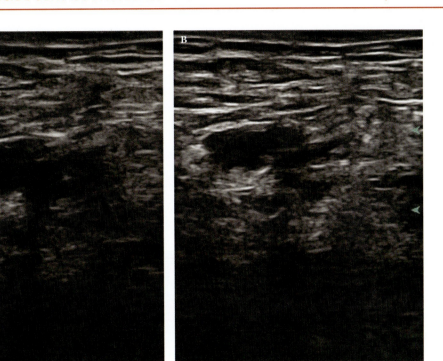

FIGURE 3.39 ■ (**A**) This uncompressed femoral vein is located medial to the femoral artery of the right leg. (**B**) With compression, the vein only partially collapses due to thrombosis. Notice, the adjacent artery is slightly collapsed, indicating adequate compressive force by the sonographer.

Pearls and Pitfalls

- Instruct the patient to relax, especially during popliteal scanning. Increased muscle tone can make compression difficult. Dependent positioning of the limb being evaluated is important.
- The walls of the vein must touch completely across the entire vessel to be considered compressible and negative for DVT. Partial collapse is abnormal.
- As with any lower extremity ultrasound exam, iliac and IVC thrombi are not effectively evaluated by physician-performed bedside ultrasound of the lower extremity.
- Sensitivity of bedside physician-performed ultrasound evaluation for DVT is dependent on the skill and experience of the operator. Scans performed in the ED should be followed closely by formal lower extremity duplex ultrasonography.

CARDIAC COMPUTED TOMOGRAPHY

Daniel Entrikin
Chadwick D. Miller

Technology/Technique

Cardiac computed tomography (CT) is used primarily to assess cardiac structure, and to a lesser extent, to evaluate cardiac function. These components can be separated if angiography is performed. Noncontrast cardiac CT exams are primarily used to obtain coronary calcium scores. The exact role of coronary calcium scoring in the evaluation of patients with chest pain is not clear. Cardiac CT angiography (CCTA) involves the use of IV contrast injection timed to optimize coronary artery opacification. Use of CCTA has proved to be a safe and cost-effective method of evaluating patients with symptoms concerning for acute coronary syndrome (ACS) and low- or intermediate-risk features. Proper patient selection is required to ensure good image quality. Image quality degrades with obesity, increasing heart rate, irregular heart rhythms, inability to perform breath-holds, and vascular calcifications.

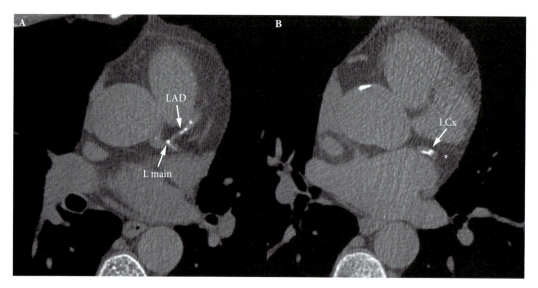

FIGURE 3.40 ■ Two axial images from a coronary artery calcium scoring scan demonstrating calcified atherosclerotic plaque in the (**A**) distal left main, left anterior descending (LAD), and (**B**) left circumflex (LCx) coronary arteries (arrows).

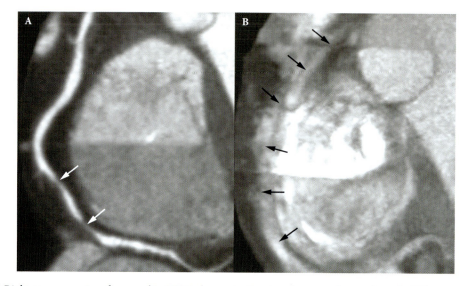

FIGURE 3.41 ■ (**A**) Right coronary artery from quality CCTA demonstrating two stenoses of approximately 25% to 50% and 50% to 75% in the mid-RCA (arrows). (**B**) Nondiagnostic CCTA because of variable heart rhythm that results in obscured proximal and mid RCA (black arrows).

Interpretation

The absence of coronary disease on CCTA, or maximal coronary stenosis ≤50% of the luminal diameter, makes it highly unlikely that ACS is the cause of the patient's symptoms. In addition to providing an assessment of luminal stenosis, CCTA also details the extent of extra-luminal vascular remodeling (ie, positive remodeling) and plaque characteristics. Such detection of subclinical coronary disease is not obtained with stress testing, and may not be detected with invasive angiography. Cardiac biomarkers of necrosis (eg, troponin) are typically used to complement the information provided with CCTA. Unexpected yet emergent causes of chest pain such as PE or aortic dissection may be detected with CCTA. However, CCTA imaging protocols are not typically optimized for assessment of these disease processes and therefore should not be relied upon for these diagnoses.

Patients with low-risk chest pain, nonelevated serial troponin measurements, and ≤50% maximal coronary stenosis on CCTA imaging should be evaluated for an alternative cause for their symptoms and appropriately treated for that condition. Patients with >50% maximal coronary stenosis on CCTA should undergo further assessment with stress testing or invasive angiography, typically in consultation with a cardiologist. All patients with coronary artery disease should be informed of this diagnosis and referred to their physician for risk factor modification and medical management.

Risk

Patients who undergo CCTA imaging are exposed to the risks of IV contrast administration including allergic reaction, contrast-induced nephropathy, and extravasation of IV contrast into soft tissues. Radiation exposure is also a risk of CCTA, but the short- and long-term consequences of this exposure are unclear. With current methods to reduce radiation doses,

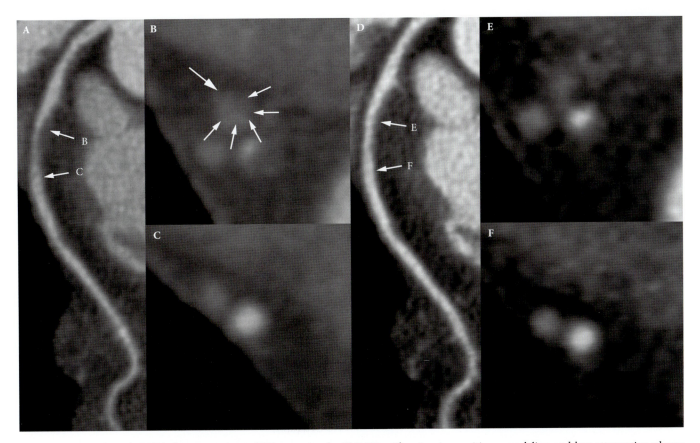

FIGURE 3.42 ■ (**A–C**) CCTA demonstrating >50% stenosis of mid-LAD with extensive positive remodeling and low attenuation plaque (small arrows in panel **B**). (**D–F**) After 18 months of statin therapy, stenosis is now <25% with resolution of positive remodeling and majority of plaque.

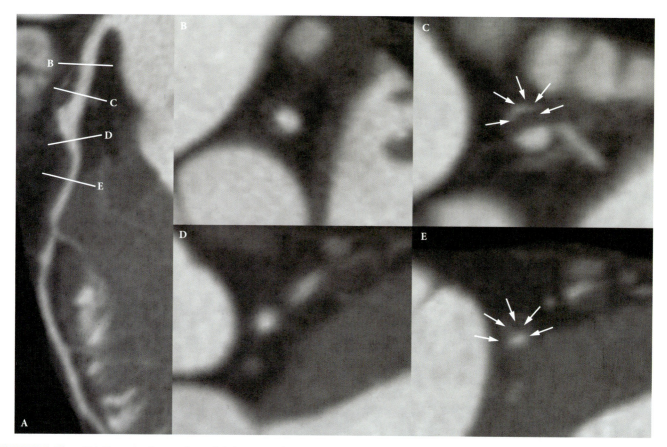

FIGURE 3.43 ■ (**A**) Curved reformat through left main and LAD with reference (**B** and **D**) and diseased (**C** and **E**) cross-sections drawn and demonstrated at right. Note extensive positive remodeling in left main and LAD (arrows in **C** and **E**).

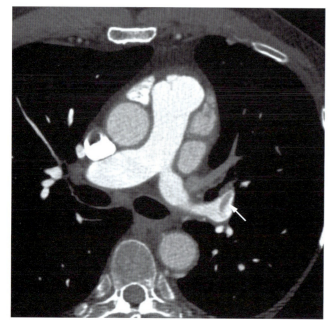

FIGURE 3.44 ■ Axial image from CCTA examination demonstrates an incidental left upper lobe pulmonary embolus (arrow). The patient had no significant coronary artery disease.

the radiation exposure during routine CCTA for adult patients is approximately 2 to 5 mSv; less than conventional thoracic CT scans. Radiation dose reduction techniques and image quality are both optimized in patients with lower heart rates (<65 vbeats/min). Heart rate control is typically accomplished through the administration of oral and/or IV β-antagonist medications.

Pearls and Pitfalls

- CCTA can fail to detect coronary stenosis in small coronary vessels that can lead to infarction. In patients with detected coronary disease in larger vessels, serial cardiac markers may be beneficial to detect MI caused by small vessel disease not visualized by CCTA.
- Poor patient selection leads to nondiagnostic CCTA results. Because suboptimal CCTA candidates often receive β-antagonist medications during the CCTA, achieving target heart rate during subsequent stress testing on the same day can be difficult.

CARDIAC MAGNETIC RESONANCE IMAGING

Chadwick D. Miller
Daniel Entrikin

Technology/Technique

Cardiac magnetic resonance (CMR) imaging can provide an assessment of cardiac structure, function, myocardial perfusion, and tissue characterization. Both rest and stress exams can be performed based on the clinical question to be addressed. CMR imaging is useful when evaluating patients with suspected ACS and intermediate to high pretest probabilities of ACS. CMR can also be used in the evaluation of myocarditis, pericarditis, cardiomyopathy, and cardiac thrombus or mass.

Evaluation for ischemic heart disease often incorporates resting images to assess wall motion, T2-weighted imaging for detection of inflammation and edema, and resting perfusion with the administration of gadolinium. If stress imaging is desired to detect inducible ischemia, a vasodilator (eg, adenosine or regadenoson) is infused followed by gadolinium administration. Alternatively, a pharmacologic stress agent (eg, dobuatmine) can be administered while assessing for wall motion changes. Resting-only imaging and rest/stress protocols both commonly conclude with delayed enhancement imaging. T2-imaging is used to detect edema, which can be an early finding of ischemia/infarction or a sign of inflammation.

Interpretation

Resting perfusion and wall motion abnormalities suggest prior or ongoing insults to myocardial perfusion. Stress perfusion or wall motion abnormalities, in the absence of resting defects, indicate inducible ischemia, suggesting the presence of hemodynamically significant coronary artery stenosis. Delayed enhancement indicates abnormal myocardium associated with scar formation, active inflammation (from acute infarction or myocarditis), or infiltrative cardiomyopathies. Edema on T2 imaging without delayed enhancement in the same anatomic distribution suggests inflammation or ischemia without infarction.

Resting CMR imaging provides accurate structural and functional information. When clinical suspicion exists, exams can be tailored to detect cardiomypathies, cardiac thrombus, and masses. Resting CMR is highly sensitive for the presence of myocarditis and can detect pericarditis. Occasionally, CMR will detect alternative causes for chest pain such as PE or aortic dissection; however, CMR is not the primary modality for these conditions. Additionally, CMR is useful to demonstrate dynamic outflow tract obstruction in patients with hypertrophic obstructive cardiomyopathy (HOCM). Patients with symptoms consistent with ACS and CMR findings suggestive of MI or unstable angina (ie, edema, new wall motion abnormality, delayed enhancement without prior infarct, or inducible ischemia) should receive a cardiology consultation and be admitted to a monitored setting.

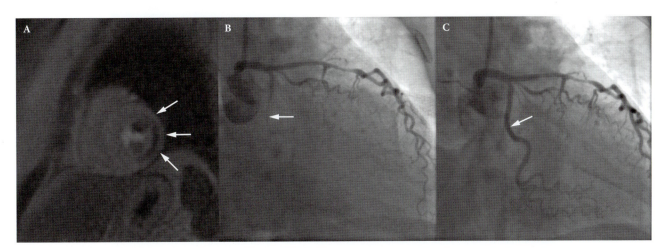

FIGURE 3.45 ■ (A) Adenosine stress perfusion defect in lateral wall (arrows) indicative of inducible ischemia. (B) This angiogram demonstrates near complete circumflex occlusion (arrow). (C) It was treated successfully with a stent (arrow).

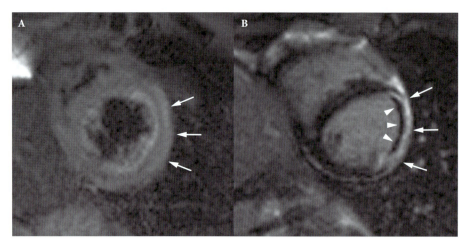

FIGURE 3.46 ■ Acute LAD territory infarction demonstrating increased signal on T2-weighted images (arrows in **A**) consistent with edema, in addition to transmural delayed enhancement (arrows in **B**) with small region of subendocardium that does not enhance (arrowheads) consistent with complete microvascular obstruction.

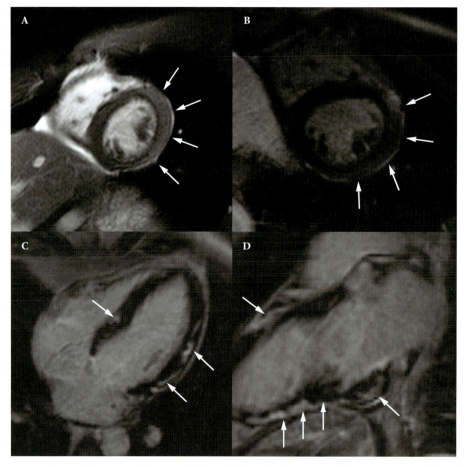

FIGURE 3.47 ■ Acute myocarditis with increased T2 signal (**A**) and delayed enhancement (**B**) in anterior and lateral walls. Panels **C** and **D** show scarring from old myocarditis with patchy delayed enhancement throughout myocardium.

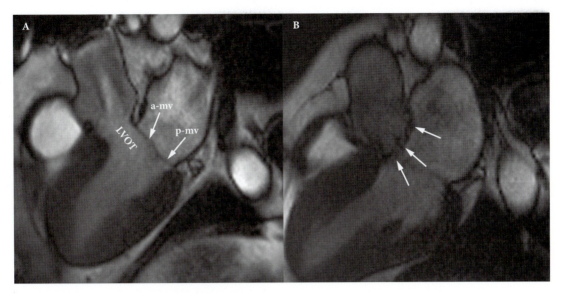

FIGURE 3.48 ■ (**A**) Normal systole with open LV outflow tract (LVOT), and closed mitral valve with apposition of the anterior (a-mv) and posterior (p-mv) leaflets. (**B**) HOCM in systole demonstrating obstruction of LVOT by anterior displacement of the anterior leaflet of the mitral valve (arrows).

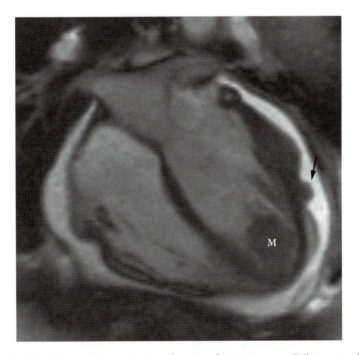

FIGURE 3.49 ■ Four-chamber white blood image demonstrating a low signal intensity mass (M) in apex of LV, as well as a small pericardial nodule (black arrow), consistent with metastatic disease.

CT ANGIOGRAM FOR PULMONARY EMBOLISM

Jon W. Schrock

Technology/Technique

CT angiography (CTA) has dramatically improved the clinical investigation of PE and is commonly used for the evaluation of PE. CT angiogram (CTA) involves a CT scan of the torso with a focus on the pulmonary vessels during simultaneous administration of an IV contrast bolus. Imaging is timed to coincide with opacification of the pulmonary arterial system. A PE will result in a perfusion or filling defect(s) within the pulmonary vasculature. Newer generations of CT technology have improved the ability to detect smaller, subsegmental emboli. Sixty-four row detector scanners have shown the ability to identify clots as small as 2 mm with accuracy similar to pulmonary angiography. The risks of pulmonary CTA include reactions to or complications from contrast dye administration (eg, contrast-induced nephropathy) and radiation exposure.

An additional benefit of pulmonary CTA is the potential to identify alternative life-threatening diagnoses. In up to 25% of cases, pulmonary CTA will reveal alternative diagnoses including lung cancer, aortic dissection, pneumothorax, and pneumonia. Dual-energy CT can be used to generate lung perfusion images (similar to the perfusion portion of a ventilation/perfusion scan [V/Q scan]) at the same time the CTA is performed. These scans can show the location of emboli and the extent of decreased perfusion. CT venography (CTV) of the pelvis can also be used to investigate thromboses in the pelvis and thighs that can identify a potential source of pulmonary emboli. However, an additional dose of radiation (6 mSv) is required to perform this imaging study and the diagnostic yield is modest. The use of CTA for the diagnosis of PE is reserved for patients who have no allergy to IV contrast agents and have no significant renal impairment.

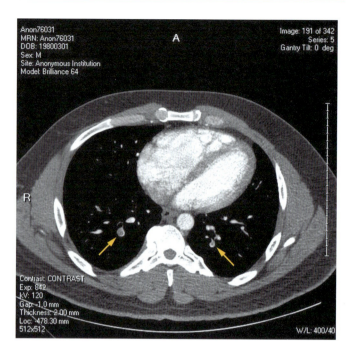

FIGURE 3.51 ■ A pulmonary CTA showing subsegmental filling defects in the bilateral lower lobes of the lungs (yellow arrows).

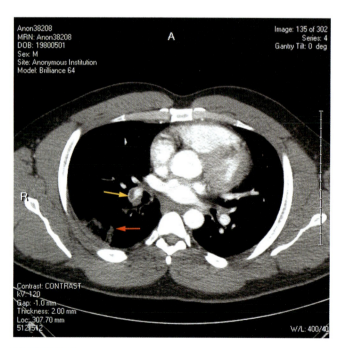

FIGURE 3.50 ■ This pulmonary CTA shows a right lower lobe pulmonary artery filling defect (yellow arrow) with a wedge shaped pulmonary infarction (Hampton's hump; red arrow).

Interpretation

Imaging with CTA allows the clinician to quantify clot burden, pinpoint embolism location, and help identify patients with circulatory compromise caused by a large or massive PE. Patients with CT evidence of right heart strain may benefit from more aggressive therapeutic strategies including pharmacologic thrombolysis or mechanical embolectomy.

CT ANGIOGRAM FOR PULMONARY EMBOLISM (CONTINUED)

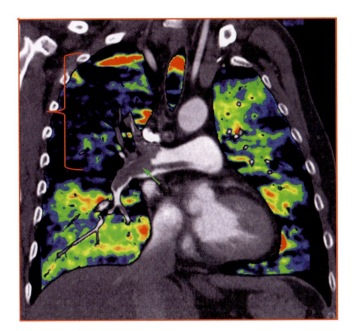

FIGURE 3.52 ■ This is an example of a coronal dual-energy CTA showing a large right pulmonary artery embolism (green arrow) with decreased perfusion to the right upper and middle lobes (red bracket). Reproduced, with permission, from Chae EJ, Seo JB, Jang YM, et al. Dual-energy CT for assessment of the severity of acute pulmonary embolism: pulmonary perfusion defect score compared with CT angiographic obstruction score and RV/LV diameter ration. *Am J Roentgenol.* 2010;194:604-610.

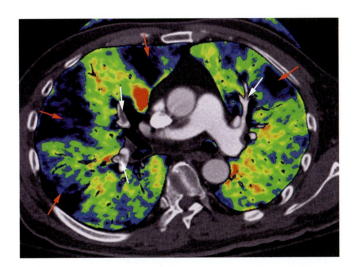

FIGURE 3.53 ■ This axial dual-energy CTA reveals multiple sub-segmental emboli (3 white arrows) with associated perfusion defects in both lungs (4 red arrows). Reproduced, with permission, from Chae EJ, Seo JB, Jang YM, et al. Dual-energy CT for assessment of the severity of acute pulmonary embolism: pulmonary perfusion defect score compared with CT angiographic obstruction score and right ventricular/left ventricular diameter ratio. *Am J Roentgenol.* 2010;194:604-610.

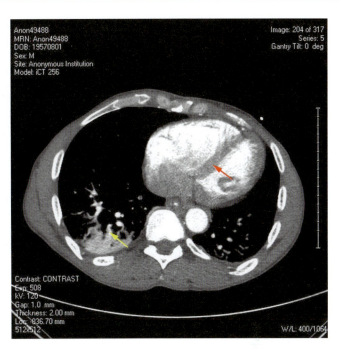

FIGURE 3.54 ■ This pulmonary CTA shows right heart strain with bowing of the interventricular septum (red arrow) and a pulmonary infarction of the right lower lobe (yellow arrow).

A recent study (PIOPED II) of CTA for the investigation of PE demonstrated a 83% sensitivity, 96% sensitivity, negative predictive value 95%, and positive predictive value 86%. Positive predictive value was 97% for main or lobar artery emboli. The rate of technically poor studies is 2% to 6% and is commonly due to poor bolus timing, obesity, and motion artifact from tachypnea. In these patients, alternative imaging such as V/Q studies or venous duplex imaging of the lower extremities may be employed to evaluate for thomboembolic disease. The diagnostic gold standard for PE is pulmonary angiography but this study is invasive and not commonly used.

Pearls and Pitfalls

- The risk of contrast-induced nephropathy is increased in elderly patients and in those with anemia, preexisting renal dysfunction, diabetes, and heart failure.
- Incidental findings that require future studies, such as pulmonary nodules, should be to the disclosed patient and the need for follow-up imaging should be discussed in the discharge instructions and documented in the medical record.
- In patients with significant central clot burden, echocardiography may be considered to evaluate the presence and/or degree of RV strain.

VENTILATION/PERFUSION SCAN (V/Q SCAN)

Michael Schinlever

Technology/Technique

Although pulmonary CTA has become the diagnostic modality of choice for the evaluation of PE in recent years, V/Q scan remains a viable diagnostic option. The V/Q scan is a form of phased scintigraphy. Gamma cameras detect radiation emitted by specific radioisotopes and display the emissions as two-dimensional images. The first phase is typically the ventilation assessment that involves inhalation of a radionuclide, such as xenon-133 or technetium-99m (Tc99m; DTPA aerosol or Technegas). At that time, six to eight planar images are obtained in order to adequately view each pulmonary lobe. Next, the perfusion analysis is initiated with an IV injection of Tc99m macro aggregated albumin. Similar planar images are obtained once the Tc99m has reached the pulmonary arterial circulation. The entire study typically takes between 30 and 45 minutes.

For patients in whom PE is a concern and IV contrast infusion is contraindicated (ie, patients with significant renal dysfunction or severe contrast allergy), V/Q scan should be considered. The predominant risk of a V/Q scan is radiation exposure. However, a V/Q scan confers significantly less radiation exposure compared to CTA (1.2 – 2.0 mSv vs. 1.6 – 8.3 mSv, respectively). Therefore, V/Q scan can be considered for women of reproductive age and pregnant women.

Interpretation

The two sets of planar images are compared and analyzed for mismatching between the ventilation and perfusion phases. A mismatch is suggestive of PE.

There are a number of different criteria available for reporting V/Q scan results. Results are often broken into three or four categories based on probability of PE: high probability (80%–100%), indeterminate/intermediate (20%–80%), low probability (0%–19%), and normal or "PE absent." The overall sensitivity and specificity of V/Q scan varies widely depending on grading criteria, technique, and pretest probability. In a recent analysis, V/Q scans were interpreted definitively in 73.5% of predominantly outpatient cases with a sensitivity of 77.4% and a specificity of 97.7%.

A disadvantage of V/Q scan is diminished diagnostic utility in patients with underlying lung disease (e.g., COPD, pneumonia, ARDS, pulmonary edema), grossly abnormal chest radiographs, and/or a history of prior PE. These patients will often demonstrate

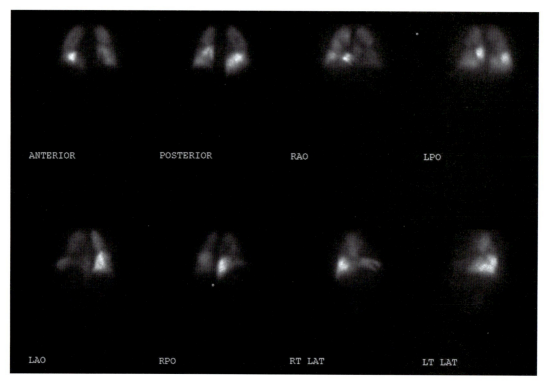

FIGURE 3.55 ■ These perfusion images show asymmetric, patchy perfusion of Tc99m consistent with multiple perfusion defects, especially in bilateral lung bases. When compared with ventilation images in Figure 3.56, these results suggest high probability for pulmonary emboli.

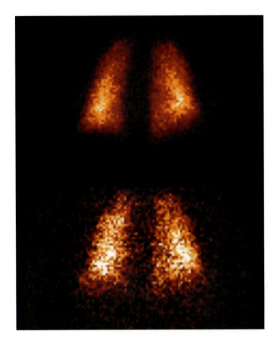

FIGURE 3.56 ■ These ventilation images show uniform distribution of inhaled xenon-133 throughout entire lung field.

evidence of a V/Q mismatch that may or may not be due to PE. When compared to CTA, V/Q scanning is often less convenient and takes longer to perform. In addition, V/Q scanning is limited to identifying ventilation–perfusion mismatching, whereas CTA can assess alternative diagnoses, locate filling defects, and identify smaller, more peripheral emboli.

Pearls and Pitfalls

- With proper patient selection, V/Q scan can be an appropriate diagnostic tool for the investigation of PE when pulmonary CTA is not feasible or appropriate. Its advantages over CTA include lower radiation dose and lack of iodinated contrast administration.
- Patients must cooperate with the ventilation phase and tolerate sitting upright or lying supine for the duration of the scan.
- Despite a V/Q scan with a low-probability result, if the clinical suspicion or pretest probability for PE is high, the diagnosis of PE is not excluded.
- A high rate of indeterminate results (up to 75% of scans, but less in typical outpatient ED patient populations) often necessitates additional diagnostic evaluation that can lead to delayed diagnosis as well as increased radiation exposure and cost.

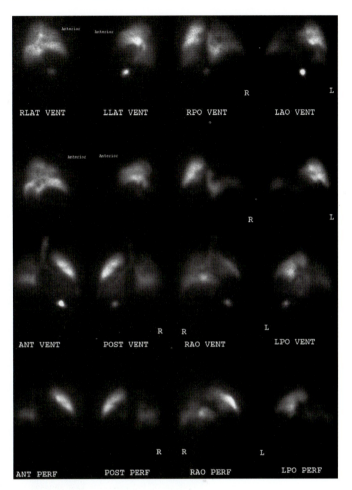

FIGURE 3.57 ■ Ventilation (VENT) and perfusion (PERF) results show good delivery of inhaled radionuclide but significant patchiness and asymmetry in the perfusion scan. The perfusion defects involve multiple lobes in both left and right lung fields. This scan suggests high probability for pulmonary emboli.

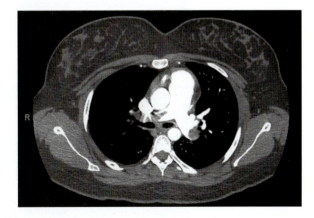

FIGURE 3.58 ■ This correlating CTA image of the same patient shows large clot burden in the proximal right and left pulmonary arteries. This patient had significant right heart strain secondary to large bilateral pulmonary emboli and underwent thrombolytic therapy.

DOPPLER ULTRASOUND OF PERIPHERAL VENOUS SYSTEM

Thomas D. Conlee

Technology/Technique

Ultrasound examination of the peripheral venous system is typically performed to investigate DVT. Lower frequency, curvilinear transducers (3–5 MHz) are used to evaluate vessels within deeper tissues, whereas higher frequency, linear array transducers (5–10 MHz) are used for more superficial tissue examination such as in the extremities. To evaluate the lower extremities for DVT, it is important to position the patient in a supine position with 10° to 20° of reverse Trendelenberg to augment venous filling. B-mode, pulsed Doppler, and color-flow imaging may be used to determine vessel patency. In contrast to B-mode and color-flow imaging, pulsed Doppler uses a static image to evaluate flow at a specific depth. Vessel patency is established by four characteristics on ultrasound examination including compressibility, spontaneity, phasicity, and distal augmentation. In a transverse plane, compressibility is determined by the ability to coapt opposing walls of a vein with pressure from the transducer. Compression should be done with care in patients with an acute DVT for concern of dislodging the thrombus. Color-flow imaging may be used to help identify the vein being evaluated. Normal venous flow has spontaneous velocity changes that depend on pressure gradients and are present without distal augmentation. Phasicity is best evaluated

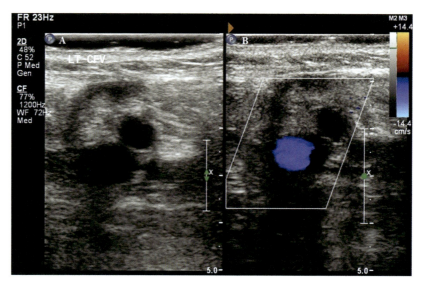

FIGURE 3.59 ■ This is an ultrasound image of a normal common femoral vein in B-mode and with color flow.

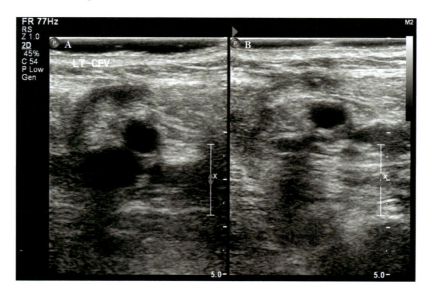

FIGURE 3.60 ■ This split image shows an uncompressed (**A**) and compressed (**B**) patent common femoral vein in B-mode.

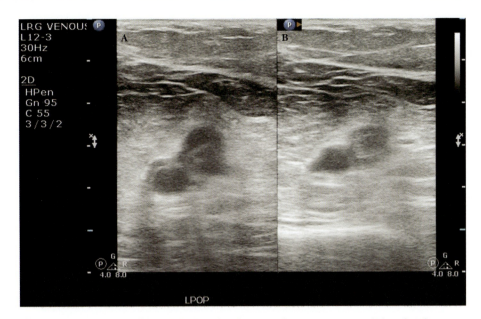

FIGURE 3.61 ■ This split image shows a partially occluded popliteal vein without compression (**A**) and with compression (**B**). Wall apposition is not achieved with compression in this thrombosed vein.

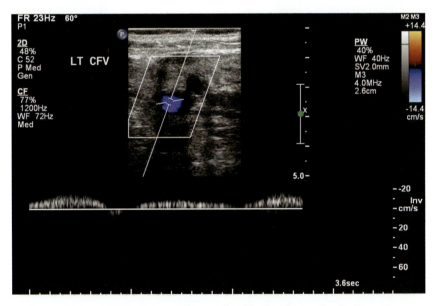

FIGURE 3.62 ■ Spontaneity of this common femoral vein is illustrated with color-flow and pulsed Doppler.

using the pulsed Doppler mode and appears as cyclical, low-amplitude fluctuations of flow that are driven by the respiratory cycle. Augmentation is an abrupt increase in flow induced by the return of blood by squeezing a distal muscle belly.

Interpretation

Thrombosed veins lack compressibility, spontaneity, phasicity, and augmentation. Although acute and chronic DVTs may exhibit overlapping sonographic characteristics, there are a number of factors that help to determine the age of the clot. An acutely thrombosed vein tends to be distended with thin walls and slightly deformable, if not completely occluded. Acute DVTs contain an anechoic or hypoechoic thrombus and lack collateral veins. A vein with a previous thrombus may have thickened hyperechoic walls with a small, irregular shaped lumen. With damage from aprior DVT, the patient may develop evidence of collateral veins and incompetent valves.

68 ■ DOPPLER ULTRASOUND OF PERIPHERAL VENOUS SYSTEM (CONTINUED)

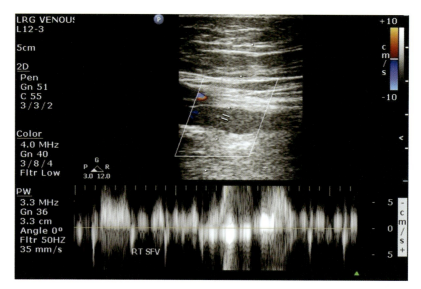

FIGURE 3.63 ■ Pulsed Doppler imaging of the superficial femoral vein illustrates spontaneous, phasic flow with distal augmentation.

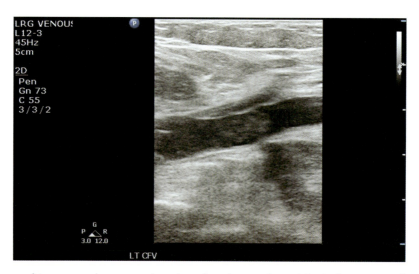

FIGURE 3.64 ■ This ultrasound image reveals an acute thrombus of moderate echogenicity in the common femoral vein that is somewhat dilated and without thickened vessel walls.

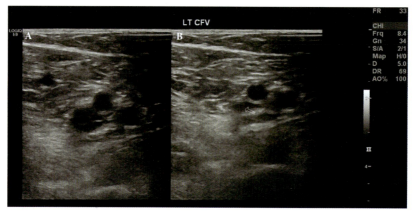

FIGURE 3.65 ■ This split image shows an uncompressed (**A**) and compressed (**B**) common femoral vein illustrating the incompressibility and thickened vessel wall of a chronic DVT.

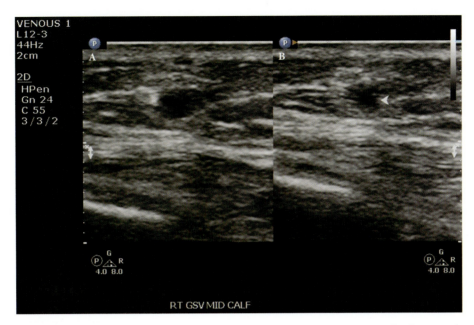

FIGURE 3.66 ■ An uncompressed (**A**) and compressed (**B**) greater saphenous vein illustrates a superficial venous thrombosis (superficial to the fascia) and inability to oppose the vessel walls.

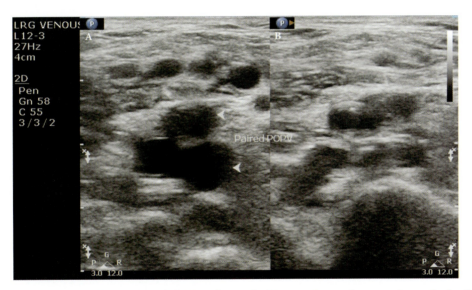

FIGURE 3.67 ■ This ultrasound image shows a chronic DVT of the popliteal vein with paired veins and superficial collateral vessels.

Pearls and Pitfalls

- When searching for a vein during ultrasound examination, start with the transducer in the transverse position and use color-flow imaging to identify the vessel. B-mode may offer better detail once the vein is localized.
- Superficial veins can be differentiated from deep veins by their position relative to the fascia of the extremity.
- Spontaneous flow is more pronounced in proximal veins and may be difficult to detect at more distal locations.
- Most named arteries distal to the knee and elbow are accompanied by a pair of adjacent veins. Proximal veins may be duplicated, but it is the exception rather than the rule.
- Differentiate arteries from the veins by their pulsatility and relative incompressibility compared to normal veins. Avoid relying on color patterns while in the color-flow mode as the transducer is easily reversed and venous flow may appear red.
- Definitive treatment decisions should be based on a study performed by a certified vascular laboratory and a registered vascular technician whenever possible.

DOPPLER ULTRASOUND OF PERIPHERAL ARTERIAL SYSTEM

Jason W. Christie
Justin B. Hurie

Technology/Technique

Doppler and duplex ultrasound of the peripheral arterial system can be obtained to investigate the presence or absence of blood flow in the setting of acute limb ischemia. When acute arterial occlusion is suspected, a pulse check should be performed. When performing a vascular evaluation, bilateral physical examination can help distinguish acute versus chronic disease because the contralateral limb may serve as the patient's reference. In a patient with chronic limb ischemia, an examination of the contralateral limb would be expected to be similar to the side in question. Strong palpable pulses in one limb and the absence of pulses in the symptomatic leg suggest acute limb ischemia.

After diminished or absent pulses are noted on physical examination, Doppler and duplex ultrasound are employed. The hand-held continuous Doppler probe offers audio output that is quickly obtained and easily interpreted. With duplex imaging, a color-flow mode can be used to determine the presence or absence of blood flow. The determination of a low flow state involves comparison of the waveforms or velocities to the proximal segment.

Interpretation

The key to Doppler and duplex ultrasound interpretation is waveform evaluation. With a hand-held Doppler, evaluation relies on acoustic interpretation. A normal artery will demonstrate a triphasic signal composed of brisk forward systolic flow followed by a short reversed flow phase in diastole. Most peripheral arteries will exhibit a small forward flow component in late diastole. The presence of a triphasic waveform rules out obstructive disease at or above the level being examined. A preocclusive "thump" may be heard just proximal to a site of occlusion.

AUDIO 3.1 ■ Monophasic waveform. *Available at* http://mhprofessional.com/sites/lefebvre

AUDIO 3.2 ■ Triphasic waveform. *Available at* http://mhprofessional.com/sites/lefebvre

When using duplex ultrasound, interpretation is accomplished by evaluating key waveform characteristics. The distinguishing elements in extremity arterial duplex include peak systolic velocity, end diastolic velocity, acceleration time (upstroke), and waveform phase. Reference criteria are used to determine the degree of occlusion or flow abnormality (Tables 3.2 and 3.3). Velocity criteria are often unique to each laboratory due to subtle variations in equipment. Therefore, the clinician should use site-specific reference criteria when performing a duplex ultrasound examination.

TABLE 3.2 ■ CRITERIA FOR DUPLEX INTERPRETATION OF LOWER EXTREMITY ARTERIAL DISEASE

Disease Severity	Waveform Characteristics
Normal	• Triphasic Waveform • Normal Peak Systolic Velocity (PSV) • No filling in of clear area under systolic peak (spectral broadening)
0%–49% Diameter Reduction	• PSV <100% increase relative to proximal segment • No evidence of poststenotic turbulence
50%–99% Diameter Reduction	• PSV ≥ 100% increase relative to proximal segment • Distal monophasic waveform may be present • Poststenotic turbulence present
Complete Occlusion	• No flow in imaged artery

TABLE 3.3 ■ GENERAL GUIDELINES FOR INTERPRETATION OF UPPER EXTREMITY ARTERIAL DUPLEX*

Disease Severity	Waveform Characteristics
Normal	• Triphasic waveform • Clear window beneath systolic peak
Complete Occlusion	• No flow detected

*No specific velocity criteria exists for upper extremity.

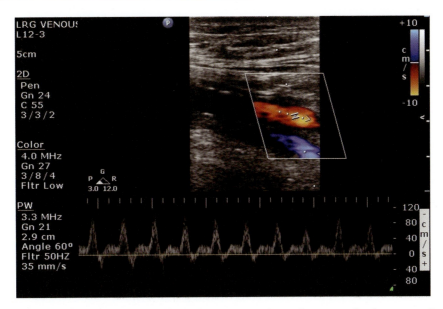

FIGURE 3.68 ■ This is an example of a normal, triphasic femoral artery spectral waveform. Note the clear area under the systolic peaks, sharp upstroke on the systolic wave, normal peak systolic velocity, reverse flow component, and forward flow at end diastole.

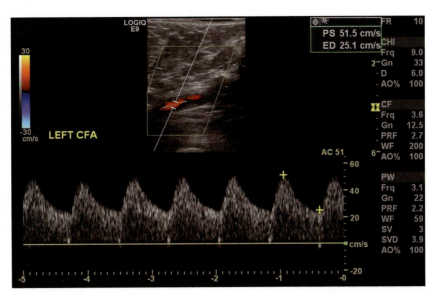

FIGURE 3.69 ■ This is an example of an abnormal, monophasic waveform of the common femoral artery. Note the "filling-in" of the clear area under the systolic peaks (spectral broadening), gentle upstroke on the systolic wave, decreased peak systolic velocity, loss of reverse flow component, and forward flow throughout the cardiac cycle.

Pearls and Pitfalls

- The presence of a pulse does not necessarily equal presence of adequate flow.
- Angle of insonation must be as close as possible to 60° and probe should be longitudinal to artery being imaged.
- Color gain must be set properly for an accurate color Doppler examination. The clinician should increase the color gain until noise appears in region of flow, then decrease slightly.
- Red and blue can represent either arterial or venous flow in color Doppler. Color assignment is based upon the direction of the probe.

ULTRASOUND GUIDED VASCULAR ACCESS

Manoj Pariyadath

Indications

Central Venous Access

Central venous access if often required in the critically ill patient to monitor hemodynamic measurements, for aggressive fluid resuscitation, and to administer medications and nutrition that otherwise would not be delivered safely or effectively through a peripheral IV. The consistent location of the internal jugular vein, subclavian vein, and femoral vein make them easy to cannulate when central access is needed. While a landmark technique has been traditionally utilized for this procedure, an ultrasound device can be used to facilitate central venous access by improving preprocedure planning, decreasing complications, and decreasing procedure time.

Peripheral Venous Access

Peripheral venous access may be difficult to obtain in patients who are obese, dehydrated, have peripheral edema, or upon whom multiple prior attempts at peripheral access have been made. Ultrasound guidance allows for visualization of veins that are more proximal and thus not palpable for traditional peripheral access techniques. Accessing these veins under ultrasound guidance prevents the need for central access when peripheral venous access is adequate.

Technique

Central Venous Access

Prior to the procedure, ultrasound may be utilized to determine the ideal vessel to cannulate, as well as the side to attempt cannulation, by determining and comparing the size of the vessels, identifying the relationship of adjacent structures, and determining other factors that may complicate the procedure, such as the presence of DVT.

Ultrasound guidance is typically accomplished with a high-frequency linear array transducer with the ultrasound device in a vascular mode. Commercial sterile transducer covers are utilized so that the ultrasound probe may be used during the sterile procedure. The probe is aligned either perpendicular (transverse) or parallel (longitudinal) to the vessel being cannulated. With the probe in the transverse orientation, the vessel is centered on the screen to provide a target for the introducer needle. The needle is advanced along the long axis of the vessel and perpendicular to the axis of the probe. Only

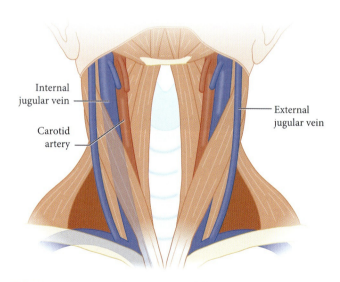

FIGURE 3.70 ■ Vascular anatomy of the neck. Reproduced, with permission, from Wyatt CR. Chapter 33. Venous and intraosseous access in adults. In: Tintinalli JE, Stapczynski J, Ma O, Cline DM, Cydulka RK, Meckler GD, eds. *Tintinalli's Emergency Medicine: A Comprehensive Study Guide*. 7th ed. New York, NY: McGraw-Hill; 2011.

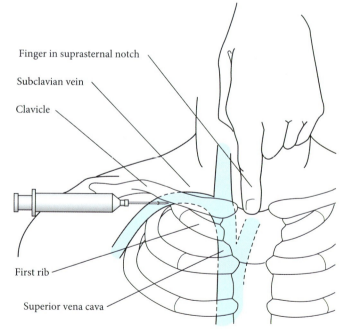

FIGURE 3.71 ■ Technique for the catheterization of the subclavian vein. Reproduced, with permission, from Chapter 13. Bedside procedures. In: Gomella LG, Haist SA, eds. *Clinician's Pocket Reference: The Scut Monkey*. 11th ed. New York, NY: McGraw-Hill; 2007.

ULTRASOUND GUIDED VASCULAR ACCESS (CONTINUED) ■ 73

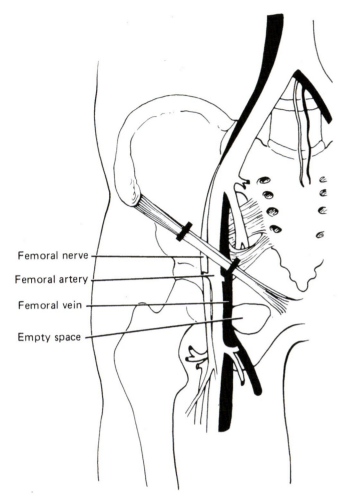

FIGURE 3.72 ■ Anatomic relationships of the femoral vein at the inguinal ligament. Reproduced, with permission, from Partin W, Dorroh C. Chapter 7. Emergency procedures. In: Stone C, Humphries RL. eds. *Current Diagnosis & Treatment Emergency Medicine*. 7th ed. New York, NY: McGraw-Hill; 2011.

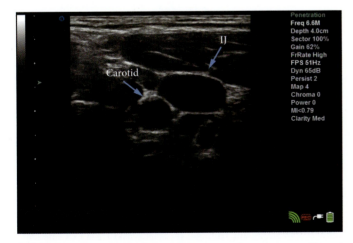

FIGURE 3.73 ■ Relationship of right internal jugular vein (IJ) and carotid artery with probe in a transverse orientation.

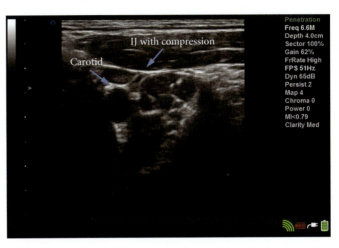

FIGURE 3.74 ■ Veins can be differentiated from arteries by their compressibility. Here the internal jugular vein is easily compressed by the probe.

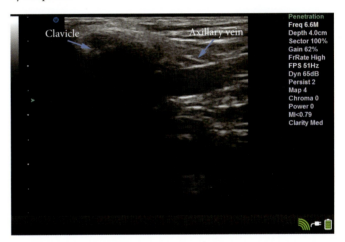

FIGURE 3.75 ■ Axillary vein as it becomes subclavian vein. Ultrasound can help determine the relationship of subclavian vein and clavicle and can guide needle entry.

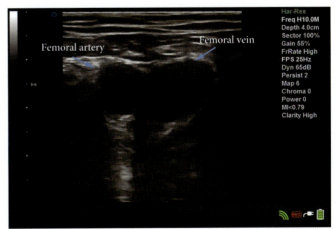

FIGURE 3.76 ■ Right femoral vein and femoral artery with the probe in a transverse orientation.

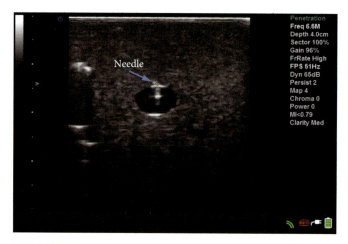

FIGURE 3.77 ■ Transverse view of vein with needle tip seen entering vein.

spans the entire length of the monitor and is seen at its widest diameter. The needle is advanced along the long axis of the vessel, which is now parallel to the axis of the probe. In this fashion, the needle is seen in its entirety and visualized during entry into the vessel. While the needle is more easily seen in this probe orientation, adjacent structures are not visualized.

Peripheral Venous Access

A tourniquet is placed near the axilla with the upper extremity abducted and externally rotated. The arm is scanned with a high-frequency linear array transducer for potential

the cross-section of the vessel under the probe is visualized. Therefore, in order to visualize the needle on ultrasound, the needle must enter the skin at a distance from the probe such that the needle enters the vessel directly underneath the probe. Knowledge of the depth of the vessel will help estimate the entry point of the needle on the skin surface. The probe may be tilted backward toward the entry point of the needle in order to find the needle tip, and then returned to a perpendicular position relative to the skin surface as the needle is advanced. The tip of the needle is then visualized as it enters the vessel. Visualization of the needle tip prevents puncturing through the back of the vessel wall and other complications such as arterial puncture and pneumothorax.

With the probe in the longitudinal orientation, the probe is aligned with the long axis of the vessel such that the vessel

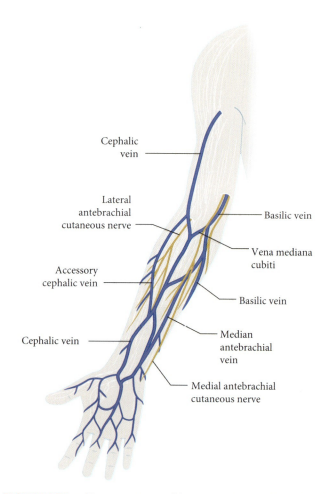

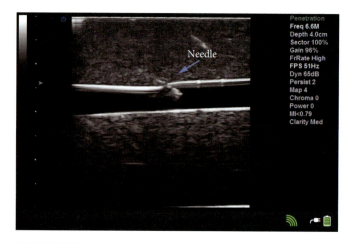

FIGURE 3.78 ■ Longitudinal view of vein with needle seen entering vein.

FIGURE 3.79 ■ Venous anatomy of the upper extremity. Reproduced, with permission, from Wyatt CR. Chapter 33. Venous and intraosseous access in adults. In: Tintinalli JE, Stapczynski J, Ma O, Cline DM, Cydulka RK, Meckler GD, eds. *Tintinalli's Emergency Medicine: A Comprehensive Study Guide*. 7th ed. New York, NY: McGraw-Hill; 2011.

access sites starting in the antecubital fossa and proceeding proximally. Veins in the antecubital fossa, the basilic vein, or cephalic vein are typically utilized for access. The brachial vein may also be utilized but is more difficult to cannulate due to its depth and close proximity of the brachial artery. Once an appropriate vein is visualized, it is accessed with the probe in a transverse or longitudinal orientation in relation to the vein as previously described. Attention must be placed on finding and following the tip of the needle so that the back of the vessel is not punctured, as this will compromise the vein and increase the likelihood of catheter failure.

Pearls and Pitfalls

- Ultrasound guidance for peripheral access allows for placement of IV catheters in peripheral veins that are not palpable for traditional techniques and can prevent the need for central access.
- The transverse probe orientation allows for visualization of structures adjacent to the target vein, but does not allow for visualization of the entire needle.
- The longitudinal probe orientation allows for visualization of the entire needle, but does not allow for visualization of adjacent structures.

Chapter 4
DEVICES

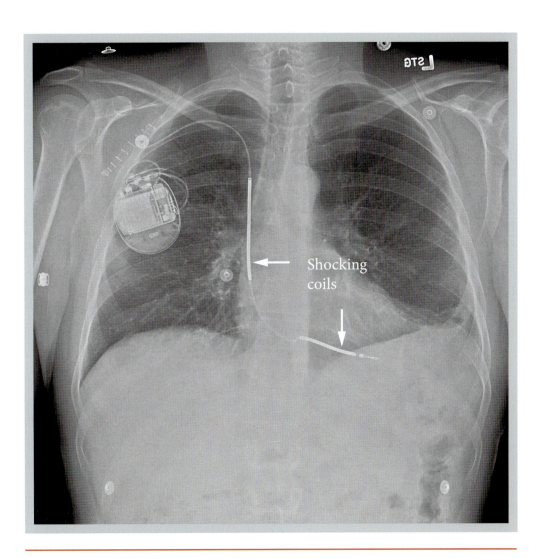

TRANSCUTANEOUS PACEMAKER

Benjamin C. Smith III

Indications

Symptomatic Bradyarrhythmias

Unstable bradycardic patients who do not respond to a trial of atropine should be considered candidates for transcutaneous pacing. One important exception is hypothermia-induced bradycardia, where pacing may induce more unstable rhythms.

Recalcitrant Tachyarrhythmias

Patients who have tachyarrhythmias recalcitrant to one or more pharmacological interventions can be considered for transcutaneous overdrive pacing. In particular, patients with torsades recalcitrant to magnesium may respond to overdrive pacing. Use caution, however, overdrive pacing ventricular dysrhythmias can induce ventricular fibrillation.

Technique

Pacer pads preferably should be placed on the left anterior and posterior chest wall, or the less desirable left and right anterior chest walls. To enable the defibrillator to sense the patient's intrinsic rhythm, the three-pacer electrocardiogram (ECG) leads should be placed on the patient's chest.

The pacing function should be enabled at a rate of 70 to 80 beats per minute when treating bradycardia, and the current (in milliamperes, mA) should be increased until 100% electromechanical capture is verified. Mechanical capture should be verified by palpating a coincident central pulse, verifying distal flow with Doppler ultrasound, or performing a bedside echocardiogram. Transcutaneous pacing causes muscle twitches of the thorax and upper extremities that can cloud the reader's visualization of ventricular capture on the rhythm strip, so electrical capture alone is insufficient to verify cardiac stimulation. Demand pacemaker mode should be used unless significant artifact is present that falsely inhibits pacing. This mode is usually on by default and senses the patient's intrinsic rhythm, inhibiting pacing unless the patient's ventricular rate drops below the set threshold.

When treating recalcitrant tachyarrhythmias, the pacer mode should be in "nondemand" mode. The rate should be set at, or just above, the patient's intrinsic ventricular rate and the current should be increased until mechanical capture is obtained. The pacer rate can then slowly be lowered to a normal level over several minutes.

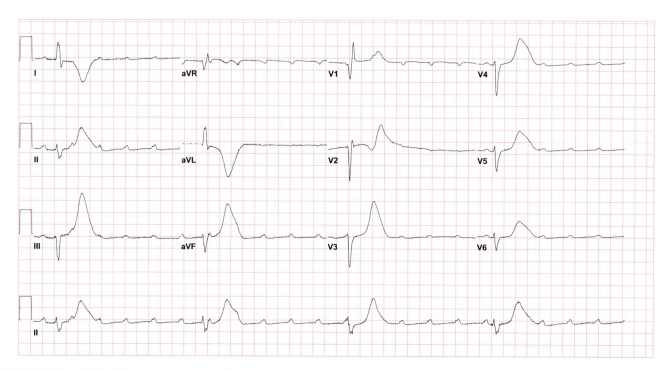

FIGURE 4.1 ■ ECG of third-degree heart block with a ventricular escape rhythm.

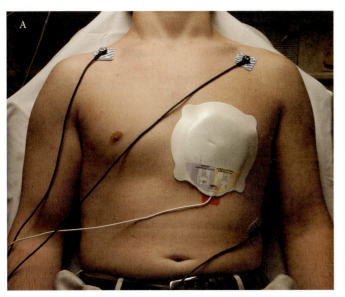 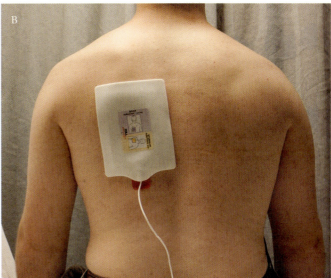

FIGURE 4.2 ■ Preferred anterior (**A**)/posterior (**B**) pacer pad placement with three-monitor leads for demand mode.

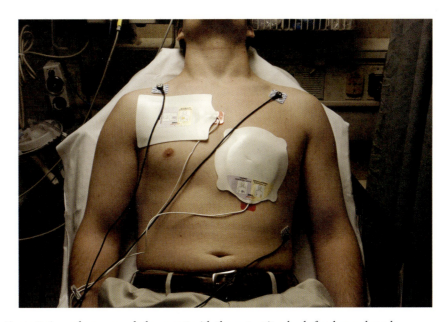

FIGURE 4.3 ■ Alternative anterior only pacer pad placement with three-monitor leads for demand mode.

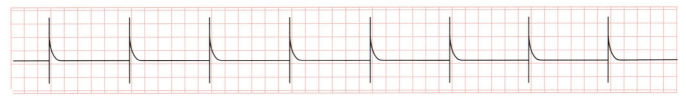

FIGURE 4.4 ■ Monitor strip of transcutaneous pacing without ventricular capture. Note the typical appearance of artifact following the pacer spike.

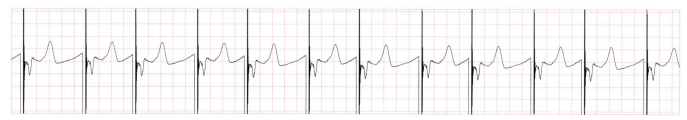

FIGURE 4.5 ■ Strip of transcutaneous pacing with ventricular capture. Note the left bundle branch block appearance to the QRS complex, as well as the presence of a T wave.

Complications

Because transcutaneous pacing impulses must traverse the chest wall to simulate the heart, higher currents are required as compared with internal pacemakers. Sedation and analgesia are almost universally necessary, with intubation for pain control sometimes a requirement. Patients without readily reversible etiologies or patients without adequate capture from transvenous pacing should be considered for transvenous pacer placement (see later).

Pearls and Pitfalls

- Small changes in the patient's physiologic status (eg, worsening acidosis and hypoxemia) can increase their capture threshold. Therefore, the patient being paced should have 1:1 nursing care to verify continuing pacing capture until definitive treatment can be instituted.
- Most 12-lead ECG machines handle the large pacing current very poorly, rendering the resultant ECG uninterpretable. The defibrillator monitor strip should be used instead.
- Prolonged transcutaneous pacing should be avoided to prevent cutaneous burns.
- Overdrive pacing can induce secondary arrhythmias, including ventricular tachycardia and fibrillation, so the clinician should be at the bedside during this procedure ready to treat those conditions should they arise.
- All the patients who require transcutaneous pacing should have an emergent cardiology consult and should be considered critically ill.

TRANSVENOUS PACEMAKER

Benjamin C. Smith III

Indications

Unstable bradycardic patients who do not respond to a trial of atropine should be considered candidates for pacing. Initially, transcutaneous pacing should be instituted for its ease in application. Patients who are expected to require pacing for a significant duration, or fail transcutaneous pacing, should be considered for transvenous pacing emergently. Ultimately, the underlying etiology of bradycardia should be corrected, or a permanent implantable pacemaker should be inserted.

Technique

First, placement of a transvenous pacemaker involves obtaining central venous access with an introducer sheath in either the left subclavian vein or the preferred right internal jugular vein. These sites provide the most direct anatomical path for right ventricle (RV) pacer wire placement, although the femoral vein is an acceptable alternative. The proximal pacer wire lead should be connected to the V1 lead of an ECG machine, while the patient should be connected to the limb leads. The pacer wire can then be inserted into the introducer, and once in the superior vena cava, the pacer wire balloon should be inflated; thereafter, direct the pacer lead toward the RV. Monitoring the V1 lead setup created above will help determine the location of the pacer wire. Confirmation of placement in the RV can be made under real-time guidance with ultrasound or fluoroscopy, or statically with a chest x-ray.

Once adequate position is verified, the balloon should then be deflated and the pacer wire should be attached to the transvenous pacing unit. Pacing function should be enabled

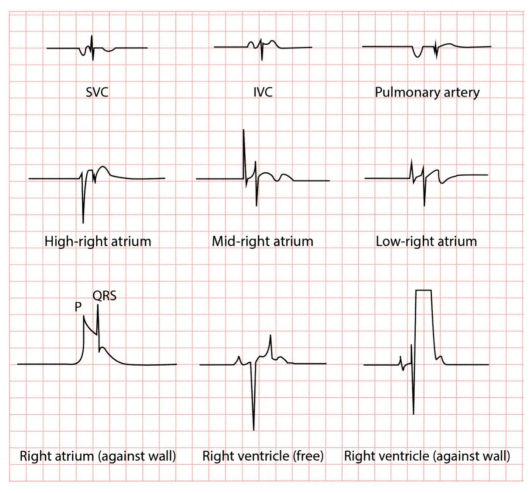

FIGURE 4.6 ■ Transvenous pacemaker wire ECG tracings as the lead passes from the superior vena cava (SVC) to the RV.

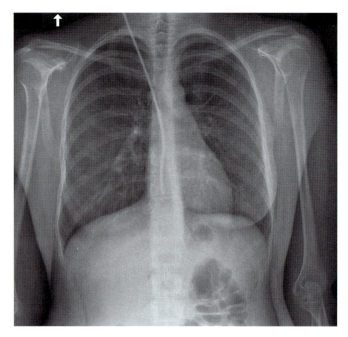

FIGURE 4.7 ■ Chest x-ray, posterior–anterior (PA) view, showing a transvenous pacemaker wire properly placed in the RV.

at a rate of 80 beats per minute, and the current should be set to the maximum, usually 20 mA. Mechanical capture should be verified by palpating a coincident central pulse, verifying distal flow with Doppler ultrasound, or performing a bedside echocardiogram. Electrical capture alone is insufficient to verify cardiac stimulation. The current should then be decreased until electromechanical capture ceases, this value is the capture threshold. The current should then be set to two to three times the capture threshold. If insufficient capture is initially obtained at the maximum current, the pacer wire needs repositioning. To enable the pacemaker unit to sense the patient's intrinsic rhythm, it should be placed in demand mode.

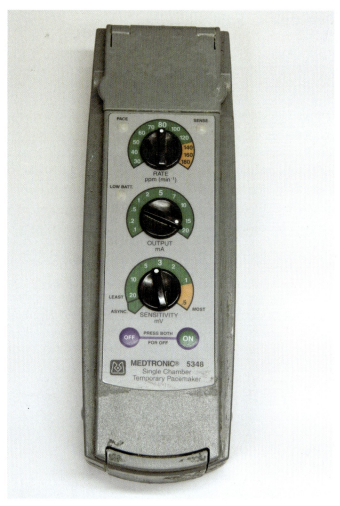

FIGURE 4.8 ■ Temporary transvenous pacing generator with knobs for rate, output (current), and sensitivity (for demand mode).

Complications

Placement complications include arterial puncture, pneumothorax, venous thrombosis, pulmonary embolism, arrhythmias due to RV stimulation, and cardiac perforation.

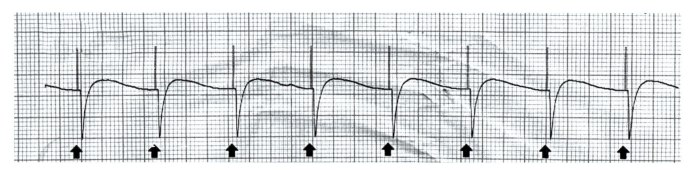

FIGURE 4.9 ■ ECG monitor strip of pacing impulses (arrows) with failed capture. Note artifact following the pacer spike; this does not represent capture.

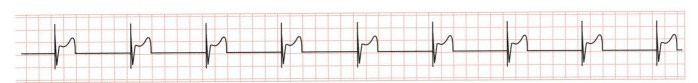

FIGURE 4.10 ■ ECG monitor strip of pacing impulses with successful capture. Note T-wave following successful capture.

Pearls and Pitfalls

- A subxiphoid ultrasound view usually allows adequate visualization of the right heart for real-time guidance of pacer wire placement without breaking the sterile field.
- Patients who have cardiac ischemia as the etiology of their symptomatic bradycardia are more likely to have an irritable myocardium that is particularly prone to catheter-induced arrhythmias.
- Low cardiac output states will make proper placement of the pacer wire more difficult because there will be little forward venous flow to direct the inflated catheter tip. Using the optimal right internal jugular approach is of particular importance in this situation.

COMPLICATIONS OF IMPLANTED PACEMAKERS

Bryon E. Rubery
Glenn M. Brammer

Indications

Symptomatic bradycardia due to nonreversible causes, requiring prolonged intravenous pacing of the heart, most commonly due to sick sinus syndrome, atrioventricular block, and, less frequently, carotid sinus hypersensitivity.

Technique

After initial implantation, the cardiologist will determine the function of the pacemaker by checking the pacing capture threshold, lead impedance, native rhythm sensing, resulting ECG, and position on chest x-ray.

Complications

Investigation of pacemaker dysfunction in the Emergency Department (ED) typically requires an ECG looking for expected pacemaker spikes/significant changes and a chest

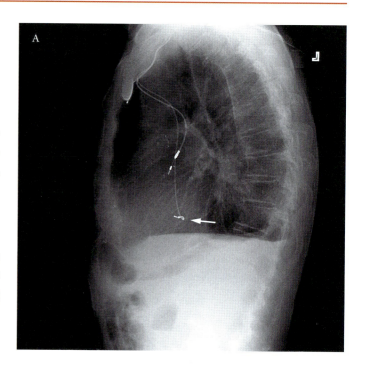

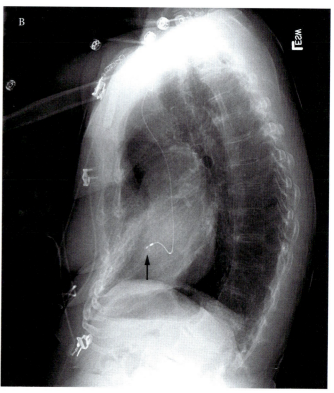

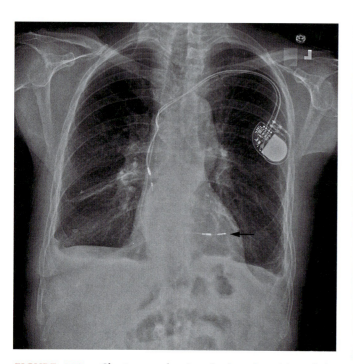

FIGURE 4.11 ■ Chest x-ray showing the lateral position of the RV pacemaker lead tip (arrow). In this case, an unsuspected VSD allowed the lead to enter the left ventricle (LV).

FIGURE 4.12 ■ (A) The lateral chest x-ray of the same patient in Figure 4.11; the tip of the right ventricular lead (arrow) is clearly posterior (territory of the LV). (B) Compare A with the normal anterior position of the RV lead (arrow) in B.

COMPLICATIONS OF IMPLANTED PACEMAKERS (CONTINUED)

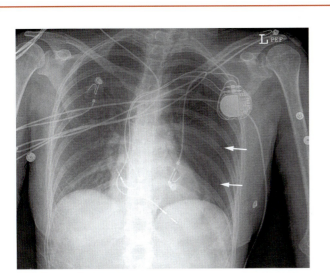

FIGURE 4.13 ■ Left-sided pneumothorax one day after dual-chamber pacemaker insertion. Note the lateral margin of the left lung (arrows) with the absence of lung markings lateral to the lung edge.

x-ray to compare with the postprocedure chest x-ray. Other tests should only be ordered as indicated by chief complaint or past medical history. Interrogation of the device and disposition typically requires discussion with the patient's cardiologist.

Pneumothorax

Occasionally, this complication will not be seen until the day following implantation. Patients typically present with pleuritic chest pain, with or without shortness of breath.

Lead Dislodgement

The patient may experience syncope, recurrence of the original symptoms that prompted placement of the pacemaker, pacing of chest muscles or the diaphragm, or the patient may experience subtle symptoms such as fatigue or "ill" feeling.

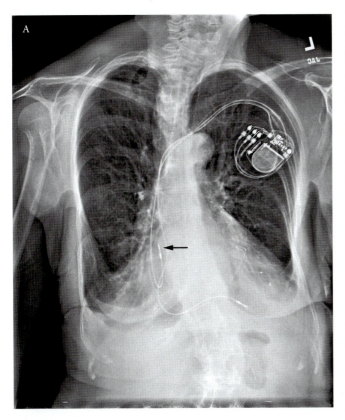
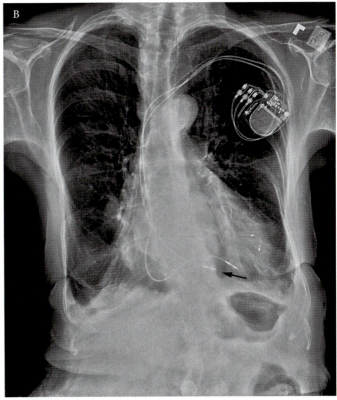

FIGURE 4.14 ■ (A) Chest radiograph showing a biventricular pacemaker with properly positioned atrial (arrow) and ventricular leads. (B) Repeat chest radiograph after the onset of generalized malaise, the atrial lead (arrow) has migrated into the RV. Interrogation of the pacemaker confirmed loss of atrial capture due to improper placement.

Lead Fracture

Pacemakers may fail to capture due to lead fracture (breakage of the lead) or damage to the insulation surrounding the wire causing leakage of the electrical signal.

Lead Perforations

Pacemaker lead perforations may present with symptoms of chest pain, from mild to severe, and vital signs may be normal, or present with hypotension due to pericardial

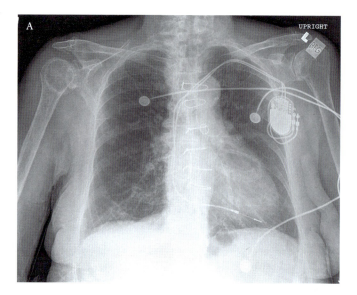

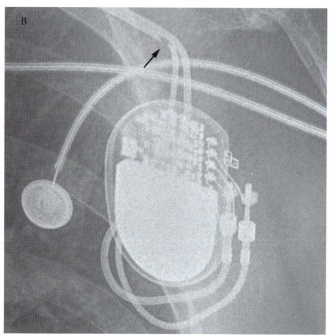

FIGURE 4.15 ■ (A) Chest radiograph of patient with pacemaker wire fracture. The patient suddenly experienced fatigue which prompted the investigation of pacemaker function, including this chest radiograph. The broken wire can be seen near the pacemaker unit, at the bend in the wire. (B) Enlargement of the fracture point (see arrow).

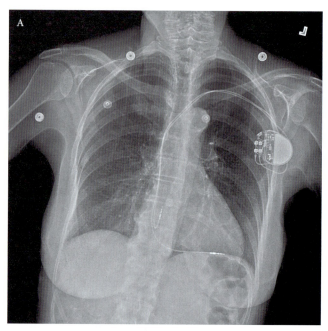

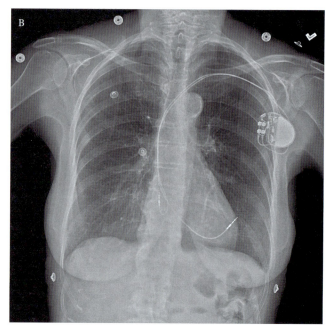

FIGURE 4.16 ■ (A) Chest x-ray after initial pacemaker implant. The RV lead perforation through the ventricle went undiagnosed. (B) Chest x-ray three days later; the perforation is more obvious. The tip of the RV lead is clearly outside the ventricle.

tamponade. The patient may have a pericardial friction rub. Typically when the pacemaker is interrogated, the device shows abnormalities of lead pacing, sensing, or impedance; rarely these lead parameters are normal. Occasionally, a perforation is missed on initial implant, but may become more obvious over time.

Other Complications

Infections at the pacemaker insertion site are not uncommon; typical skin organisms should be covered, device removal may be required. Hematoma may follow insertion or trauma to the area. Skin erosion occasionally occurs, often the result of pocket infection.

Pearls and Pitfalls

- Pacemaker dysfunction may present with subtle symptoms such as fatigue or "ill" feeling.
- Old records or a device card in the patient's wallet should help with the investigation of potential dysfunction.

IMPLANTED CARDIOVERTER-DEFIBRILLATOR: COMPLICATIONS

Bryon E. Rubery
Glenn M. Brammer

Indications (Class I)

Survivors of cardiac arrest due to ventricular fibrillation or unstable ventricular tachycardia (excluding reversible causes), and patients with significant left ventricular (LV) dysfunction who meet specified heart failure criteria.

Technique

After initial implantation, the cardiologist may or may not test defibrillation threshold depending on the perceived risk of testing. An implanted cardioverter-defibrillator (ICD), or combination ICD–pacemaker, can be differentiated from a pacemaker by the presence of shocking coils seen on chest x-ray (one or two will be seen). This chapter focuses on complications following implantation.

Complications

Pneumothorax

See Complications of Implanted Pacemakers section on previous page for discussion.

Inappropriate Shocks

Causes of inappropriate shocks include false sensing, unsustained tachyarrhythmia, ICD–pacemaker interactions, and component failure. The conditions that may trigger false sensing include rapid supraventricular tachycardias, muscular activity, sensing T waves, and lead fracture or migration. For a patient with repeated inappropriate shocks, it may be necessary to temporarily deactivate the ICD by placing a magnet over the device. If defibrillation is necessary, do not place either the paddle or pad directly over the ICD. Perform cardiopulmonary resuscitation (CPR) in the usual fashion. ICD shocks during CPR are neither dangerous nor painful.

Lead Dislodgement or Lead Fracture

See the Complications of Implanted Pacemakers section on page 84 for a discussion of identifying lead dislodgements or fractures.

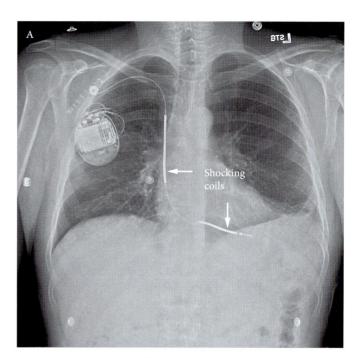

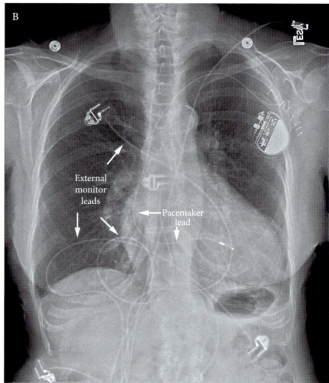

FIGURE 4.17 ■ (A) Chest x-ray of a patient with a dual-coil ICD with a characteristic shocking lead. (B) Chest x-ray showing a single-chamber pacemaker with single lead to the RV.

IMPLANTED CARDIOVERTER-DEFIBRILLATOR: COMPLICATIONS (CONTINUED)

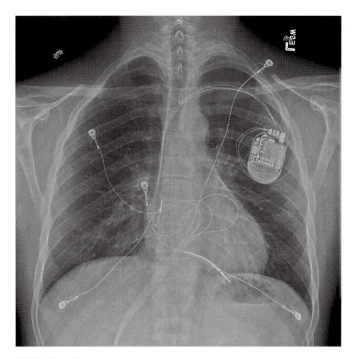

FIGURE 4.18 ■ An ICD lead that appears to be at the base of the RV, but bedside echocardiography revealed significant pericardial effusion.

Lead Perforations

In a patient with an ICD, lead perforation may present with chest pain, hypotension due to pericardial tamponade, or the patient's vital signs may be normal. The patient may have a pericardial friction rub. Typically when the ICD is interrogated, the device shows abnormalities of sensing, or impedance.

Other Complications

See the Complications of Implanted Pacemakers section above for further discussion.

Pearls and Pitfalls

- Patients with ICDs (without combined pacing function) who do not experience frequent arrhythmias may incur lead dislodgement without symptoms; this may be picked when a chest x-ray is performed for an unrelated symptom.
- Lack of symptoms does not rule out lead perforation; however, lead perforation may present with life-threatening signs.
- Patients with inappropriate shocks may suffer from severe anxiety and request to have their ICD removed or deactivated; this is a decision for the cardiologist and the patient.

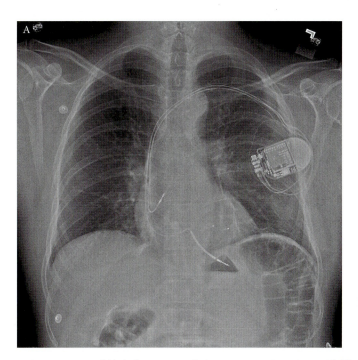
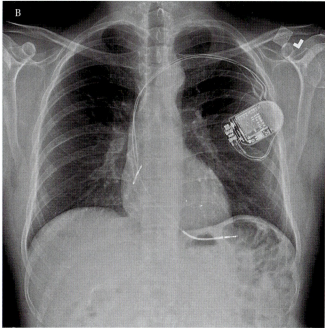

FIGURE 4.19 ■ (A) A chest x-ray of an asymptomatic patient with likely lead perforation one day after implant, yet this was not discovered. (B) Two months later, repeat chest x-ray was more obvious for perforation.

LVAD: LEFT VENTRICULAR ASSIST DEVICE

Daniel Renner
Heather Heaton
Jason N. Katz

Indications

Left ventricular assist devices (LVAD) augment LV output in patients with severe cardiomyopathy. The implanted pump transfers blood from the apex of the LV to the proximal aorta. The pump is powered by an external power source, regulated by a controller. Both the battery and controller reside outside of the body. The controller drives the pump through a driveline, connected through a surgical incision in the abdominal wall.

Most LVADs pump blood using a continuous flow mechanism (eg, axial or centrifugal flow), maintaining a normal mean arterial blood pressure in the absence of a palpable pulse. However, many patients retain some cardiac contractility; in these individuals, a pulse may be present. LVAD patients still rely upon reasonable RV function to pump blood to the lungs.

Technique

LVAD patients should have a normal mean arterial pressure. Blood pressure can be assessed by a mechanical cuff or by Doppler ultrasound. Flow may be continuous and not pulsatile. When auscultating the heart, the continuous whirr of the pump is heard. The ECG should have discernible QRS complexes. The LVAD is visible on a chest radiograph. MRI imaging is contraindicated.

The Hemodynamically Unstable LVAD Patient

If an audible "whirr" is not heard over the precordium, search for a cause of mechanical LVAD failure. Check and/or change the batteries and/or controller. Do not disconnect anything. For hypotension, give a bolus of normal saline. If hypotension persists, or in the presence of RV failure or LVAD malfunction, initiate IV pressors. Dopamine is a reasonable first-line therapy. Obtain an ECG to rule out RV myocardial infarction or strain. Obtain standard laboratory studies as clinically indicated. Bedside ultrasound can be used to assess RV function and to evaluate for pericardial effusion/tamponade. Give heparin if device thrombosis is suspected and bleeding is excluded. Ventricular tachycardia or fibrillation in an unstable patient requires defibrillation/cardioversion. Do not place defibrillator pads over the driveline. If the patient is clinically stable, give amiodarone.

Complications

Medical complications include bleeding, anemia (hemolysis), thromboembolism, or infection. LVAD patients are typically anticoagulated with an international normalized ratio (INR) target of 2 to 3. LVAD patients are also at risk for thromboembolism, such as pulmonary embolism, stroke, and mesenteric ischemia, especially in the setting of suboptimal anticoagulation. Heparin is safe and indicated for such events once bleeding has been ruled out. Infection is a common complication, especially at the driveline exit site. Treat sepsis with volume resuscitation, blood cultures, and antibiotics.

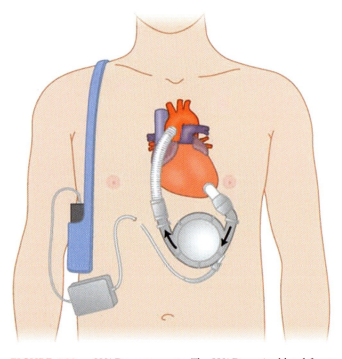

FIGURE 4.20 ■ LVAD components. The LVAD carries blood from the LV to the aorta. Reproduced, with permission, from Renner D, Heaton H, Katz JN. Left Ventricular Assist Devices, Chapter 53. The cardiomyopathies and pericardial disease. In: Tintinalli JE, Stapczynski J, Ma O, Cline DM, Cydulka RK, Meckler GD, eds. *Tintinalli's Emergency Medicine: A Comprehensive Study Guide.* 7th ed. New York, NY: McGraw-Hill; 2011.

LVAD: LEFT VENTRICULAR ASSIST DEVICE (CONTINUED)

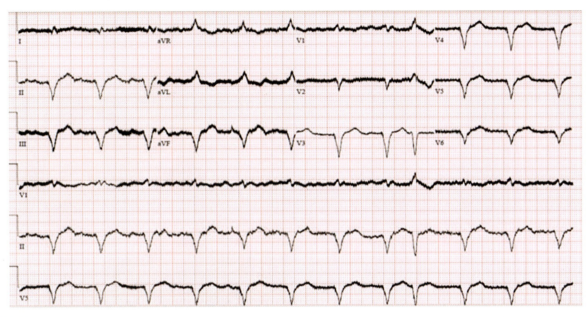

FIGURE 4.21 ■ ECG of a patient with an LVAD. QRS is evident and baseline shows some electrical interference from the pump. ECG courtesy of Daniel Renner, MD. Reproduced, with permission, from Renner D, Heaton H, Katz JN. Left Ventricular Assist Devices, Chapter 53. The cardiomyopathies and pericardial disease. In: Tintinalli JE, Stapczynski J, Ma O, Cline DM, Cydulka RK, Meckler GD, eds. *Tintinalli's Emergency Medicine: A Comprehensive Study Guide.* 7th ed. New York, NY: McGraw-Hill; 2011.

Pearls and Pitfalls

- *Never* perform chest compressions on an LVAD patient. Chest compressions can dislodge the LVAD from the heart and aorta, causing LV rupture and intractable hemorrhage.
- If the LVAD model does not provide pulsatile flow, it is difficult to obtain a reading by pulse oximetry.
- Patients and families should be involved during patient assessment and management.
- It is essential to call the patient's LVAD coordinator as soon as possible to assist with management decisions.

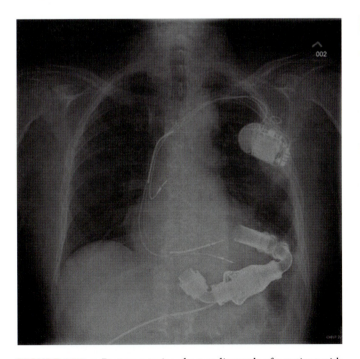

FIGURE 4.22 ■ Posteroanterior chest radiograph of a patient with an LVAD and implantable defibrillator. The outflow conduit to the proximal aorta is not radiographically visible. Reproduced, with permission, from Renner D, Heaton H, Katz JN. Left Ventricular Assist Devices, Chapter 53. The cardiomyopathies and pericardial disease. In: Tintinalli JE, Stapczynski J, Ma O, Cline DM, Cydulka RK, Meckler GD, eds. *Tintinalli's Emergency Medicine: A Comprehensive Study Guide.* 7th ed. New York, NY: McGraw-Hill; 2011.

AUTOMATED CPR DEVICE

Jeffrey W. Hinshaw

Indication

Patients in cardiac arrest require consistent and good-quality CPR. This helps maintain limited organ perfusion until definitive therapy can be performed and/or while rescue medications are administered. Although chest compressions are typically delivered by human first responders, medical personnel, and nonmedical by-standers, external automated compression devices are available to assist with this task.

Current American Heart Association (AHA) guidelines recommend that chest compressions be at least 2 inches deep (5 cm) and at a rate greater than 100 compressions per minute. Complete chest recoil should be allowed between each compression. CPR should be delivered in 2-minute intervals with limited interruptions between compression cycles to perform other tasks. CPR is physically taxing, requiring providers to switch at regular intervals to maintain vigorous compression of the chest wall. Automated compression devices can help deliver compressions in out-of-hospital settings and/or during transport, thus sparing the rescuer of physical exertion and allowing them to perform other resuscitative tasks. In addition, according to the 2010 AHA guidelines for CPR and emergency cardiovascular care, it is reasonable to employ mechanical CPR devices for cardiac arrest while continuing a percutaneous coronary intervention (recommendation class IIA, level of evidence C).

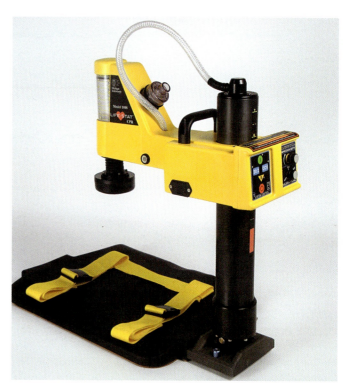

FIGURE 4.23 ■ The LifeStat system is an example of a piston compression device. (Courtesy of Michigan Instruments.)

Technique

Piston chest compression devices consist of a base plate and an arm from which a piston extends. The piston drives several inches downward into the chest wall creating compressive forces. A ventilation circuit can be added to the device to synchronize compressions with ventilation, and most models allow defibrillation without an interruption in compressions.

Proper CPR by a human rescuer or compression device depends on passive recoil of the chest. Some chest compression devices have a modified piston drive-arm attachment in the form of a suction cup that causes active return of the chest to the uncompressed position. Another type of compression device involves a load-distributing band. This device compresses the entire anterior chest via a compression band that is

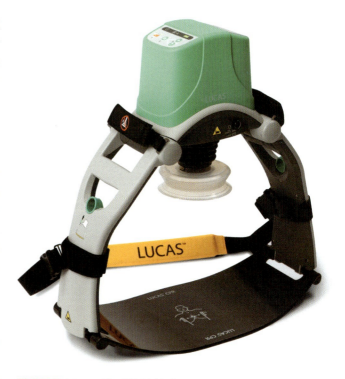

FIGURE 4.24 ■ The LUCAS® chest compression system employs a suction cup at the end of the piston to provide active chest recoil. (Courtesy of PhysioControl, Inc.)

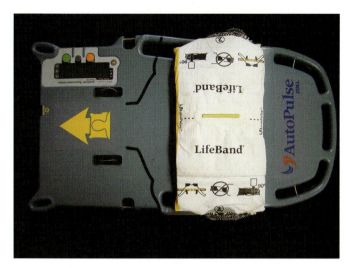

FIGURE 4.25 ■ The AutoPulse CPR device employs a load-distributing band to generate chest compression.

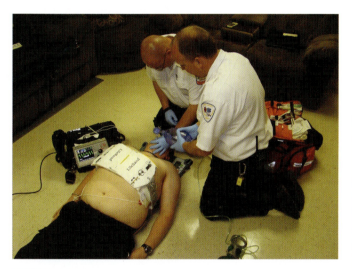

FIGURE 4.26 ■ In this pre-hospital cardiac arrest scene, an automated CPR device has been applied to the victim.

driven by a motor. The band tightens during compression and releases to allow for chest expansion.

Complications

Traumatic injury to the chest wall and thoracic structures is a potential complication of automated CPR devices.

Pearls and Pitfalls

- Automated CPR devices are capable of delivering good-quality CPR for long periods of time and may be particularly

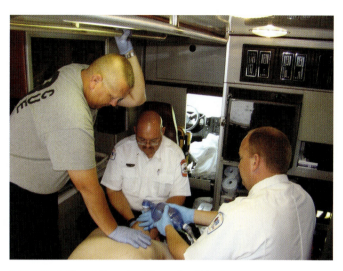

FIGURE 4.27 ■ Manual CPR can be difficult to perform in a moving vehicle. As shown here, manual CPR is attempted with one hand on the patient's chest and the other on a hand rail to maintain balance. The emergency medical services (EMS) provider is in danger because he is not restrained and chest compressions are likely to be suboptimal in this case.

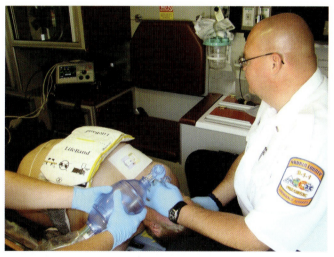

FIGURE 4.28 ■ Use of an automated CPR device in this scenario allows EMS personnel to remain seated and restrained during transport to a medical facility. Chest compressions are more likely to be consistent in this case.

useful during pre-hospital vehicular transport when effective manual CPR can be physically challenging.
- Investigational data have not demonstrated an increase in survival to hospital discharge when comparing automated and manual CPR.
- Cost, battery life, and clinical efficacy of automated CPR devices should always be considered before use.

EXTERNAL RHYTHM RECORDER: HOLTER MONITOR AND KING OF HEARTS

Joshua T. James

Technique

Ambulatory ECG, or external rhythm recorder, is a commonly used modality to evaluate cardiac rhythm disturbances. The AHA Practice Guidelines have released class I indications for the use of ambulatory ECGs: the evaluation of unexplained syncope or near syncope, episodic dizziness, or recurrent unexplained palpitations. As opposed to the standard 12-lead ECG, ambulatory ECGs typically use no more than five leads to monitor for arrhythmias for an extended period of time. There are two types of ambulatory ECG: continuous and intermittent. Holter monitor, a continuous monitor, is typically worn for 24 to 48 hours and provides continuous monitoring of the cardiac cycle. King of Hearts, an intermittent monitor, is worn by the patient for longer periods of time, often weeks, and is activated in response to symptoms.

There are two types of intermittent recorders: event type and loop recorders. Event type recorders store a brief moment of activity when activated by the patient. Loop recorders record continuously but store only brief recordings when activated. Ambulatory ECGs can be analyzed rapidly by transferring data over conventional telephone lines or online via microprocessors.

Interpretation

As there can be motion artifact due to normal daily activities, the data are analyzed by an experienced technician or physician. The patient is asked to record daily events and symptoms in a timed diary. Detection of particular arrhythmia may aide

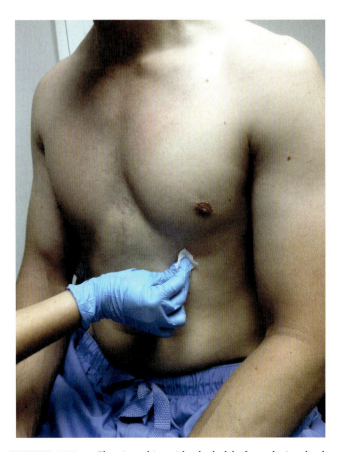

FIGURE 4.29 ■ Cleaning skin with alcohol before placing leads. If the skin is not adequately cleaned and dried, there is significant chance of lead-adherence failure.

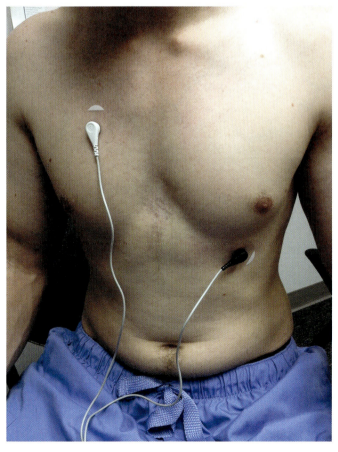

FIGURE 4.30 ■ King of Hearts monitor lead placement. Note that there are only two leads.

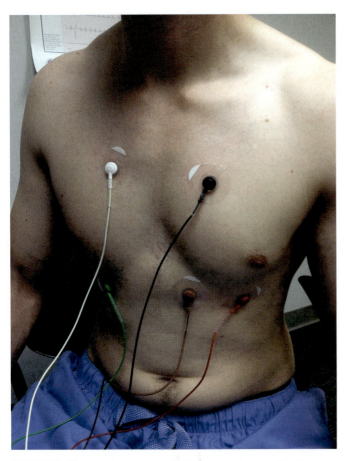

FIGURE 4.31 ■ Holter monitor lead placement. Note that there are five leads.

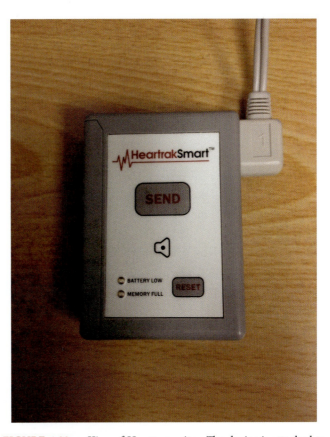

FIGURE 4.32 ■ King of Hearts monitor. The device is attached to the patient and easily activated when symptoms arise. Record button is on top; out of view. The send button transmits event data; reset button clears memory.

in determining an abnormal rhythm diagnosis. Symptoms may occur simultaneously with a documented arrhythmia that may guide therapy. Another helpful finding is significant symptoms in the absence of an arrhythmia, effectively ruling out a rhythm disturbance as the etiology. Arrhythmias may be noted in the absence of symptoms; this finding, however, is equivocal as asymptomatic arrhythmias may or may not be clinically significant. An arrhythmia may not be detected and the patient may remain asymptomatic. This is of no value.

Pearls and Pitfalls

- Consider continuous monitoring for patients who would not be able to activate the device, such as in the evaluation of a patient with syncope.
- Consider an intermittent monitor for symptoms that occur less frequently.
- Due to normal variability in arrhythmia frequency, a 65% to 95% reduction in arrhythmia frequency is required to prove treatment effect.
- Data suggest the Holter monitor to have sensitivity as low as 22% for detecting arrhythmias.

EXTRACORPOREAL MEMBRANE OXYGENATION

Sydney Larken Ware

Indications

Acute severe cardiac or pulmonary failure that is potentially reversible and unresponsive to conventional management. Patients with hypoxemic respiratory failure despite optimal ventilator management may benefit from venovenous ECMO (VV ECMO), such as patients with severe pulmonary contusions after trauma or severe pneumonia. Patients in refractory cardiogenic shock or post-cardiac arrest may benefit from venoarterial ECMO (VA ECMO). ECMO should not be initiated in patients who have contraindications to anticoagulants. Patients with advanced age, neurological dysfunction, and poor preexisting functional capacity are not suitable candidates for ECMO.

Technique

ECMO was first used as a means to provide oxygenation, now ventilation (removal of CO_2) and pressure support can be accomplished as well. In VV ECMO, blood is removed

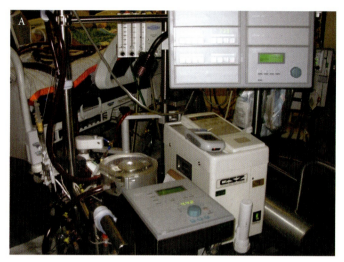

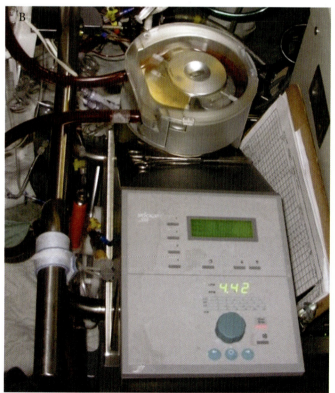

FIGURE 4.34 ■ Flow monitor (**A**) and flow adjustor (**B**). The monitor that rates the flow through the ECMO device and back to the patient is shown. In a patient on VA ECMO, cardiac output is generated by the device. When flow settings are increased, the rotating oscillator speed increases, spinning faster to deliver a higher cardiac output.

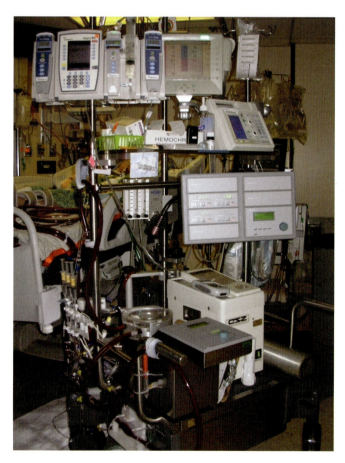

FIGURE 4.33 ■ ECMO machine. The ECMO device shows all the operating parts of ECMO device. Cardiac output (flow), ventilation (CO_2 removal), and oxygenation (O_2 enrichment) can be adjusted by the clinician.

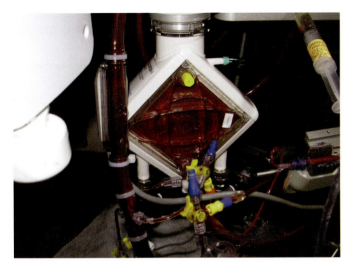

FIGURE 4.35 ■ The ECMO oxygenator. Blood flows across a membrane increasing the oxygen tension. Increasing premembrane pressures may signal clot formation in the oxygenator circuit. When clots are recognized, the membrane should be changed quickly to prevent oxygen desaturations.

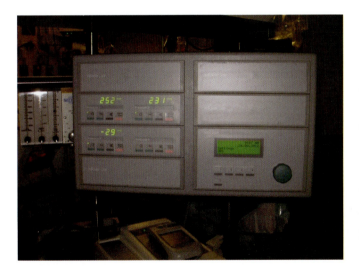

FIGURE 4.36 ■ ECMO in and out flow pressure monitor. This figure shows the measured pressures in the circuit. With proper setup, this value can be used to estimate patient's approximate fluid status.

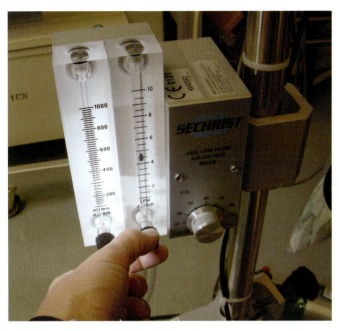

FIGURE 4.37 ■ ECMO sweep monitor, or ventilation (CO_2 removal) monitor. Ventilation can be adjusted based on the patient's pCO_2 reading. Despite full implementation of ECMO, a ventilator may still be used to prevent or reduce reducing atelectasis.

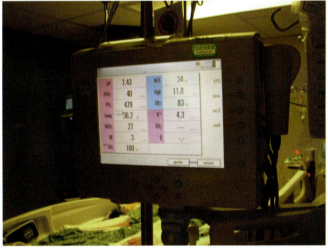

FIGURE 4.38 ■ Laboratory monitor shows the continuous display of blood gas parameters in the circuit. This measurement is highly accurate.

from the right atrium or vena cava and then returned to the right atrium. Therefore, oxygen-poor blood is removed and oxygen-rich blood is returned to the venous system. With this method, cardiac output is dependent on the patient's heart, while the patient's lungs need not provide any oxygenation or ventilation. In VA ECMO, oxygen-poor blood is removed from the venous system and oxygen-rich blood is returned to the arterial system with pressure support. VA ECMO is capable of providing the required cardiac output and oxygenation/ventilation support for the patient.

While successful ECMO programs have trained teams to provide support, the physician who initiates ECMO is responsible for adjusting the machine's settings to match the needs of the patient. The oxygenator determines the intensity of oxygen support for the patient. Increasing premembrane pressures may signal clot formation in the oxygenator circuit. A monitor displays continuous readings of blood gas parameters. Ventilation can be adjusted, which is termed sweep. Despite full implementation of ECMO support, patients frequently remain connected to a ventilator to prevent alveolar collapse. Cardiac output is provided with VA circuits and is termed the "flow" while on ECMO. Clinician-determined flow adjustments are based on lactate levels, blood pressure readings, and mixed venous oxygen saturation. If the patient's heart is not providing any detectable cardiac output, only a mean arterial pressure will be measurable and the patient will not have a pulse. ECMO patients require continued optimization of blood flow, intravascular volume, and hemoglobin concentration. Anticoagulation typically is obtained via heparin infusion. Platelets are consumed with time and require monitoring and replacement.

Complications

Complications include brain injury, sepsis, bleeding, access vessel injury, pulmonary hemorrhage, and thromboembolism including cardiac thrombosis.

Pearls and Pitfalls

- Failing to recognize patients with respiratory or cardiovascular failure unresponsive to optimal management may be candidates for ECMO, which may require transfer to an ECMO center.
- Although ECMO access and monitoring equipment makes examination challenging, failure to reexamine the patient regularly may prevent early detection and treatment of complications such as bleeding, thromboembolism, pulmonary hemorrhage, sepsis, and brain injury.
- The patient must be carefully monitored and ECMO settings adjusted accordingly to maximize respiratory and hemodynamic benefit while preventing complications.

Chapter 5
ARRHYTHMIAS

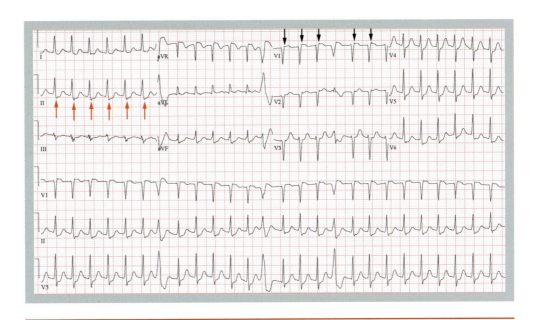

Sinus Arrhythmias

SINUS BRADYCARDIA/TACHYCARDIA INCLUDING RESPIRATORY VARIABLITY

Scott Goldston

Sinus Tachycardia

Clinical Highlights

Normal adult heart rates are 60 to 100 beats per minute (bpm). See Chap. 8, section on Normal ECG at Age Intervals for discussion of childhood norms. Sinus tachycardia is a rapid heart rate that originates from the sinus node. Diagnostic criteria include normal P-wave morphology (normal for the patient), normal PR intervals (0.12–0.2 s), and a 1-to-1 P wave to QRS relationship. Rate is usually less than 160 except in critically ill patients. Occasionally, sinus tachycardia cannot be confirmed and other rhythm diagnoses must be considered. There are numerous causes, including fever, dehydration, hypoxia, stimulants (ie, coffee, nicotine, and illicit drugs), pulmonary

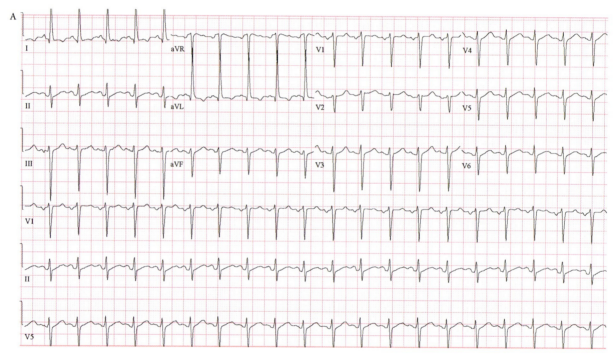

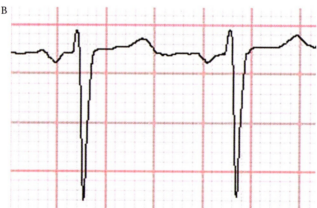

FIGURE 5.1 ■ (A) ECG showing sinus tachycardia with the rate of 123 bpm. If there is suspicion that the P-wave morphology is abnormal on the tachycardic rhythm, compare the P wave with the patient's normal resting ECG. (B) ECG lead V1 detail of P wave and QRS morphology from the same patient in A at a rate within the normal range. The P wave and QRS complexes are identical in V1 leads

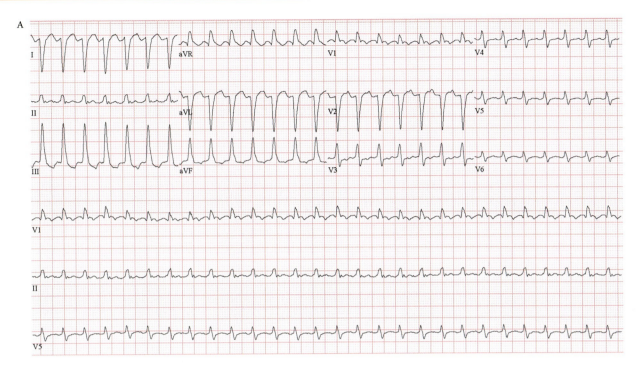

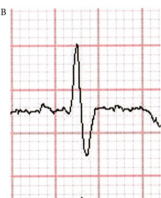

FIGURE 5.2 ■ (A) ECG showing rhythm of 169 bpm in a patient with a prior episode of atrial flutter complaining of palpitations and generalized weakness. The computer, the emergency physician, and the cardiologist initially read the ECG as sinus tachycardia (look at lead V3). (B) An ECG lead V3 from an ECG 2 months before presentation. Only after ruling out other causes was the patient successfully slowed with diltiazem, and cardioverted to normal sinus rhythm from atrial flutter.

embolism, anemia, anxiety, hyperthyroidism, hypotension/shock, sepsis, and many more.

ED Care and Disposition

Sinus tachycardia may be perceived as a fast or "pounding" heartbeat. Usually symptoms are felt if there is underlying cardiac disease. Treating the underlying disorder will typically resolve the tachycardia and success can be gauged by the trend toward a normal rate. Consider airway, breathing, and circulation first; oxygen, fluids, airway intervention, or specific therapy are often required.

Pearls and Pitfalls

- Sinus tachycardia is always 1:1 P wave to QRS conduction.
- There is no specific treatment for sinus tachycardia, treat the underlying cause.
- If you have trouble identifying P waves in rhythms over 120/minute, consider running the electrocardiogram (ECG) at double speed.
- If workup and treatment of suspected sinus tachycardia fail to prove useful, pursue other rhythm diagnoses.

Sinus Bradycardia

Clinical Highlights

Sinus bradycardia is a heart rate that is below 60 bpm originating from the sinus node. In addition to rate, diagnostic criteria include normal P-wave morphology (normal for the patient), normal PR intervals (0.12–0.2 s), and a 1-to-1 P wave to QRS relationship. There are multiple causes including normal physiology (athletes, sleep, etc.), increased vagal activity (cough, vomiting, Valsalva, etc.), or sudden exposure to cold. Several medications cause sinus bradycardia, including beta-blockers, digoxin, calcium channel blockers, amiodarone (and many other antiarrhythmic drugs), and clonidine. There are also many pathologic causes, such as increased intracranial pressure, acute myocardial infarction (AMI), hypothyroidism, and carotid sinus hypersensitivity. Although frequently asymptomatic, the patient may have fatigue or symptoms of presyncope or syncope.

ED Care and Disposition

If asymptomatic, no treatment is indicated. Treatment is usually aimed at finding and correcting the source. If required, first-line treatment is almost always atropine. Temporary transcutaneous or transvenous pacing may be required.

Pearls and Pitfalls

- Sinus bradycardia is the most common presenting arrhythmia in an AMI (up to 15%–25%).
- Sinus bradycardia is usually a response to an underlying disease process from medication use or pathology.

Sinus Arrhythmia

Clinical Highlights

Sinus arrhythmia is a normal variant of sinus rhythm, most commonly due to respiratory effect. The criterion is variation in sinus node discharge larger than 0.12 seconds between the shortest and longest intervals (measured by the R-to-R interval). During normal respiration there are changes in the autonomic tone. Inspiring causes a decrease in vagal tone, thus increasing a sinus rate. The opposite is true with expiration, causing the sinus rate to decrease.

Pearls and Pitfalls

- Sinus arrhythmia is a normal variant of sinus rhythm, and no treatment is required.

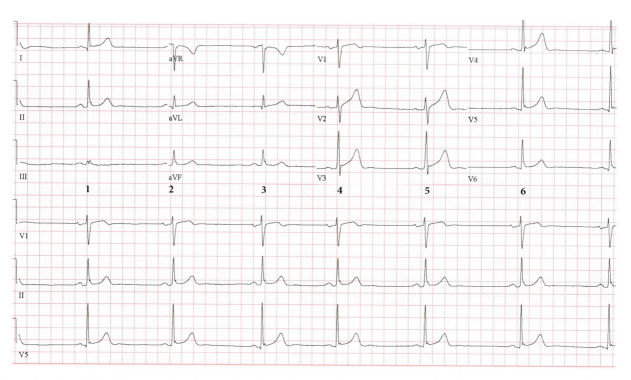

FIGURE 5.3 ■ ECG showing sinus bradycardia rate of 41 bpm; P wave and QRS are normal; each QRS is preceded by a P wave. This ECG also demonstrates sinus arrhythmia; compare the R–R interval between the third and fourth QRS to the interval between the fifth and sixth QRS. The variation in R–R intervals is 360 milliseconds.

Atrial Arrhythmias
PREMATURE ATRIAL CONTRACTIONS (PAC)

Jackson Henley

Clinical Highlights

A premature atrial complex (PAC) is an atrial depolarization that originates from an ectopic focus anywhere in the atria outside of the sinoatrial (SA) node. They occur earlier in the cardiac cycle than those originating from the SA node. The patient may present with a chief complaint of palpitations, or they may incidentally be found to have PACs on an ECG or on telemetry monitoring while in the emergency department (ED). PACs are generally benign heart arrhythmias that rarely lead to clinically significant arrhythmias unless the patient has a history of significant arrhythmia such as atrial fibrillation. PACs may be caused by abnormal automaticity within the atria or from a reentry phenomenon. PACs can occur in isolation or may occur as frequently as every other beat, as in atrial bigemeny.

On ECG interpretation, an ectopic P wave will occur in a shorter interval after the prior T wave, indicating that it is premature. It will also have a different morphology than a

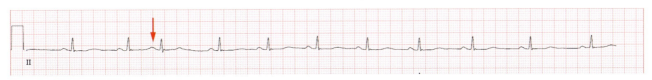

FIGURE 5.4 ■ This rhythm strip demonstrates a premature atrial complex (PAC; arrow). This P wave has a different shape and occurs earlier than the other P waves.

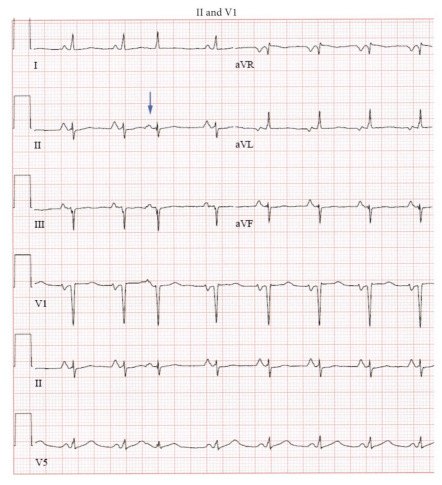

FIGURE 5.5 ■ This ECG reveals a PAC (arrow). Note the shortened interval after the preceding T wave. The unique P-wave morphology associated with the PAC is most notable in leads II and V1.

103

regular P wave. The P wave of the ectopic focus may have different polarity PR interval compared to the normal P wave. Depending on when the PAC occurs, it may not lead to ventricular depolarization. If the PAC occurs early enough during the cardiac cycle, the atrioventricular (AV) node being in its refractory period may not conduct the signal.

ED Care and Disposition

As PACs rarely lead to clinically significant arrhythmias, PACs usually do not require further workup or intervention. If PACs are accompanied by concerning symptoms such as chest pain or shortness of breath in a patient with underlying cardiopulmonary disease, further testing may be warranted such as cardiac biomarkers, serum electrolytes, or a toxicology screen. Because PACs may be related to a toxin, such as caffeine, alcohol, or tobacco, the patient should be encouraged to stop the potential offending agent. Beta-blockers may improve symptoms associated with PACs by reducing their frequency. These medications can be considered if the symptoms are bothersome to the patient and are interfering with daily activities.

Pearls and Pitfalls

- PACs are generally considered a benign arrhythmia.
- PACs are observed on an ECG as an early atrial depolarization after a preceding T wave with a different morphology than other P waves.
- If there is a suspected underlying cause of PACs, especially if it is easily reversible (toxin), this should be addressed. If symptoms persist and interfere with the patient's life significantly, the use of a beta-blocker may be considered.

WANDERING ATRIAL PACEMAKER

Cedric Lefebvre

Clinical Highlights

Wandering atrial pacemaker (WAP) is an electrophysiological phenomenon in which multiple areas, or ectopic foci, within the atria initiate action potentials and temporarily serve as the dominant pacemaker. The constantly shifting location of impulse origin gives the impression of "wandering" foci. Each electrical impulse is transmitted from the atria to the ventricles. This signal conduction leads to ventricular depolarization, and the resulting QRS complexes are narrow and uniform. The overall rhythm is usually irregularly irregular. Each QRS complex will be preceded by a P wave but because the origin of the atrial impulses varies from beat to beat, P-wave morphology will not be uniform. P waves can differ in size, shape, and vector. Typically, WAP will demonstrate at least three different P-wave morphologies on the ECG. The PR interval is generally normal (0.12–0.20 milliseconds) but may vary from beat to beat. The heart rate will be less than 100 bpm. If the heart rate exceeds 100 bpm, the term "multifocal atrial tachycardia" applies.

The causes of WAP include increased vagal tone, digoxin toxicity, chronic lung disease, valvular disease, and coronary disease or ischemia. Certain sympathomimetic medications can induce arrhythmias including WAP. WAP can also occur in normal, healthy patients and during sleep. Patients with WAP may experience palpitations. If the overall heart rate is slow, WAP may cause fatigue or dizziness. At times, WAP is identified incidentally on an ECG.

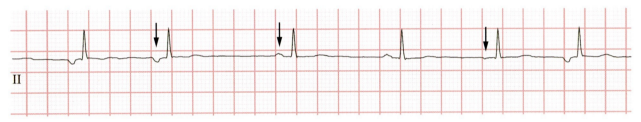

FIGURE 5.6 ■ This ECG segment demonstrates wandering atrial pacemaker. Note the three morphologically distinct P waves (arrows). A dominant pacemaker (P wave) is not identified. The QRS complexes are narrow.

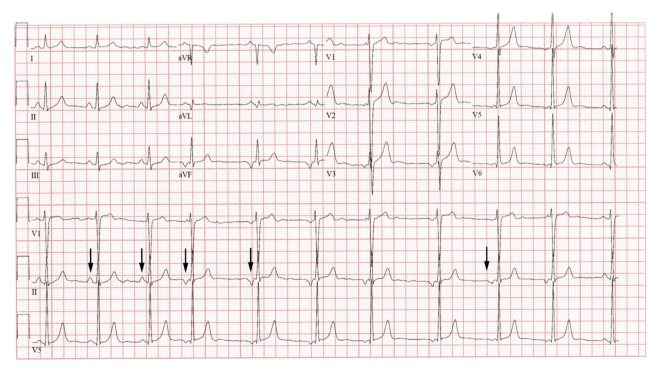

FIGURE 5.7 ■ On this ECG from a patient with wandering atrial pacemaker, the R–R intervals vary from beat to beat, creating an irregularly irregular rhythm. Note the difference in shape and vector of the P waves (arrows) in rhythm strip lead II.

ED Care and Disposition

WAP is generally a benign condition, is usually transient, and rarely requires treatment. However, the etiology of WAP includes serious underlying medical diseases (ie, lung disease); therefore, an investigation into such conditions should be pursued when indicated. The significance of WAP is most likely related to the condition of the patient in which it is noted. In an asymptomatic young athlete, WAP may stem from increased vagal tone, whereas in a patient with lung disease, WAP may suggest acute illness. In an elderly patient, WAP may be an indication of sinus node malfunction or disease. In rare instances, if the symptoms associated with WAP are persistent or severe, atrial pacing may be necessary.

Pearls and Pitfalls

- Unlike PACs, a dominant P wave is not identified in WAP and periods of RR interval regularity are not seen.
- WAP should not be confused with atrial pauses, atrial arrest, or a junctional escape rhythm with reemergence of sinus beats. Unlike WAP, these arrhythmias are clinically significant and require immediate attention or intervention.
- For a patient with a history of respiratory disease found to have WAP, the patient should be assessed for an acute respiratory illness or an exacerbation of chronic respiratory disease and treated accordingly.

CLASSIFICATION AND MECHANISMS OF SUPRAVENTRICULAR TACHYCARDIA

David M. Cline

Supraventricular tachycardia (SVT) is a broad category of rapid cardiac rhythms that originate above the bifurcation of the bundle of His or that have mechanisms dependent on the bundle of His (see also Chap. 2, Electrocardiography: Normal Heart, Acute Ischemia, and Chronic Disease, section on Normal Cardiac Conduction). Therefore, SVT can be used to describe sinus tachycardia and atrial tachycardias (AT) including atrial flutter and fibrillation. However, clinicians generally use the term "SVT" to describe paroxysmal, narrow complex tachycardias that start abruptly and end abruptly. Over the last 30 years, the classification of SVT has advanced with the advent of diagnostic and therapeutic cardiac electrophysiology. The two major mechanisms of SVT are reentry and increased automaticity, with reentry accounting for the majority of SVT rhythms.

Clinical Highlights

Patients most commonly complain of sudden onset of palpitations, but may experience anxiety, fatigue, chest pain, near-syncope, or syncope. The most common cause of SVT is AV nodal reentrant tachycardia (AVNRT), the second most common cause of SVT is AV reciprocating, or reentrant tachycardia (AVRT). Table 5.1 lists the major AV node-dependent causes of SVT. Table 5.2 lists the causes of SVT

TABLE 5.1 ■ AV NODE-DEPENDENT SUPRAVENTRICULAR TACHYCARDIAS

SVT Type	Mechanism
AV nodal reentrant tachycardia (AVNRT)	Reentry circuit including the AV Node (AV node is in one arm of the circuit), there is a fast arm with longer refractory period, and slow arm with a short refractory period.
AVNRT slow–fast conduction	The typical mechanism (80%–90%) involves slow–fast conduction, an ectopic beat initiates the reentry circuit, and the impulse finds the fast arm refractory from the last normal sinus node impulse; therefore, it travels down the slow arm but then is able to arc back up the fast arm (which has now completed its refractory period), creating the circus movement of the propagated conduction and resulting tachycardia. Most commonly the P wave is hidden in the QRS, but may be found at the end of the QRS complex as a pseudo r' wave.
AVNRT fast–slow conduction	The atypical mechanism (10%), involving fast–slow conduction, an ectopic beat initiates the reentry circuit, the impulse travels down the fast arm, and arcs back up the slow pathway to create the circus movement of the propagated conduction and resulting tachycardia. The QRS is narrow, and the retrograde P wave appears after the corresponding QRS.
AV reciprocating tachycardia (AVRT)	Two or more conducing pathways: the AV node and one or more bypass tracts that serve as accessory pathways. See WPW syndrome and Mahaim fiber tachycardia on next page.
Orthodromic AV reciprocating tachycardia	The impulse travels down (anterograde) via the AV node and His bundle and back up (retrograde) via the accessory pathway creating circus conduction.
Wolf–Parkinson–White (WPW) syndrome with narrow complex SVT	The bundle of Kent is the accessory pathway associated with the WPW syndrome. During sinus rhythm, patients with manifest WPW have a *delta wave* on the ECG: a short PR interval, and a slurred R wave upstroke ("manifest" because the delta wave is visible on the resting ECG). During sinus rhythm, there is anterograde conduction near simultaneously down both the bundle of Kent and the through the AV node. The most common mechanism for SVT in association with WPW is a narrow complex orthodromic reciprocating tachycardia triggered by a PAC (or PVC). During this common form of reentrant tachycardia, conduction is anterograde though the AV node, and retrograde up through the bundle of Kent perpetuating reentry producing a narrow complex tachycardia. WPW has also a "concealed" form, where anterograde conduction is blocked down the accessory pathway during sinus rhythm, but retrograde conduction is possible during AVRT. In these patients, no delta wave is visible during sinus rhythm, but AVRT occurs. The diagnosis of concealed WPW is made with confirmation of the accessory pathway during electrophysiology study.
Antidromic AV reciprocating tachycardia	The impulse travels down the accessory pathway (anterograde) and back up (retrograde) the His-Purkinje system and the AV node to create circus conduction. There may be more than one accessory pathway, which may participate in doubling either anterograde or retrograde impulse propagation. This creates a wide complex tachycardia that may be indistinguishable from VT.

TABLE 5.1 Continued	
SVT Type	Mechanism
WPW syndrome with wide complex SVT	Five to ten percent of patients with WPW sustain reentrant tachycardia with antegrade conduction down the accessory pathway, and retrograde back up the through the AV node, creating the reentrant circuit. The resulting tachycardia is wide complex, and typically indistinguishable from VT. The onset of atrial fibrillation in these patients may yield a VF like rhythm and poor perfusion.
Mahaim fiber tachycardia	Most likely the accessory pathway is atriofascicular fibers that arise from the right atrium close to the annulus, inserting into the apical part of the right ventricle close to a fascicular branch of the right bundle branch. The accessory pathway conducts anterograde and the AV node conducts retrograde completing the circuit. Resting ECG is usually normal. Reentrant tachycardias are typically wide, with a left bundle branch pattern, a rate between 130 and 270 bpm, but variants exist. This rhythm may be indistinguishable from VT.
Lown–Ganong–Levine syndrome	This diagnosis is now being abandoned but is included for historical reasons. The ECG findings are explained by enhanced AV nodal conduction.
Junctional ectopic tachycardia	Abnormal automaticity of the AV nodal region sustains this uncommon tachycardia. Typically the ventricular and atrial rates are identical; in some cases, the ventricular rate is faster than the atrial rate in the setting of ventriculoatrial block. The resulting tachycardia is a narrow complex rhythm.

that are not dependent on the AV node for perpetuation of the abnormal rhythm.

ED Care and Disposition

Detailed management of these tachycardias is described in the individual chapters named for each of the different rhythms. In general, for stable patients with narrow complextachycardias where sinus tachycardia can be excluded, a step-wise approach is used in an attempt to abort the tachycardia: vagal maneuvers, adenosine, calcium channel blockers, beta-blockers, and then amiodarone. If at any point the patientbecomes unstable, direct current (DC) cardioversion is recommended; sedate the patient if the clinical circumstances allow time for drug administration. See specific chapters below for treatment recommendations corresponding to the rhythms listed in Table 5.2. The exception is sinus node reentry tachycardia (SNRT), which is treated with vagal maneuvers; adenosine can also be used.

TABLE 5.2 AV NODE-INDEPENDENT SUPRAVENTRICULAR TACHYCARDIAS	
SVT Type	Mechanism
Sinus node reentrant tachycardia (SNRT)	Reentry circuit involving the sinus node, or the surrounding tissues. QRS often indistinguishable from sinus tachycardia, but may be recognized by sudden onset and offset. Direct comparison of P waves during and before tachycardia may aid diagnosis.
Ectopic atrial tachycardia or focal atrial tachycaria	Abnormal impulse formation from atrial source. P waves during the tachycardia are different from those arising from the sinus node, but differences may be subtle.
Multifocal atrial tachycardia	Variable mechanism including severe COPD, digoxin toxicity, sepsis, heart failure, and certain drugs (ie, theophylline) . Resulting rhythm is over 100 bpm, irregular with three or more P-wave morphologies.
Atrial fibrillation	Mechanism is a chaotic atrial depolarization secondary to microreentry or automatic triggered activity. Resulting rhythm is irregularly irregular.
Atrial flutter	Macroreentry of the right atria (rarely the left atria). The AV node determines the ventricular rate depending on the degree of AV block, but perpetuation of the rhythm is not AV node dependant.

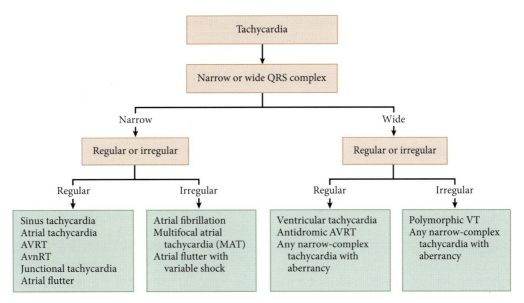

FIGURE 5.8 ■ Systematic approach for initial evaluation of tachycardia. AvnRT = atrioventricular nodal reentrant tachycardia; AVRT = atrioventricular reentrant tachycardia; VT = ventricular tachycardia. Reproduced, with permission, from Chapter 22. Piktel JS. Cardiac rhythm disturbances. In: Tintinalli JE, Stapczynski J, Ma O, Cline DM, Cydulka RK, Meckler GD, eds. *Tintinalli's Emergency Medicine: A Comprehensive Study Guide*. 7th ed. New York, NY: McGraw-Hill; 2011.

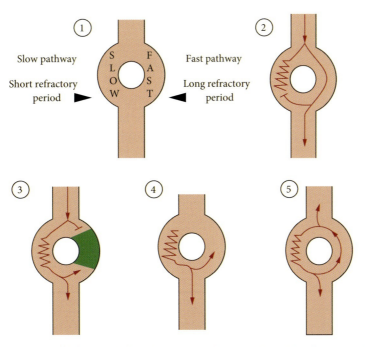

FIGURE 5.9 ■ Schematic drawing showing dual AV nodal conduction. (1) The two AV nodal pathways are shown, one with fast conduction and a relatively long refractory period and a second with slower conduction and shorter refractory period. (2) During sinus rhythm, impulses are conducted over both pathways but reach the bundle of His through the fast pathway. (3) A premature atrial impulse finds the fast pathway still refractory and is conducted over the slow pathway. (4 and 5) If the fast pathway has enough time to recover excitability, the impulse may reenter the fast pathway retrogradely and establish reentry, initiating AV Nodal Reentrant Tachycardia. Reproduced, with permission, from Chapter 41. Calkins H. Supraventricular tachycardia: atrioventricular nodal reentry and Wolff–Parkinson–White syndrome. In: Fuster V, Walsh RA, Harrington RA, eds. *Hurst's The Heart*. 13th ed. New York, NY: McGraw-Hill; 2011.

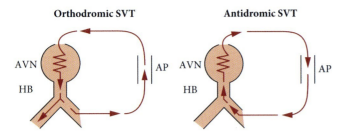

FIGURE 5.10 ■ Schematic representation of the patterns of conduction through an accessory pathway (AP) and the normal conduction system (AVN HB) during orthodromic atrioventricular reciprocating tachycardia (AVRT) and antidromic AVRT. During orthodromic SVT, impulse conduction is anterograde through the AV node and specialized conduction system, and the resulting QRS is normal. During antidromic SVT, impulse conduction is anterograde though the accessory pathway generating a wide QRS tachycardia. AVN = AV node; HB = bundle of His; SVT = supraventricular tachycardia. Reproduced, with permission, from Chapter 41. Calkins H. Supraventricular tachycardia: atrioventricular nodal reentry and Wolff–Parkinson–White syndrome. In: Fuster V, Walsh RA, Harrington RA, eds. *Hurst's The Heart*. 13th ed. New York, NY: McGraw-Hill; 2011.

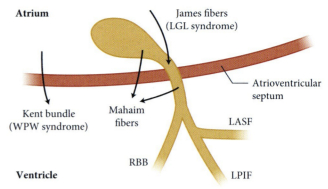

FIGURE 5.11 ■ Illustrated are the most common bypass tracts associated with atrioventricular reciprocating tachycardia (AVRT): from left to right, the Kent bundle associated with the WPW syndrome, Mahaim fibers associated with Mahaim fiber tachycardia, and James fibers associated with the Lown–Ganong–Levine syndrome. Anatomic sites of bypass tracts. AVRT = atrioventricular reciprocating tachycardia; LASF = left anterior superior fascicle; LGL = Lown–Ganong–Levine; LPIF = left posterior inferior fascicle; RBB = right bundle branch; WPW = Wolff–Parkinson–White syndrome. Reproduced, with permission, from Chapter 22. Piktel JS. Cardiac rhythm disturbances. In: Tintinalli JE, Stapczynski J, Ma O, Cline DM, Cydulka RK, Meckler GD, eds. *Tintinalli's Emergency Medicine: A Comprehensive Study Guide*. 7th ed. New York, NY: McGraw-Hill; 2011.

Pearls and Pitfalls

- Wide complex tachycardia should always be first treated as ventricular tachycardia (VT) unless the diagnosis of SVT with aberrant conduction is 100% certain.
- Palpitations secondary to SVT are frequently misdiagnosed as anxiety.
- Patients should be warned that adenosine transiently pauses their heartbeat and yields a brief but uncomfortable feeling in many patients.

Atrioventricular Tachycardias
AV NODAL REENTRY TACHYCARDIA SLOW-FAST CONDUCTION, FAST-SLOW CONDUCTION

David M. Cline

Clinical Highlights

Patients with AV nodal reentrant tachycardia (AVNRT) most commonly complain of sudden onset of palpitations, but may experience anxiety, fatigue, near-syncope, or syncope. AVNRT is the most common cause of SVT. The section earlier, Classification and Mechanisms of SVT, illustrates the AVNRT reentry mechanism. The AVNRT reentry circuit includes the AV node (AV node is in one arm of the circuit); there is a fast arm usually situated along the septal portion of the tricuspid annulus with a longer refractory period, and a slow arm situated posteriorly, close to the coronary sinus ostium, with a short refractory period. The typical mechanism (80%–90% of cases) involves slow–fast conduction, an ectopic beat initiates the reentry circuit, and the impulse finds the fast arm refractory from the last normal sinus node impulse; therefore, it travels down the slow arm but then is able to arc back up the fast arm (which has now completed its refractory period), creating the circus movement of the propagated conduction and resulting tachycardia. Most commonly the P wave is hidden in the QRS, but may be found at the end of the QRS complex as a pseudo r' wave most commonly in lead I, or a pseudo S wave in leads II and III.

The atypical mechanism (10% of cases) of AVNRT involves fast–slow conduction, an ectopic beat initiates the reentry circuit, the impulse travels down the fast arm, and arcs back up the slow pathway to create the circus movement of the propagated conduction and resulting tachycardia. The QRS is narrow, and the retrograde P wave appears after the corresponding QRS, often in the ST segment. A retrograde P wave following the QRS is also common in AVRT with a concealed pathway (see section AV Reciprocating Tachycardia).

Slow–slow AVNRT is the least common form, accounting for 1% to 5% of cases. In this form of AVNRT, the impulse is first conducted antegrade down the slow AV nodal pathway

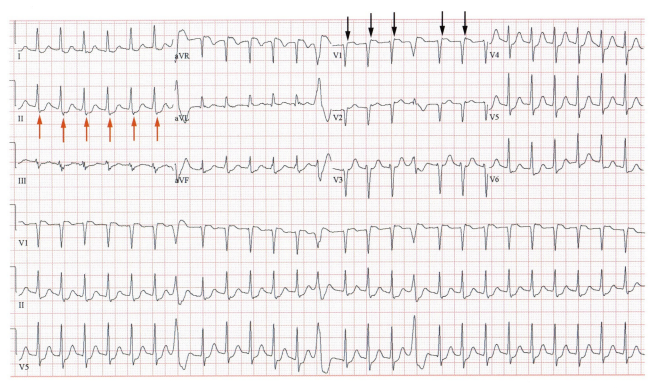

FIGURE 5.12 ■ ECG shows AV nodal reentrant tachycardia (AVNRT), rate of 160 bpm, with several PVCs, QRS duration of 90 milliseconds. Pseudo r' waves, representing P-wave deflections, are seen in V1 (black arrows) before and after the PVC. Pseudo S waves are seen in lead II (red arrows). This tachycardia was confirmed as AVNRT during electrophysiology investigation the day following.

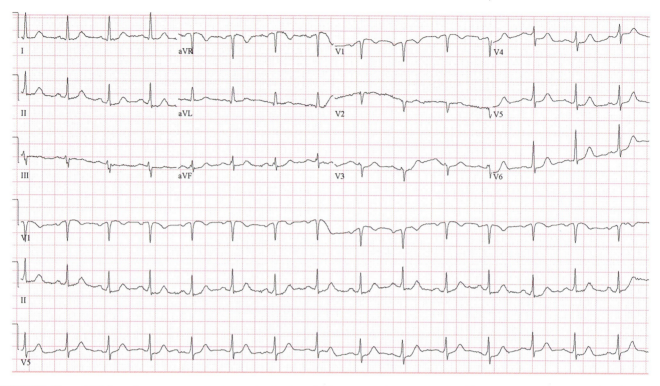

FIGURE 5.13 ■ ECG from the same patient as Figure 5.12, sinus rhythm rate of 89 bpm, after the administration of adenosine that broke the tachycardia. Note the absence of pseudo r' waves in V1, and the absence of pseudo S waves in lead II.

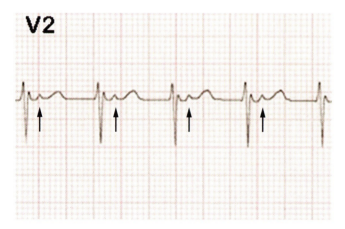

FIGURE 5.14 ■ ECG lead V2 showing P waves following the QRS complexes (arrows) in a patient with fast–slow conduction of AVNRT documented subsequently in the electrophysiology laboratory.

and then retrograde up the slow left atrial fibers approaching the AV node. The P wave may appear just before the QRS complex, and this makes it hard to distinguish the rhythm from sinus tachycardia.

ED Care and Disposition

For stable patients with AVNRT, a step-wise approach is recommended in an attempt to abort the tachycardia: vagal maneuvers, adenosine, calcium channel blockers, beta-blockers, and then amiodarone. If at any point the patient becomes unstable, DC cardioversion is recommended; sedate the patient if the clinical circumstances allow time for drug administration.

Pearls and Pitfalls

- Palpitations secondary to AVNRT (the most common cause of SVT) are frequently misdiagnosed as anxiety.
- Patients should be warned that adenosine transiently stops their heartbeat and yields a brief but uncomfortable feeling in many patients.

AV RECIPROCATING TACHYCARDIA, ORTHODROMIC AVRT, ANTIDROMIC AVRT

John D. Wofford
Cedric Lefebvre

Clinical Highlights

AV reciprocating (or reentrant) tachycardia (AVRT) is the second most common type of SVT, accounting for 20% to 30% of SVT cases. It is more likely to affect younger male patients in whom sudden onset of palpitations, chest pain, anxiety, dyspnea, and dizziness may be experienced. AVRT involves an accessory pathway outside of the AV node that enables an electrical signal to bypass the AV node from atria to ventricle. A bypass tract may conduct impulses in both directions, whereas a concealed accessory pathway conducts signals exclusively in a retrograde direction from ventricle to atria. See section Classification and Mechanisms of Supraventricular Tachycardia for a discussion of the mechanism of the reentry in AVRT. When the reentry circuit conducts anterograde though the AV node to the ventricle and retrograde through the accessory pathway back to the atrium, *orthodromic AVRT* is established, yielding a narrow complex tachycardia, which is the most common pattern (85% of AVRT). Conversely, if the activation signal follows the accessory pathway in an anterograde direction to the ventricle and returns to the atrium via the AV node, *antidromic AVRT* occurs (15% of AVRT), yielding a wide complex tachycardia.

Anterograde conduction through the accessory pathway is typically more rapid than AV nodal transmission; therefore, the ventricles may be activated early (varies with location of the pathway). Such ventricular preexcitation can generate a delta wave on ECG. A symptomatic patient with an accessory pathway that manifests as a delta wave on ECG has Wolf–Parkinson–White (WPW) syndrome (discussed in section WPW Syndrome). Accessory pathways that conduct anterograde may permit unrestricted conduction of rapid atrial impulses, as in atrial fibrillation, resulting in ventricular rates exceeding 300 bpm. This may mimic ventricular tachycardia (VT) or ventricular fibrillation (VF).

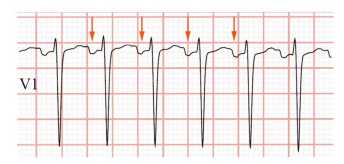

FIGURE 5.16 ■ This regular, narrow complex tachyarrhythmia with inverted P waves (arrows) is suggestive of orthodromic AVRT.

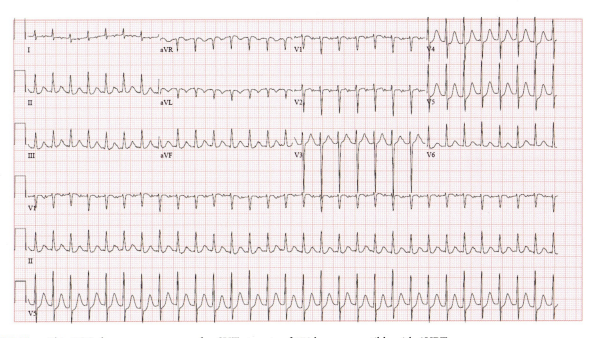

FIGURE 5.15 ■ This ECG shows a narrow complex SVT at a rate of 178 bpm compatible with AVRT.

114 ■ AV RECIPROCATING TACHYCARDIA (CONTINUED)

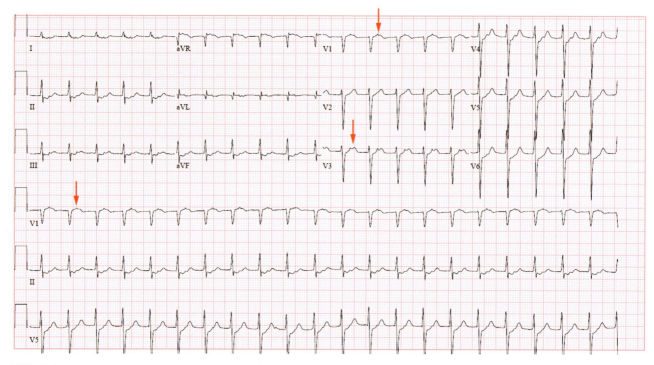

FIGURE 5.17 ■ This SVT is characterized by narrow QRS complexes and retrograde P waves (arrows) suggesting AVRT.

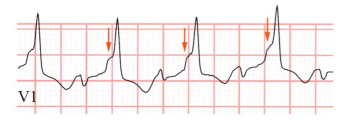

FIGURE 5.18 ■ Lead V1 reveals a wide complex rhythm with delta waves (arrow), consistent with ventricular preexcitation physiology via an accessory pathway, or the WPW syndrome.

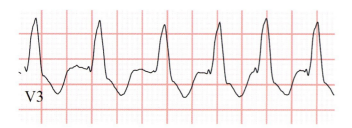

FIGURE 5.19 ■ SVT with a conduction abnormality such as a BBB (pictured here) can produce a wide complex tachycardia. When the heart rate is fast enough, it can be difficult to differentiate from ventricluar tachycardias VT.

ED Care and Disposition

In most cases of AVRT, the ECG reveals a narrow complex tachycardia at a rate of 160 to 300 bpm. P waves may be "buried" in the QRS complex or retrograde P waves can appear after each QRS complex. In orthodromic AVRT, inverted P waves can be seen with a RP interval of less than one half the RR Interval. In antidromic AVRT, a wide complex tachycardia is noted with inverted P waves and a RP interval greater than one half the RR interval.

In general, for stable patients with narrow complex tachycardias, a step-wise approach is used in an attempt to abort the tachycardia: vagal maneuvers, adenosine, calcium channel blockers, beta-blockers, and then amiodarone. If at any point the patient becomes unstable, DC cardioversion is recommended; sedate the patient if the clinical circumstances allow time for drug administration.

Patients with ventricular preexcitation physiology require special consideration because they are at risk for VF induced by rapidly conducted atrial impulses. Adenosine can be considered for SVT in the presence of WPW syndrome if the QRS complexes are narrow. For wide complex tachycardias, adenosine and especially other AV nodal–blocking agents should be avoided. Amiodarone, or procainamide, can be used for hemodynamically stable patients; these drugs are typically successful for either VT or SVT with aberrancy. Use DC cardioversion for unstable patients.

After appropriate measures have been employed to stabilize the patient, cardiology consultation should be obtained for reentry tachycardias. For patients with an easily terminated tachyarrhythmias, mild symptoms, and no comorbidities, close outpatient cardiology follow-up may be reasonable. Long-term management of these conditions can be achieved with medication (often beta-blockers) or potentially with radiofrequency ablation.

Pearls and Pitfalls

- SVT with a heart rate ≥250 bpm should prompt consideration of the presence of a preexcitation syndrome.
- AVRT with widened QRS complexes should not be treated with adenosine or other AV nodal–blocking medications as this could provoke VF in a patient with an accessory pathway.
- If there is a doubt concerning the possibility of VT versus SVT with aberrancy in a stable patient, the treatment algorithm for VT should be followed.
- Unstable patients with suspected SVT (or VT) should receive DC cardioversion.

WOLFF–PARKINSON–WHITE SYNDROME AND PRE-EXCITATION SYNDROMES

J. Stephan Stapczynski

Clinical Highlights

Preexcitation occurs when the ventricular myocardium is depolarized via an alternative electrical connection between the atria and ventricles that bypasses part or all of the normal AV conduction system. The anatomic basis for the WPW syndrome are bundles of myogenic tissue that transverse the AV annulus (termed Kent bundles), directly linking the atria to the ventricles. During sinus rhythm, the atrial depolarization can be conducted down to the ventricles by both the accessory tract and the normal conducting system. In manifest (visible delta wave) WPW syndrome, ventricular activation is produced by a fusion of both pathways and appears on the surface ECG as a short PR interval and a slurred initial portion of the QRS complex (termed the delta wave). The delta wave represents anterograde conduction through the accessory pathway; the remainder of the QRS represents normal conduction through the AV node to His-Purkinje fibers.

SVT are common in patients with WPW syndrome. The most common arrhythmia is paroxysmal reentrant SVT sustained when electrical depolarization is conducted around a loop composed of the bypass tract and the AV conducting system, with the impulse traveling down one and up the other. If reentrant impulses conduct down (anterograde) the AV node His-Purkinje system and back up the accessory pathway, the SVT is narrow and is termed orthodromic AVRT. If the reentrant impulses conduct down the accessory pathway and back up the His-Purkinje system to AV node, the SVT is wide complex and is termed antidromic AVRT (see Classification and Mechanisms of SVT section earlier).

About 5% to 10% of patients with WPW syndrome develop atrial fibrillation or flutter. In these arrhythmias, the predominant pathway for ventricular activation depends on the refractory period of Kent bundle and AV node; the path with the shorter refractory period conducts. New-onset atrial fibrillation in most patients with the WPW syndrome is conducted through the AV node yielding narrow QRS complexes; however, if the accessory pathway conducts primarily, the QRS complexes will be wide and the rate may be excessively rapid. With atrial flutter, 1:1 AV conduction is possible, with ventricular rates of 300 bpm. With atrial fibrillation, very rapid and irregular ventricular rates are possible and excessive stimulation of the ventricles may precipitate ventricular fibrillation (VF).

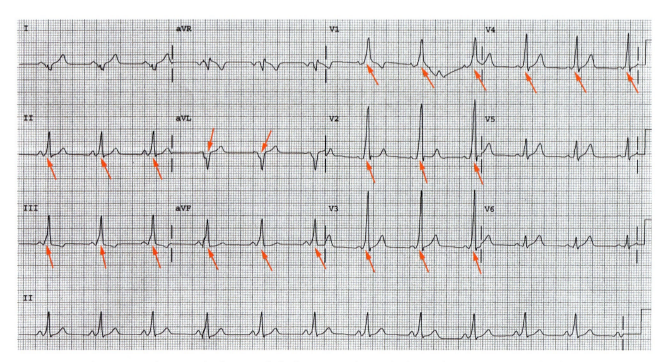

FIGURE 5.20 ■ The WPW syndrome, 12-lead ECG with rhythm strip, and sinus rhythm. Delta waves are marked with red arrows. Based on dominant R wave in lead V1, the accessory pathway is likely left sided.

WOLFF–PARKINSON–WHITE SYNDROME AND PRE-EXCITATION SYNDROMES (CONTINUED)

ED Care and Disposition

Unstable patients with WPW syndrome tachyarrhythmias should be treated with urgent synchronized cardioversion, starting at 100 J, with pharmacologic sedation if time permits.

Stable patients with WPW syndrome and narrow complex SVT can be treated with vagal maneuvers or drugs (adenosine, verapamil, diltiazem, or beta-blockers) that slow conduction through the AV node and break the reentry cycle.

Wide complex tachycardias in patients with WPW syndrome are at risk for rapid ventricular rates and degeneration into VF. Avoid beta-blocking agents, calcium channel blockers, and adenosine that can shorten the refractory period of

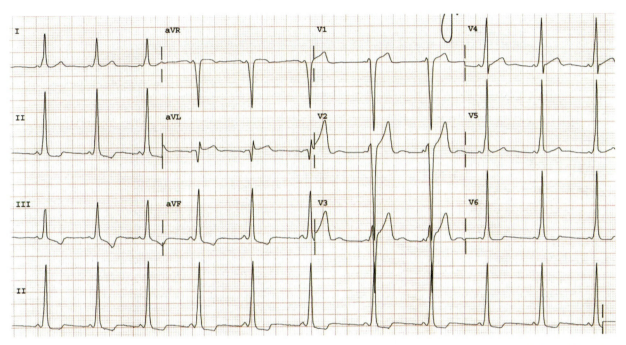

FIGURE 5.21 ■ The WPW syndrome, 12-lead ECG with rhythm strip, sinus rhythm. Delta waves are evident in the lateral leads. Based on negative QRS in lead V1, the accessory pathway is likely right sided.

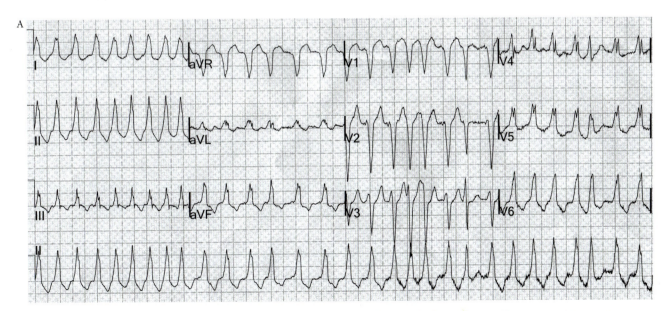

FIGURE 5.22 ■ (A) The WPW syndrome, 12-lead ECG with rhythm strip, and atrial fibrillation with wide irregular QRS complexes.

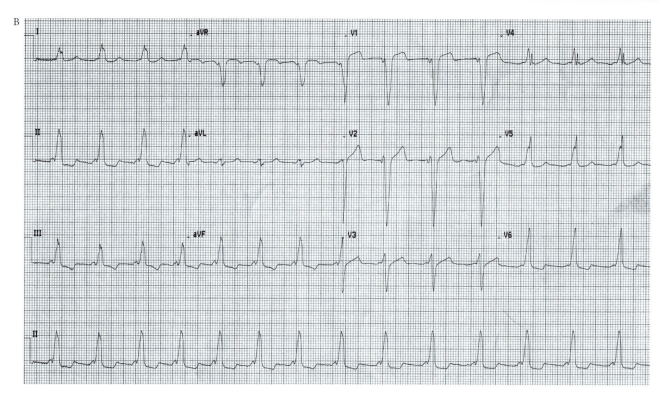

FIGURE 5.22 ■ Continued. **(B)** Same patient as in 5.22A, now in sinus rhythm after treatment; delta waves are evident in the inferior and lateral leads.

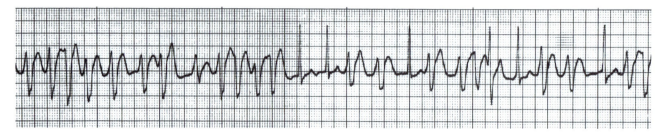

FIGURE 5.23 ■ The WPW syndrome, lead II rhythm strip, atrial fibrillation, ventricular rate 191 bpm, and variation in the QRS complexes due to ventricular activation via the bypass tract or AV node.

the Kent bundle and accelerate the ventricular rate. Therefore, wide complex tachycardias in patients with WPW syndrome—antidromic SVT, atrial flutter, or atrial fibrillation with a rapid ventricular response—are best treated with cardioversion. Alternatively, agents that prolong the refractory period of the accessory tract, such as intravenous (IV) procainamide or amiodarone, can be used.

Patients with WPW syndrome and tachyarrhythmias should be referred to a cardiologist with electrophysiology capability; admission to the hospital is required for unstable patients and persistently tachycardic or symptomatic patients. Asymptomatic patients with a new WPW pattern on ECG testing need routine follow-up.

Pearls and Pitfalls

- The ECG in patients with WPW syndrome may mimic the QRS complex, ST segment, and T wave changes of myocardial ischemia and the delta wave may be difficult to appreciate amid such abnormalities.
- A ventricular rate >250 bpm should raise the suspicion of preexcitation syndrome.
- Avoid beta-blocking agents, calcium channel blockers, and adenosine in WPW syndrome patients with wide complex tachycardias.

LOWN–GANONG–LEVINE SYNDROME

Laura Yoder

Clinical Highlights

The Lown–Ganong–Levine (LGL) syndrome is now believed to be due to enhanced AV nodal conduction. The proposed mechanism is an intranodal bypass tract or atrionodal tracts formerly known as James fibers. This diagnosis has been largely abandoned in the era of electrophysiology. Syndrome diagnostic criteria classically have been: a short PR interval (less than 0.12 s) and a normal QRS complex on ECG, and the clinical history of intermittent palpitations or episodes of paroxysmal SVT, atrial flutter, or atrial fibrillation.

The most important differential diagnosis is that of the WPW syndrome that has a specific treatment. The ECG finding that differs is the delta wave leading into the QRS complex seen with WPW; this is not found in LGL.

FIGURE 5.25 ■ Short PR interval, normal QRS complex, but shortened PJ interval (LGL syndrome). Reproduced, with permission, from Goldschlager N, Goldman MJ. *Principles of Clinical Electrocardiography*. 13th ed. Originally published by Appleton & Lange. Copyright © 1989 by McGraw-Hill.

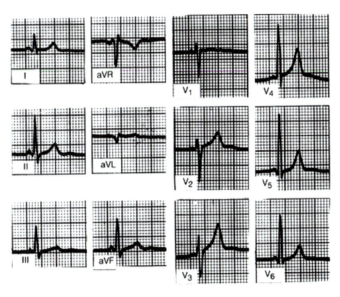

FIGURE 5.24 ■ ECG compatible with the Lown–Ganong–Levine syndrome. There is a short PR interval, the QRS complexes are normal. Reproduced, with permission, from Goldschlager N, Goldman MJ. *Principles of Clinical Electrocardiography*. 13th ed. Originally published by Appleton & Lange. Copyright © 1989 by The McGraw-Hill Companies, Inc.

ED Care and Disposition

If a patient carries this historical diagnosis, their tachycardia should be treated as other tachycardias, differentiating narrow complex tachycardias from wide complex tachycardias. Unstable patients should undergo emergent synchronized cardioversion. For stable patients with narrow-complex tachycardias, adenosine can be used diagnostically, as well as attempted therapeutically. Wide complex tachycardias should first be treated as VT until proven otherwise.

Pearls and Pitfalls

- The LGL syndrome is largely a historical diagnosis; patients who have undergone prior electrophysiology testing may carry the diagnosis of enhanced AV nodal conduction that may yield the ECG findings formerly used in the diagnosis of LGL syndrome.
- An abnormal QRS pattern or the presence of delta wave should trigger concern for WPW, and should be managed as WPW.

Atrial Tachycardias
MULTIFOCAL ATRIAL TACHYCARDIA

Jennifer Mitzman

Clinical Highlights

Multifocal atrial tachycardia (AT) occurs when three or more nonsinus atrial foci conduct though the AV node. On an ECG, this presents as more than three distinct P-wave morphologies preceding the QRS complex. The QRS complex is narrow as ventricular conduction through the AV node His-Purkinje system is normal. It is differentiated from Wandering Atrial Pacemaker based on the rate; the rate must be over 100 bpm to meet criteria for Multifocal AT.

Multifocal AT is most commonly seen in patients with chronic lung disease with worsening dyspnea as the chief complaint. However, as a result of the excessive heart rates, patients may present with palpitations, dizziness, or syncope. In patients with other risk factors for myocardial ischemia, MI or acute congestive heart failure can also occur. It has also been documented with metabolic disturbances, septic shock, and historically with theophylline toxicity.

ED Care and Disposition

Treatment of multifocal AT relies foremost on identifying and addressing the underlying condition. Hypoxia associated with chronic comorbidities is the single most frequent cause and should always be addressed first. Verapamil 5 mg IV

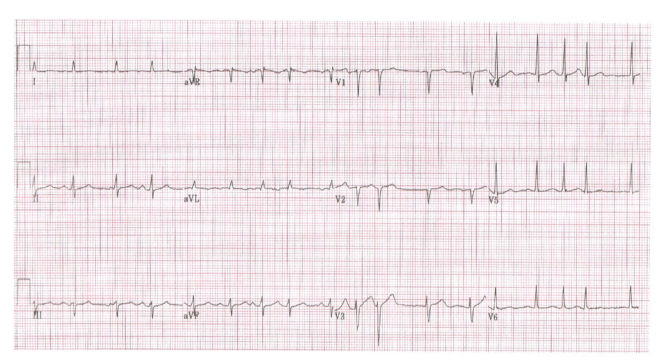

FIGURE 5.26 ■ ECG demonstrating multifocal atrial tachycardia (MAT). This irregularly, irregular rhythm with a rate of approximately 105 bpm meets MAT criteria with lead II illustrating three different P waves.

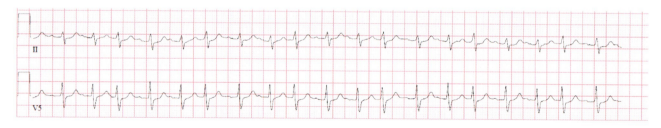

FIGURE 5.27 ■ Leads II and V5 rhythm strip demonstrating multifocal atrial tachycardia. Rhythm strip leads are particularly helpful in identifying multiple foci as demonstrated by the variable P-wave morphologies.

is considered the first-line therapy when a specific cause is unknown, but should be used with caution in hypotensive patients. Metoprolol is also effective though can cause undesirable bronchospasm.

Pearls and Pitfalls

- Consider multifocal AT in all patients with irregularly irregular heart rhythms. It is most commonly misdiagnosed as atrial flutter or atrial fibrillation.
- The need for cardioversion in multifocal AT is rare. If hemodynamic instability dictates this therapy, shocks should be synchronized at 50 to 100 J.

ECTOPIC (UNIFOCAL) ATRIAL TACHYCARDIA

David M. Cline

The term "atrial tachycaria" (AT) encompasses several types of uncommon tachycardias that originate in the atria (right or left) and do not require the participation of the AV node to sustain the arrhythmia. These tachycardias have differing arrhythmia mechanisms and are often related to anatomical structures. Mechanisms include abnormal automaticity, triggered activity, and microreentry.

Clinical Highlights

Focal AT or ectopic AT sustains atrial rates between 130 and 250 bpm. Age of onset is typically 10 to 39 years. Younger patients sustain higher heart rates. P-wave morphology is usually different than sinus rhythm (if a prior ECG is available for comparison), and the P-wave axis changes during the tachycardia. One confounding factor is that abnormal atrial foci may be responsive to autonomic tone and vary with activity making clinical differentiation from sinus tachycardia difficult. Patients experience a variety of symptoms, including palpitations, dizziness, chest pain, dyspnea, fatigue, and syncope.

Key ECG findings in ectopic AT are atrial rate >100 bpm, P-wave morphology differs from P waves originating from the SA node, at least three consecutive ectopic P waves, and typically abnormal or a change in P-wave axis, usually an inferior P-wave axis. Often normal inverted P waves in V1 are upright during the tachycardia; normal upright P waves in the inferior leads are inverted during the tachycardia.

ED Care and Disposition

Patients with acute ectopic AT respond differently to medications than other forms of SVT. Vagal maneuvers may not be effective. Ectopic AT secondary to triggered activity or microreentry may respond to adenosine, calcium channel blockers, or beta-blockers. While synchronized cardioversion is recommended for unstable patients with SVT, it may not be successful in patients with ectopic AT. Agents that block the AV node

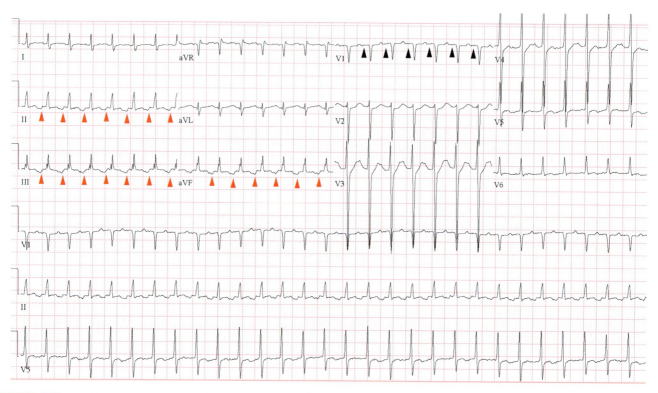

FIGURE 5.28 ■ ECG demonstrating ectopic AT or focal AT with a rate of 176 bpm. Notice that the P waves in V1 are part positive, part negative (black arrowheads). Notice that the P waves in the inferior leads (red arrowheads) are primarily negative. Review of the same patient's subsequent ECG in the next figure verifies that the P-wave findings are unique to this tachycardia suggesting ectopic AT.

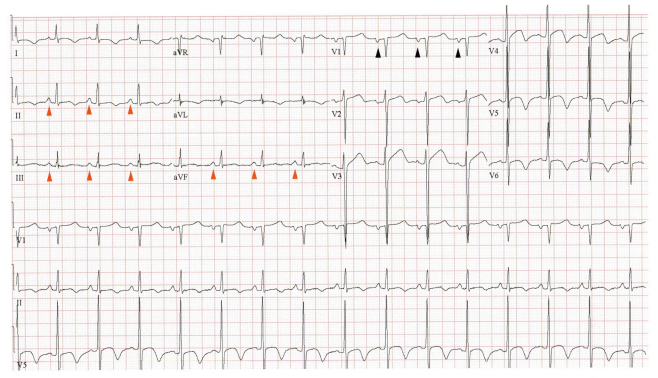

FIGURE 5.29 ■ ECG of the same patient as previous figure immediately after a dose of IV beta-blocker broke the ectopic AT. Compare previous figure to this ECG; the P waves in V1 (black arrowheads) are normally primarily inverted in V1, reflecting chronic left atrial enlargement, and the P waves in the inferior leads (red arrowheads) are normally upright. The differences between the this baseline ECG and the ECG taken during tachycardia shown in Figure 5.28 support the diagnosis of ectopic AT. Electrophysiology testing can confirm the diagnosis.

generally slow the rhythm and improve hemodynamics until a cardiologist can be consulted. Patients who sustain ectopic AT due to abnormal automaticity may be resistant to drug therapy. Consultation with a cardiologist may be required for resolution.

Pearls and Pitfalls

- Classic pharmacologic or electrical treatments for SVT may not break the tachycardia in patient with ectopic AT; however, beta-blockers or calcium channel blockers generally slow the rhythm and improve patient symptoms.
- The most common mechanism of ectopic AT that is resistant to acute treatment is abnormal automaticity, which causes approximately 20% of EAT cases.
- The most common mechanism of ectopic AT is microreentry that typically responds to pharmacologic or electrical therapy.

ATRIAL FLUTTER

J. Stephan Stapczynski

Clinical Highlights

Atrial flutter is a cardiac arrhythmia with regular atrial depolarizations at rates of between 240 and 400 bpm, usually with an AV nodal block, typically at 2:1 ratios or greater. The most common form (type I, or typical, or classic) is due to counterclockwise reentry encircling the tricuspid valve annulus. In this common form, atrial rates are generally 250 to 350 bpm, producing prominent downward deflections, negative "flutter waves," in the inferior ECG leads and positive flutter waves in the V1 lead. A less common form, atypical atrial flutter, is due to clockwise macroreentry that produces positive flutter waves in the inferior leads and negative flutter waves in lead V1. However, ECG findings frequently fail to predict the correct reentry direction, and experts do not agree which flutter waves are negative or positive. Observed precipitants of new-onset atrial flutter include open heart surgery (typically with atrial incisions), heavy alcohol consumption ("holiday heart syndrome"), hypoxia, and pulmonary embolism.

ED Care and Disposition

Unstable patients should be treated with urgent synchronized cardioversion, starting at 100 J, with pharmacologic sedation if time permits. For hemodynamically stable patients with atrial flutter of less than 48-hour duration, consider synchronized electrical cardioversion that converts about 95% to sinus rhythm. Typically, a small amount of energy is required for conversion; as little as 50 J. Techniques to enhance success are to (1) utilize a biphasic waveform, (2) employ wide electrode separation (right anterior and left posterior positions), and (3) apply pressure to the electrodes to diminish thoracic impedance.

Chemical conversion can be successful in about 60% of patients with recent-onset atrial flutter using an IV ibutilide infusion. Ibutilide can cause QT prolongation and torsade de pointes, so the patient should be on continuous ECG monitoring during the infusion and for 4 hours afterward.

For atrial flutter of uncertain duration or greater than 48 hours, initiate ventricular rate control with IV drugs that

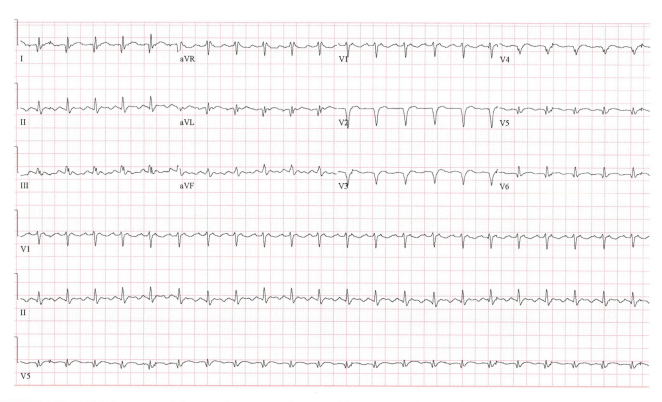

FIGURE 5.30 ■ ECG showing atrial flutter with 2:1 AV conduction yielding a ventricular rate of 136. The flutter waves are best seen in the inferior leads. The patient was cardioverted with 100 J. The resulting rhythm was biventricular paced rhythm. He was taken to the electrophysiology lab where his rhythm was confirmed to be "typical" counterclockwise reentrant atrial flutter.

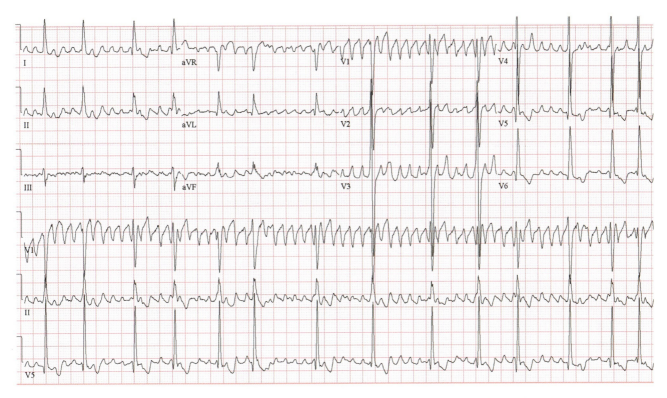

FIGURE 5.31 ■ ECG showing atrial flutter with variable AV block yielding a ventricular rate of 82 bpm. This ECG is from a 19-year-old patient with a history of tricuspid atresia repair while an infant. The atrial rate is over 300 bpm.

block the AV node, such as verapamil, diltiazem, or beta-blockers. With adequate control and symptom relief, patients are typically admitted to the hospital and transitioned to oral maintenance therapy. If conversion occurs while receiving IV AV nodal–blocking agents, the infusion should be stopped and the patient monitored for recurrence. The patient can be discharged in a few hours if there is no recurrence. If atrial flutter has been present for more than 48 hours, anticoagulation is indicated. For patients with persistent or paroxysmal atrial flutter, long-term anticoagulation is recommended if risk-stratification tools indicate that the patient is at increased risk for systemic embolism. Elective radiofrequency ablation can produce a permanent conduction block within the atrial flutter reentry circuit and both abolish the arrhythmia and prevent its recurrence (95% success rate).

Pearls and Pitfalls

- Atrial flutter with a 2:1 AV block can mimic the appearance of sinus tachycardia.
- The risk for clinical systemic embolism after conversion to sinus rhythm varies with the duration of the abnormal rhythm; from about 1% when the duration of atrial fibrillation is less than 48 hours to 5% to 7% when the duration is longer.

ATRIAL FIBRILLATION WITH/WITHOUT RVR, WITH ABERRANCY

J. Stephan Stapczynski

Clinical Highlights

Atrial fibrillation is a cardiac arrhythmia with irregular, disorganized, electrical activity of the atria that results in chaotic atrial contractions. The electrocardiographic characteristics are rapid oscillations or fibrillatory waves that vary in size, shape, and timing occurring at a rate greater than 300 bpm, typically best visualized on the V1 lead. The rapid and disorganized atrial impulses affect the AV node but are limited by the AV node refractory period yielding an irregularly irregular ventricular rhythm. Normally, the ventricular rate is 160 to 180 bpm before treatment. A ventricular rate less than 120 bpm implies impaired AV node conduction due to drugs, aging, or disease. A ventricular rate greater than 250 bpm implies enhanced atrial-ventricular conduction, as sometimes occurs in patients with the WPW syndrome (see section WPW syndrome). If the infranodal conducting system has not fully recovered when the next impulse gets through the AV node, it may be conducted in an aberrant manner, often with right bundle branch block (RBBB) morphology.

Common symptoms of atrial fibrillation include palpitations and symptoms due to depressed cardiac output, such as lightheadedness, syncope, and dyspnea. Ischemic chest pain can occur if the oxygen demand associated with the rapid ventricular rate exceeds the ability of coronary perfusion to supply. Complications include systemic emboli and heart failure.

ED Care and Disposition

Unstable patients, such as those in circulatory shock, with acute pulmonary edema, or with acute ischemic chest pain, should be treated with urgent synchronized cardioversion, starting at 100 J, with pharmacologic sedation if time permits.

In stable patients, rate control (below 100 bpm) with IV diltiazem, beta-blocker, or digoxin is appropriate. With

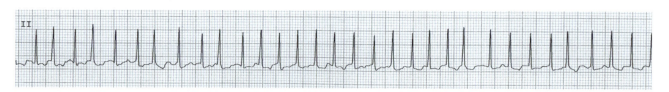

FIGURE 5.32 ■ Lead II rhythm strip showing atrial fibrillation with a ventricular rate of 208 bpm. Careful review is needed to determine that the rhythm is irregularly irregular, characteristic of atrial fibrillarin.

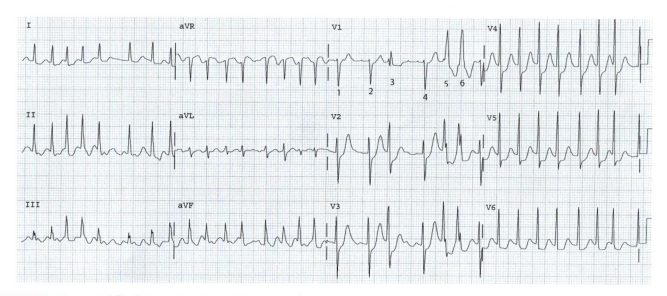

FIGURE 5.33 ■ Atrial fibrillation with 12-lead ECG. Ventricular rate of 190 bpm. Occasional aberrant conduction with RBBB morphology best seen in lead V1 (see numbered beats 3, 5, and 6).

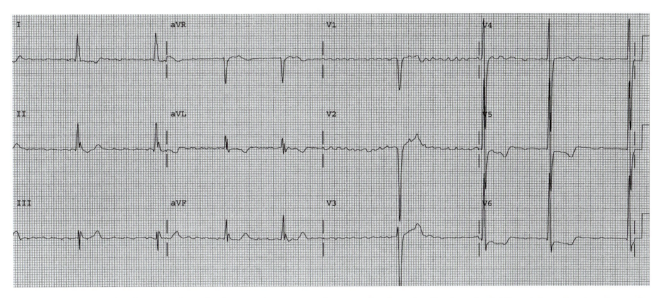

FIGURE 5.34 ■ Atrial fibrillation with 12-lead ECG. Slow ventricular rate of 49 bpm implies impaired AV nodal conduction due to drugs, disease, or age.

adequate control and symptom relief, patients are typically admitted to the hospital and transitioned to oral maintenance therapy. If conversion occurs while receiving IV rate control medications, the infusion should be stopped and the patient monitored for recurrence. If asymptomatic, the patient can be discharged.

If the atrial fibrillation onset is less than 48 hours in a patient free of significant left ventricular dysfunction, mitral valve disease, or previous embolism, restoration to sinus rhythm may be attempted with either IV antiarrhythmic medications or synchronized cardioversion. IV agents used to chemically convert atrial fibrillation include procainamide, ibutilide, propafenone, flecainide, amiodarone, and vernakalant.

For patients with duration longer than 48 hours, one option is to assess for the presence of left atrial thrombus with a transesophageal echo, and if there is no evidence of a thrombus on imaging, then proceed with electrical cardioversion. Another option is ventricular rate control and systemic anticoagulation for 4 weeks before attempting cardioversion.

Pearls and Pitfalls

- Atrial fibrillation can appear regular when the ventricular response is fast, obscuring the diagnosis.
- Spontaneous conversion to sinus rhythm with new-onset atrial fibrillation is common, occurring in 30% to 60% seen for this arrhythmia in the ED.
- Check thyroid stimulating hormone level in patients with new-onset atrial fibrillation; hyperthyroidism is found in up to 10%.
- The risk for clinical systemic embolism after conversion to sinus rhythm varies with the duration of atrial fibrillation; from about 1% when the duration of atrial fibrillation is less than 48 hours to 5% to 7% when the duration is longer.

Aberrant Atrial Conduction

ASHMAN PHENOMENA, ATRIAL FIBRILLATION WITH PREMATURE SUPRAVENTRICULAR ABERRANT BEATS

Scott Goldston

Clinical Highlights

Ashman phenomenon is a type of wide complex supraventricular aberrancy that most commonly occurs in the setting of atrial fibrillation. Ashman phenomenon is also described by the long-short rule: the earlier in the R-to-R cycle a PAC occurs, *and* the longer the preceding R-to-R cycle, the more likely a PAC will be conducted with aberration. This phenomenon occurs because the refractory period is proportional to the cycle length, which is the heart rate. The longer the cycle length, the slower the heart rate, and the longer the recovery time of the conduction system. Furthermore, in most individuals, the right bundle recovers slower than the left bundle; therefore, a critically timed PAC is more likely to conduct with RBBB aberrancy pattern, then a left bundle branch block (LBBB) pattern. The physiology predicts that following a long R-to-R cycle, if a PAC occurs early in the current cycle, the PAC is likely to be conducted with aberrancy of a RBBB pattern.

ED Care and Disposition

As stated earlier, the most common rhythm for this to occur is during atrial fibrillation due to the frequent changes in heart rate. This can occur in any type of SVT, especially with a sudden increase in the rate. It is commonly confused for a premature ventricular contraction (PVC) or an escape beat. In contrast, if the cause is of ventricular origin, then the abnormal complex usually occurs more than once and usually has fixed coupling interval. There is no treatment needed for this phenomenon.

Pearls and Pitfalls

- Ashman phenomenon usually occurs during atrial fibrillation when there are changes in R–R intervals (long to short, followed by aberrantly conducted PAC).
- Ashman phenomenon usually appears like a RBBB because the right bundle has a longer refractory period than the left bundle.

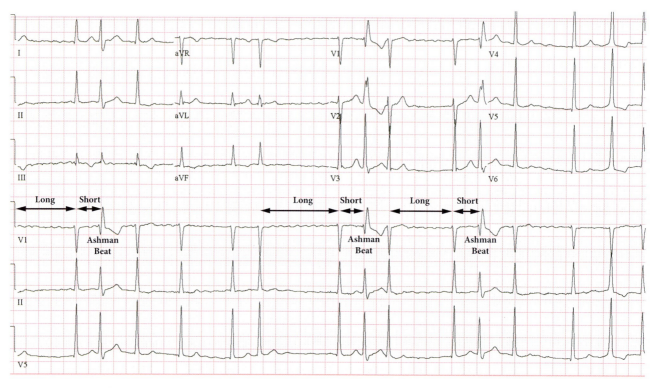

FIGURE 5.35 ■ ECG showing atrial fibrillation with three Ashman phenomenon beats. Note that the Ashman beats follow a short R-to-R interval, which was preceded by a long R-to-R interval. Also, notice that the aberration is in a right bundle branch block (RBBB) pattern with tall R wave in V1.

Junctional Rhythms
JUNCTIONAL ESCAPE RHYTHM

Jennifer Mitzman

David M. Cline

Clinical Highlights

Junctional rhythms originate from the AV junction of the heart's conduction pathway. Junctional escape rhythm occurs when the automaticity of the SA node fails or is blocked. Although in theory nearly any heart cell can generate a beat, the most common escape rhythms are junctional or AV nodal in origin. AV nodal cells generate beats at a rate of 35 to 60 bpm. Because this beat is generated at the top of the ventricle, it causes normal ventricular contraction, and the QRS is narrow and normal in appearance, unless a preexisting bundle branch block exits.

Atrial contraction can also occur in a retrograde fashion from the AV node. This contraction is initiated simultaneously with the ventricular contraction. As a result, P waves may be buried within the QRS rendering them invisible, or inverted P waves may be seen in some leads just before or just after an otherwise normal QRS. In states of abnormal automaticity of the AV node from ischemia, drug effects or electrolyte abnormalities, accelerated junctional rhythm may occur, with rates from 60 to 100 (above 100 the rhythm is called junctional tachycardia, but may still be from the same mechanism). AV dissociation may occur with this rhythm. Bradycardia may be found incidentally or may present with dizziness, weakness, fatigue, dyspnea with exertion, or syncope.

ED Care and Disposition

Junctional rhythms should be considered a consequence of bradycardia. Identifying the cause of primary bradycardia is of the utmost importance in managing these rhythm disturbances. Medications are the most common culprit including beta-blockers, calcium channel blockers, digitalis, and lithium. MI causing ischemia of the SA node resulting in its failure to generate adequate heart rate as well as postsurgical,

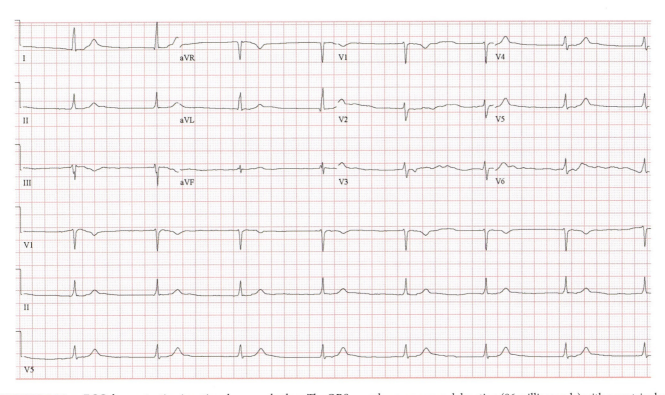

FIGURE 5.36 ■ ECG demonstrating junctional escape rhythm. The QRS complexes are normal duration (96 milliseconds) with a ventricular rate of 46 bpm and there are no P waves, typical of junctional escape rhythm in the absence of SA node conduction.

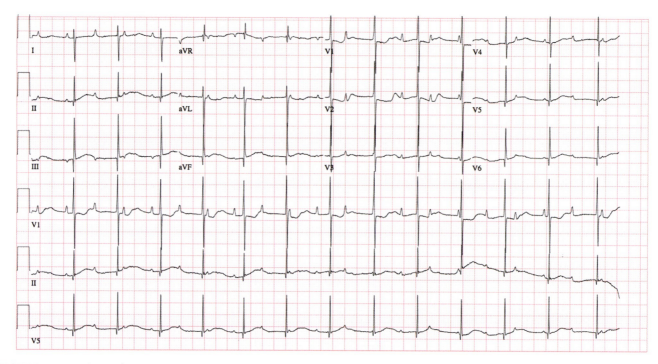

FIGURE 5.37 ■ This pediatric ECG demonstrates accelerated junctional rhythm, AV dissociation, and a sinus (or atrial) tachycardia. The junctional rate is 78 bpm, while the atrial rate is 120 bpm. There appears to be no association between the P waves and the narrow QRS complexes. The P waves are upright in leads I and II, indicating that the origin of the P waves could be sinus; however, the P waves are upright in lead V1, which is unusual for a sinus mechanism.

infectious, and age-related sick sinus syndrome should also be considered. Atropine may be effective in increasing a junctional rate. Transcutaneous or transvenous overdrive pacing may also be required in the emergency setting if pharmacologic intervention fails. Accelerated junctional rhythm usually does not require treatment; however, the underlying cause of the rhythm should be determined and treated.

Pearls and Pitfalls

- Junctional rhythms should be considered a symptom, not a diagnosis; the cause of sinus node failure yielding junctional escape rhythm or the cause of increased AV node automaticity causing accelerated junctional rhythm should be determined and treated.

JUNCTIONAL TACHYCARDIA

David M. Cline

Clinical Highlights

The term "junctional tachycardia" is used with imprecision in the medical literature; it should be distinguished from other forms of SVT that involve the AV node. This chapter discusses two rare rhythms that are more common in children and frequently incessant (lasting more than 10% of each day): permanent (persistent) junctional reciprocating tachycardia (PJRT) and junctional ectopic tachycardia (JET). PJRT is caused by an AV reentry using the AV node as the antegrade limb and a slowly conducting accessory pathway as the retrograde limb. Presentation in infants may accompany cardiomyopathy that has been caused by the tachycardia. Compromise of cardiac function is directly related to frequency and rate of the tachycardia. ECG at presentation typically reveals a narrow complex SVT with long RP interval and negative P waves in leads II, III, and aVF on the surface ECG. During sinus rhythm, the surface ECG is normal, without manifest preexcitation. The rate is more variable than most reentrant tachycardias because both limbs of the circuit are influenced by autonomic tone.

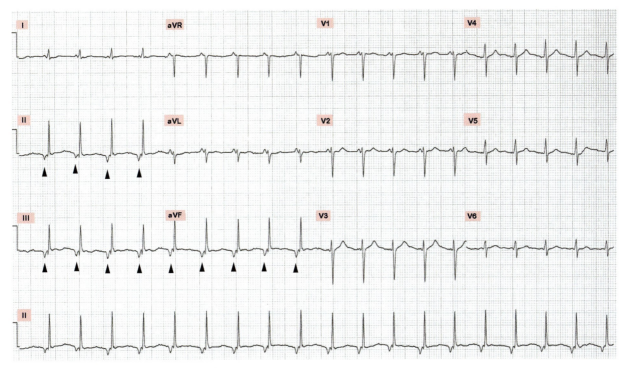

FIGURE 5.38 ■ ECG of a patient with permanent junctional reciprocating tachycarida (PJRT). Note the narrow complex tachycardia with a rate of 115 bpm with inverted P waves in the inferior leads (black arrowheads). The RP interval (from the R wave to the next P wave) is over 50% of the RR interval, meeting long RP interval criteria.

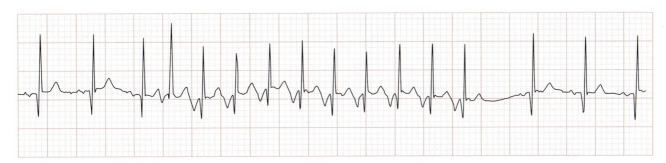

FIGURE 5.39 ■ Permanent junctional reciprocating tachycarida. Rhythm strip shows intermittent narrow complex tachycardia initiated by a premature ectopic beat. The RP interval is long (see text). Reproduced, with permission, from Chapter 10. Arrhythmias. In: Artman M, Mahony L, Teitel DF, eds. *Neonatal Cardiology*. 2nd ed. New York, NY: McGraw-Hill; 2011.

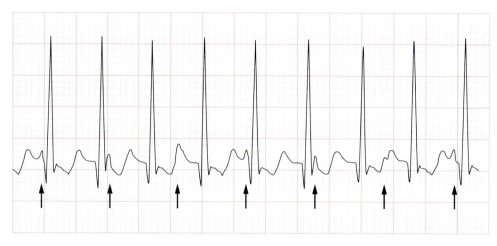

FIGURE 5.40 ■ Junctional ectopic tachycardia. AV dissociation is present. P waves are indicated by the arrows. The atrial rate is 135 bpm and the ventricular rate is 185 bpm. Reproduced, with permission, from Chapter 10. Arrhythmias. In: Artman M, Mahony L, Teitel DF, eds. *Neonatal Cardiology*. 2nd ed. New York, NY: McGraw-Hill; 2011.

JET has a congenital form that presents in the first few weeks of life and JET has a postoperative form that frequently complicates congenital heart repair. The mechanism of the JET is thought to be abnormal automaticity arising from the region of the AV junction. JET typically has gradual onset, gradual offset, and rate variability. ECG features are: (1) a narrow QRS complex with either AV dissociation and sinus capture beats or 1:1 ventricular-atrial association; or (2) a wide QRS complex with AV dissociation and sinus capture beats with the same wide QRS complex noted during tachycardia, the sinus capture beats, or sinus rhythm.

ED Care and Disposition

Both PJRT and JET are difficult to control with commonly used anti-SVT agents. For PJRT, the most efficient antiarrhythmics have been propafenone and flecainide; however, beta-blockers, verapamil, and amiodarone may be used. Rate control frequently relieves symptoms. The most effective drug for JET is amiodarone. Adenosine frequently fails to break the rhythm in both PJRT and JET, but may help to elucidate the rhythm during the temporary slowing period. Synchronized cardioversion may be required during resuscitation, but may provide only temporary relief from the tachycardia. Consultation with a cardiologist (pediatric if age <18 years) is most commonly required both initially and for ablation therapy.

Pearls and Pitfalls

- Both PJRT and JET are difficult to control; synchronized cardioversion should be available, as well as size appropriate intubation equipment.
- The rate directly affects outcome in PJRT and JET; while fatal in some because of the difficulty in finding the right drug or implementing successful ablation, if rates are well controlled and tolerated, patients may eventually do well without invasive management.

Ventricular Arrhythmias
PREMATURE VENTRICULAR CONTRACTIONS

Erin Boyd

Clinical Highlights

Prature ventricular contractions (PVCs) are one of the most common ventricular arrhythmias. ECG criteria include QRS ≥ 0.12 seconds in most leads. A retrograde P wave may be seen but this is very uncommon. The electrical activity of PVC is usually not conducted through the AV node to the atria. Therefore, the firing of the sinus node is usually not affected (this is not true for PACs that typically reset the SA node). Therefore, a PVC is usually followed by a compensatory pause, that is, the R-to-R interval straddling a PVC is the same as the R-to-R interval straddling a normal beat (corresponding to the second beat) between the first beat and the third beat in a run of normal sinus rhythm. PVCs are typically isolated, but sometimes they occur in a pattern. Bigeminy refers to a ratio of one sinus beat to one PVC. Trigeminy refers to two sinus beats for every one PVC.

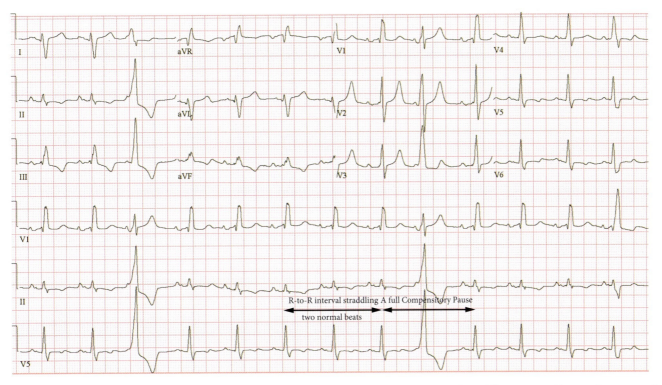

FIGURE 5.41 ■ ECG showing a PVC with a compensatory pause. Notice that the R-to-R interval straddling a normal beat is the same as the R-to-R interval straddling the PVC, which is a full compensatory pause.

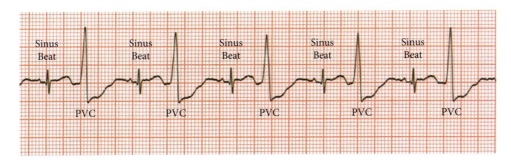

FIGURE 5.42 ■ Rhythm strip demonstrating bigeminy. Notice that every normal sinus beat is followed by a PVC: criteria for bigeminy.

134 ■ PREMATURE VENTRICULAR CONTRACTIONS (CONTINUED)

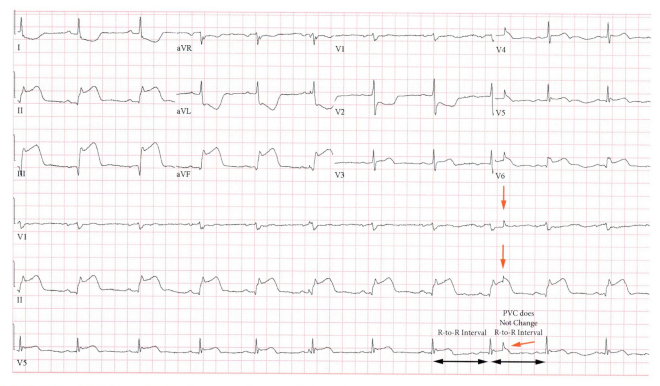

FIGURE 5.43 ■ ECG showing PVC in the setting of inferior MI. Areas of ischemic myocardium can produce PVCs (see red arrows). Notice that the PVC does not alter the normal R-to-R interval (double ended black arrows). This is a case where there is no pause; an alternative manifestation of a PVC not conducting through the AV node to the SA node.

PVCs are very common in the general healthy population as well as those with various underlying heart conditions. Symptoms can vary widely from asymptomatic to severe palpitations, chest pain, dyspnea, or syncope depending on the underlying cause. Typically there is an area of increased automaticity of the ventricles that is provoked by adrenergic stimulation such as caffeine, stress, sympathomimetic drugs, or hyperthyroidism. Cardiac ischemia, electrolyte abnormalities, especially hypokalemia and hypomagnesemia, and certain drug toxicities, such as digitalis, are other common causes.

ED Care and Disposition

The most important aspect of the treatment and care for patients with PVCs is to treat the underlying disorder. Patients with a structurally normal heart and asymptomatic PVCs do not require further treatment (but may need follow-up). Symptomatic patients should undergo an investigation in the ED to search for an underlying organic cause, which may include cardiac enzymes, potassium and magnesium levels, digitalis levels, or thyroid hormone levels. If there is an abnormality found, then treat accordingly.

Pearls and Pitfalls

- PVCs falling on the T wave of a previous beat is called the "R-on-T" phenomenon and is more likely to set off VT or VF.
- Multiform PVCs usually indicate underlying organic heart disease.
- Any PVC that occurs in the setting of an AMI should heighten concern for VT, VF, or death.

ACCELERATED IDIOVENTRICULAR RHYTHM

Joseph Hayes Calvert

Clinical Highlights

Accelerated idioventricular rhythm (AIVR) is an automatic ectopic ventricular rhythm that has at least three consecutive ventricular beats. AIVR has a regular rhythm with a prolonged (wide) QRS complex. AIVR most often has short episodes of 3 to 30 bpm and may be initiated by a fusion beat. AIVR is faster than the normal intrinsic ventricular escape rhythm of 20 to 40 bpm but does not exceed 100 bpm in most cases. AVIR most often has a single focus but can be produced from multiple foci in certain cardiac disease such as myocarditis. AVIR can be a result of myocardial ischemia, digoxin toxicity, and electrolyte abnormalities. Risk factors for developing AVIR include postresuscitation, cocaine toxicity, anesthetic agents, congenital heart disease, cardiac reperfusion, and myocarditis. Patients in AIVR most often present with hemodynamically stable vital signs. Patients in AVIR with severe heart disease can present with hypotension.

The ECG may have some degree of irregularity due to competing sinus rhythm and AIVR. The rate most often is between 80 and 100 bpm and the rate may be similar with the proceeding sinus rate. The ECG has three or more ventricular complexes and the QRS complex is greater than >120 milliseconds.

ED Care and Disposition

In most cases, there is no emergent treatment necessary for AIVR. AIVR is most often self-limited and will resolve after the sinus rate surpasses the AIVR rate. Atropine has been used to accelerate the underlying sinus rate. The most important emergency care is to identify the underlying etiology that caused the AIVR. Cardiac enzymes and electrolyte panel can be ordered to access for underlying cardiac ischemia and electrolyte abnormalities. Consider digoxin level and kidney function tests to evaluate for digoxin toxicity. Lidocaine can result in asystole if given during AIVR. Patients may be further evaluated with Holter studies or event monitors.

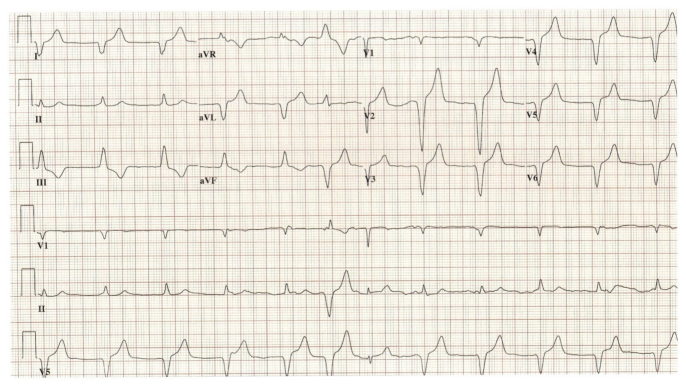

FIGURE 5.44 ■ ECG demonstrating idioventricular rhythm with a rate of 73 bpm with some fusion complexes and a QRS complex prolonged at 142 milliseconds.

136 ■ ACCELERATED IDIOVENTRICULAR RHYTHM (CONTINUED)

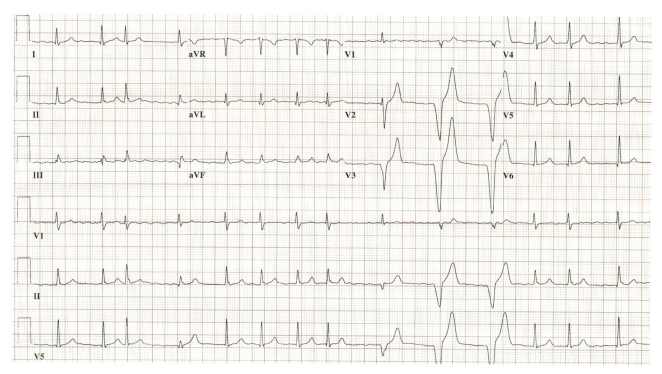

FIGURE 5.45 ■ ECG demonstrating atrial fibrillation with a rate of 87 bpm with PVCs and three beat run of AIVR.

Pearls and Pitfalls

- AIVR can rarely precipitate VT and VF.
- The most important part of the treatment of AIVR is identifying the cause.
- In most cases, AIVR is self-limiting and does not require emergency intervention.
- Lidocaine can precipitate asystole if given during AIVR.

VENTRICULAR TACHYCARDIA INCLUDING POLYMORPHIC, MONOMORPHIC

Joseph Hayes Calvert

Clinical Highlights

Ventricular tachycardia (VT) accounts for 80% of the cases of wide complex tachycardias in unselected populations. VT is defined as three or more QRS complexes of ventricular origin with a rate greater than 100 bpm. VT typically is a regular rhythm with wide QRS complexes: >140 milliseconds for RBBB pattern, or >160 milliseconds with LBBB pattern rhythms. There is evidence of AV dissociation often with fusion complexes (when a supraventricular and a ventricular impulse coincide to produce a hybrid complex). VT can be classified as either monomorphic or polymorphic. Monomorphic VT is characterized by a uniform QRS pattern usually originating from a single point. Polymorphic VT has a beat-to-beat variation in QRS morphology. Polymorphic VT can have the appearance of "twisting of points" commonly referred to as torsade de pointes (TdP; see TdP section on page 139). VT can be caused by ischemic heart disease and MI. Other causes of VT include medication toxicities such as digoxin, electrolyte abnormalities, hypoxia, blunt chest trauma, mitral valve prolapsed, alkalosis, and hypertrophic cardiomyopathy. TdP is commonly associated with long QT syndrome (see section Long QT Syndrome). Risk factors for VT are age over 35 years and prior cardiac disease, such as MI, congestive heart failure (CHF). Patients who present in VT may complain of chest pain, shortness of breath, or possible syncope secondary to poor systemic perfusion. VT can cause sudden cardiac death.

ED Care and Disposition

Emergency treatment is aimed at either terminating the VT or preventing additional episodes. The most important task to discern is whether the patient is hemodynamically stable or unstable. Patients who are pulseless or hemodynamically unstable are treated with cardioversion. A patient in pulseless VT is treated with unsynchronized cardioversion. An unstable patient with a pulse in VT is treated with synchronized cardioversion. If the patient is hemodynamically stable, recommended therapy includes IV procainamide, an amiodarone infusion, or IV

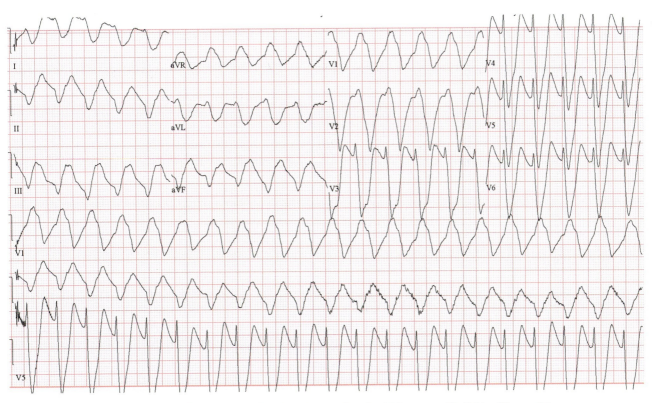

FIGURE 5.46 ■ ECG demonstrating VT with a rate of 142 bpm. Notice that the QRS is very wide (184 milliseconds).

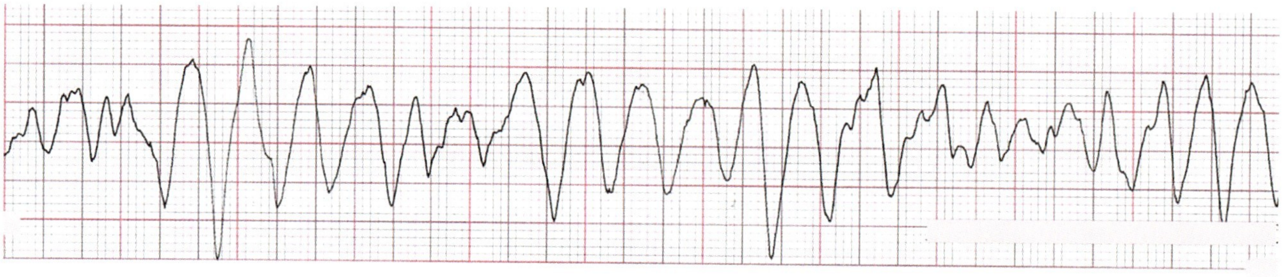

FIGURE 5.47 ■ Rhythm strip demonstrating TdP.

lidocaine. Treatment for patients who present in TdP should be magnesium sulfate infusion and/or overdrive pacing set at 90 to 120 bpm (see section Torsades de Pointes and Chap. 4, section on Transcutaneous Pacemaker). Emergency care should include identifying the underlying cause of VT. These patients must be considered for urgent revascularization because MI is a common cause. Emergency care should also include checking electrolytes (especially potassium), medication levels such as digoxin, and cardiac enzymes. All patients presenting in VT should be admitted and further evaluated.

- MI or myocardial ischemia should always be considered in a patient presenting in VT.
- A patient in pulseless VT should receive immediate unsynchronized cardioversion and an unstable patient with a pulse in VT should receive synchronized cardioversion.
- Procainamide or amiodarone are first-line therapy for stable VT.
- Consider a magnesium sulfate infusion and/or overdrive pacing in TdP.

Pearls and Pitfalls

- VT can present as either a polymorphic or monomorphic arrhythmia.

TORSADES DE POINTES

Mary A Wittler

Clinical Highlights

Torsade de pointes (TdP), translated "twisting of the points," is a polymorphic ventricular tachycardia (VT) characterized by the QRS axis twisting around the isoelectric line and occurs in the setting of a long QT interval. TdP can deteriorate into VF and sudden death. Risk factors for acquired long QT syndrome and TdP include QT-prolonging drugs (class IA, IC, and III antiarrhythmic agents; antidepressants; antipsychotics, antimicrobials, and opiate analgesics such as methadone), advanced age, electrolyte disturbances, heart disease, and bradycardia. Symptoms of TdP include palpitations, syncope, seizure-like activity, or sudden death.

The QT interval is measured from the beginning of the QRS complex to the termination of the T wave. As QT intervals shorten with tachycardia and lengthen with bradycardia, a rate-corrected QT (QTc) should be assessed.

ED Care and Disposition

For unstable TdP or VF, cardioversion or defibrillation is necessary. For stable TdP, initial therapy is magnesium sulfate and pacing. Magnesium sulfate 2 grams IV bolus, which can be repeated in 5 to 15 minutes, is a first-line therapy, regardless of magnesium levels. Additionally, pacing can be effective in terminating TdP and preventing recurrence because increasing the heart rate shortens repolarization and prevents bradycardia. Atrial pacing is preferred, with a heart rate goal of approximately 100 bpm. Alternatively, isoproterenol, a beta-adrenergic agonist, may be used temporarily to achieve the same goal, but is contraindicated in congenital long QT syndrome (LQTS). It should be used cautiously and as an interim agent while preparing for pacing. Concomitant electrolyte disturbances should be corrected. QT-prolonging drugs should be avoided, including class IA, IC, and III antidysrhythmics. Lidocaine or phenytoin may be tried, but is generally unsuccessful in terminating TdP. Acquired LQTS with a QTc greater than 500 milliseconds warrants observation until the QTc normalizes. See an up-to-date list of potential QT-prolonging drugs at www.qtdrugs.org. Urgent cardiology consultation and admission to a bed with continuous cardiac monitoring and availability of external defibrillation is warranted for all patients.

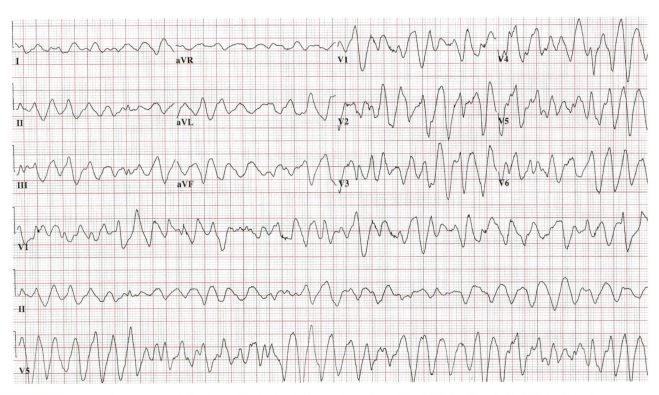

FIGURE 5.48 ■ ECG demonstrating TdP. Notice that in the rhythm strip portion of the ECG that the axis "twists" or alternates.

Pearls and Pitfalls

- TdP is a polymorphic VT associated with a long QT interval.
- Magnesium sulfate 2 grams IV bolus is a first-line therapy for TdP, regardless of magnesium levels.
- Pacing may be useful in terminating and/or preventing recurrence of TdP.
- Cardiovert or defibrillate unstable TdP.
- Eliminate exacerbating factors (electrolyte abnormalities, discontinue offending drugs, etc.).
- Monitor acquired long QT syndrome with QTc >500 milliseconds until normalized.
- Admit patients to beds with continuous cardiac monitoring, defibrillation availability, and urgent cardiology consultation.

VENTRICULAR FIBRILLATION

Benjamin C. Smith III

Clinical Highlights

Ventricular fibrillation (VF) is a cardiac arrhythmia that results in random uncoordinated contractions of the ventricles, pump failure, and loss of systemic perfusion. It is the most common arrhythmia identified in patients during cardiac arrest and the most common cause of sudden cardiac death. VF can occur without warning, often resulting in syncope as the only presenting symptom. However, there may also be a prodrome of chest pain, dyspnea, fatigue, palpitations, or near syncope.

The ECG or rhythm strip is diagnostic in patients presenting in VF. There is a classic appearance of disordered electrical activity generated by the random firing of ventricular myocytes. In the patient presenting with VF that is resuscitated, an acute coronary syndrome including ST-segment elevation MI (STEMI) must be suspected and fully ruled out.

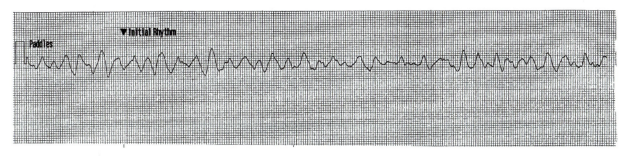

FIGURE 5.49 ■ ECG monitor strip of coarse VF.

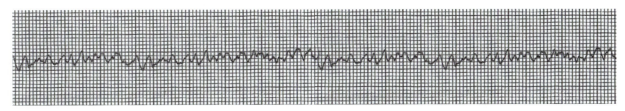

FIGURE 5.50 ■ ECG monitor strip of fine VF.

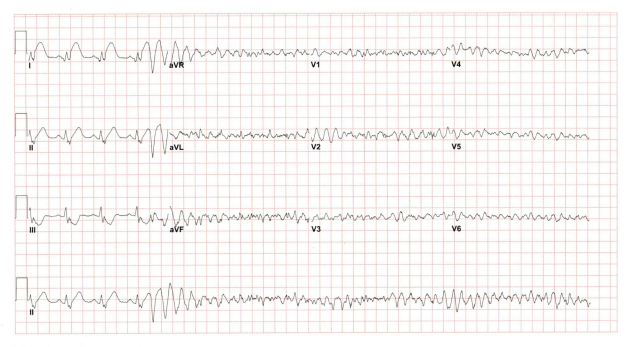

FIGURE 5.51 ■ ECG of an STEMI that degenerates into VF.

VENTRICULAR FIBRILLATION (CONTINUED)

ED Care and Disposition

The mainstay of treatment is electrical defibrillation and should be performed as soon as possible. Electrical defibrillation is the delivery of one large electrical pulse to the myocardium, simultaneously resetting all uncoordinated myocyte impulses. This will allow the patient's native cardiac pacemaker to restart its job of coordinating contractions.

If a bystander-witnessed cardiac arrest occurs in a prehospital setting, an automated external defibrillator (AED), if available, should be attached and activated. If no AED is present, Cardio Pulmonary Resusitation (CPR) should continue until Emergency Medical Services (EMS) arrives.

If VF occurs in a medical setting, a defibrillator should be placed on the patient's chest while CPR continues per Advanced Cardiac Life Support guidelines. An unsynchronized shock should be delivered as soon as possible, typically starting at 200 J for monophasic defibrillators. If unsuccessful, higher energy shocks may be delivered up to 360 J. Biphasic defibrillators have the advantage that they use lower defibrillation energies, resulting in less myocardial injury. The biphasic defibrillator manufacturer's recommended energies should be used.

For patients with VF recalcitrant to defibrillation, consider giving amiodarone 300 milligrams IV push and/or lidocaine

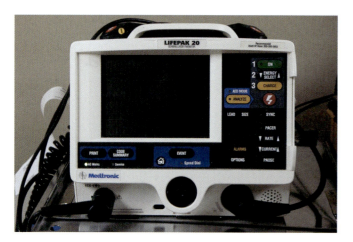

FIGURE 5.52 ■ Typical defibrillator with buttons: On, Energy Select, Charge, and Shock.

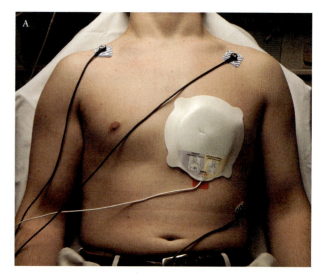

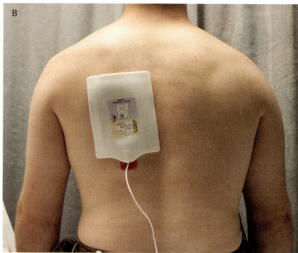

FIGURE 5.54 ■ Anterior (**A**)/posterior (**B**) placement of defibrillation pads.

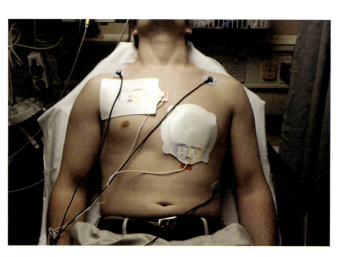

FIGURE 5.53 ■ Anterior placement of defibrillation pads.

VENTRICULAR FIBRILLATION (CONTINUED)

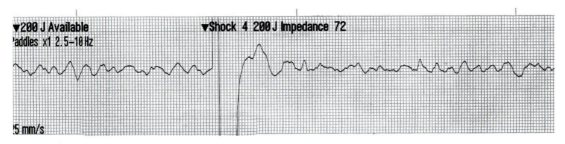

FIGURE 5.55 ■ Unsuccessful defibrillation.

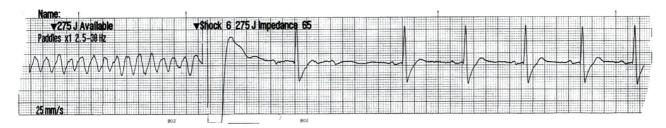

FIGURE 5.56 ■ Successful defibrillation.

1.5 milligrams/kg IV push. All the patients who have return of spontaneous circulation (ROSC) after a VF cardiac arrest should be admitted for monitoring and further testing.

Pearls and Pitfalls

- Ensure that the cardiac leads are well attached and noise free. The monitor strip should fit the clinical picture of VF: a pulseless and unconscious patient.
- Patients may present with seizure activity (convulsive syncope) when they enter VF.
- Torsades is frequently confused with VF and should be suspected in episodic VF that appears to spontaneously resolve.
- There is evidence to support 1 to 3 minutes of chest compressions prior to defibrillation if the VF patient has been down for 4 to 5 minutes without CPR.
- Patients who have ROSC after a VF arrest should remain attached to the defibrillator, as the unresolved underlying etiology of VF puts them at risk for recurrent VF.

BRUGADA SYNDROME

Ron Buchheit

Clinical Highlights

The Brugada syndrome occurs from a genetic mutation, most commonly the cardiac sodium channel SCN5A gene. These mutations are thought to cause changes in the chemical gradients of the cardiac cell leading to ventricular arrhythmias. Cocaine, alcohol intoxication, fever, increased vagal tone, and electrolyte abnormalities are thought to uncover or aggravate Brugada syndrome. Patients are most likely to be healthy young Asian men with a mean age of 41 years. Clinical features of Brugada syndrome include unexplained syncope, ventricular arrhythmias, or sudden death. Family history of sudden death may also be seen and can help identify patients at increased risk.

ECG findings for Brugada syndrome show a pseudo-RBBB and ST-segment elevation in V1 to V3. There are three patterns described. Type I is considered classic and has ST-segment elevation of 2 mm or more descending in a coved pattern from the J-point to an inverted T wave. Type II has ST-segment elevation of 1 mm or more in a saddle back pattern. Type III has ST-segment elevation of less than 1 mm in saddle back or coved pattern.

ED Care and Disposition

Emergency care is directed toward ruling out other conditions and cardiology consultation. As ECG changes can mimic STEMI, workup should include cardiac markers. Cardiac markers are negative in Brugada syndrome but findings of Brugada, such as ECG changes, warrant further evaluation by

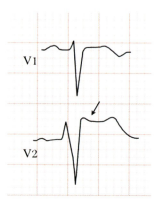

FIGURE 5.58 ■ Type II Brugada ECG pattern. Leads V1 and V2 demonstrating the findings of type II Brugada ECG pattern, with ST-segment elevation of 1 mm in a saddle back pattern.

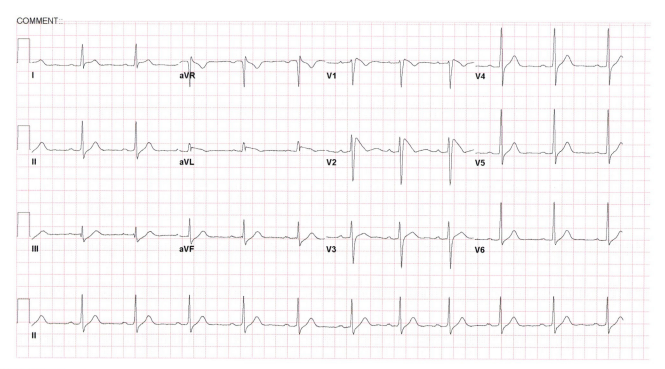

FIGURE 5.57 ■ Type I Brugada ECG pattern. Twelve-lead ECG demonstrates the findings of type I Brugada ECG pattern. Note ST-segment elevation, in a coved pattern from J point to an inverted T wave, seen in leads V1 and V2.

BRUGADA SYNDROME (CONTINUED)

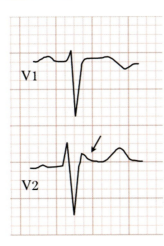

FIGURE 5.59 ■ Type III Brugada ECG pattern. Leads V1 and V2 demonstrate Brugada type III ECG pattern with ST-segment elevation of less than 1 mm in a saddle back pattern consistent with Brugada syndrome type III.

a cardiologist. Patients should be instructed to avoid cocaine, alcohol, antiarrhythmic drugs, beta-blockers, antianginal drugs, phenothiazines, psychotropic drugs, calcium channel drugs, selective serotonin reuptake inhibitors, and dimenhydrinate until they are instructed otherwise by a cardiologist.

Pearls and Pitfalls

- Young patients who present with syncope should have an ECG done with close examination of the precordial leads for findings consistent with the Brugada syndrome.
- Patients suspected to have Brugada pattern should have an evaluation by a cardiologist.
- Physical activity should be restricted, as it may increase ventricular arrhythmias in recovery or at rest from increased vagal tone.

Conduction Disorders
FIRST-DEGREE ATRIOVENTRICULAR BLOCK

Stacie Zelman

Clinical Highlights

First-degree atrioventricular (AV) block is a term used to describe delayed electrical conduction from the atria to the ventricles. While there are several degrees of AV block (first, second, and third), first-degree AV block is defined by slow AV conduction with a normal rhythm and no missed beats. This delay in transmission results in a PR interval greater than 200 milliseconds. The block is considered extremely elongated when the PR interval exceeds 300 milliseconds.

In the majority of cases, the AV node is the site of intraventricular delay. However, reduced transmission may occur in the atrium, bundle of His, or infra-Hisian conduction system. First-degree heart block with a normal QRS complex usually results from conduction delay from the AV node or above. A widened QRS complex usually means the block originates from the AV node or below, often involving the bundle of His or the bundle branches. A widened QRS complex may indicate two areas of conduction delay and is associated with potential to progress to higher levels of heart block. There are many etiologies of first-degree AV block. The majority of cases are idiopathic, but first-degree AV block can also be a result of medications (antidysrhythmics, digoxin, etc.), electrolyte disturbances (hypokalemia), infection (myocarditis, endocarditis, etc.), AMI, increased vagal tone, and coronary artery disease (CAD).

ED Care and Disposition

In the majority of cases, the finding of first-degree AV block requires no specific ED intervention. It is important to recognize and address any potential underlying etiologies of

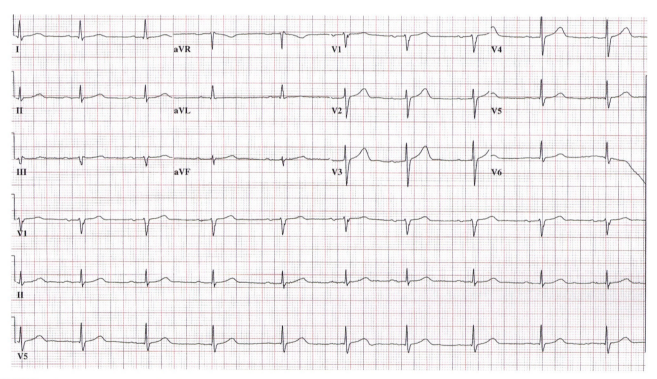

FIGURE 5.60 ■ First-degree AV block with normal QRS.

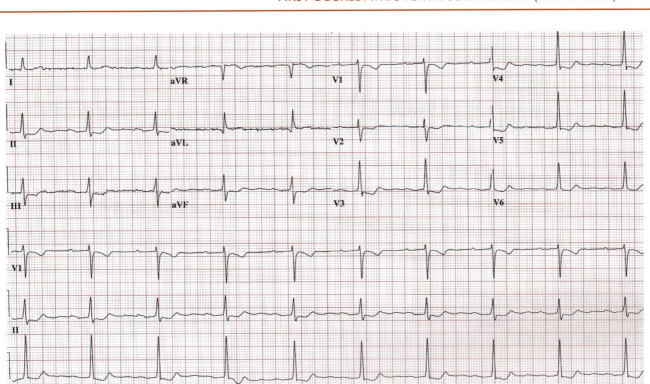

FIGURE 5.61 ■ First-degree AV block with normal QRS.

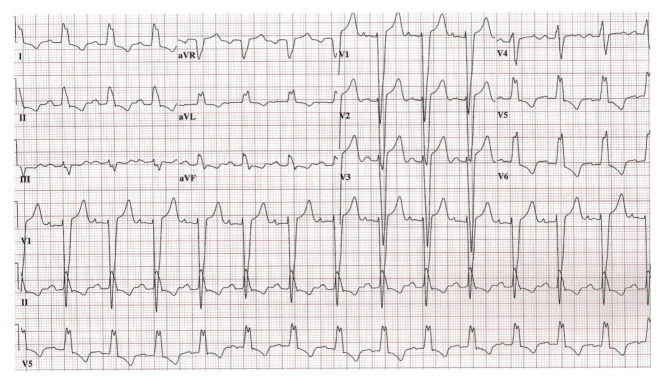

FIGURE 5.62 ■ First-degree AV block with widened QRS.

the conduction delay (AMI or endocarditis). A pacemaker is rarely indicated, but may be considered in patients at risk for future progression to higher degrees of heart block. All the patients with a new finding of first-degree AV block should be made aware of this finding and subsequent need for follow-up by their primary care physician or a cardiologist.

Pearls and Pitfalls

- AV block in the setting of AMI is often associated with inferior infarction and higher in-hospital mortality.
- Many cases of first-degree AV block have a benign course, but there may be an increased risk of developing atrial fibrillation or needing pacemaker placement later in life.
- The finding of first-degree heart block in young healthy adults (especially athletes) during an initial ED visit is usually not a cause for concern at that time. They may be safely discharged to the care of their primary care physician.

SECOND-DEGREE-ATRIOVENTRICULAR BLOCK, MOBITZ TYPE I

Kim Askew

Clinical Highlights

Patients presenting with second-degree atrioventricular (AV) block type I (Mobitz I or Wenckebach) can have a variety of symptoms based on the underlying etiology of the heart block and associated cardiac output. Patients with a low resting heart rate or increased vagal tone (eg, athletes) may be without symptoms at time of recognition. Some patients may present with a perception of an irregular heartbeat, while others may experience weakness, dizziness, syncope, or near syncope if associated with a significantly lower cardiac output. Finally, if a patient develops this type of block from ischemia, then the patient may have symptoms such as chest pressure, shortness of breath, etc. Therefore, there is no one classical presentation for second-degree type I block.

The classic finding second-degree AV block type I on an ECG is a gradually increasing PR interval until ultimately a QRS complex is not generated after the P wave. Other findings include a shortening R–R interval, groups of conducted beats, and an R–R interval including the nonconducted P wave that is less than twice the preceding R–R interval.

There are multiple causes for second-degree block type I, including medication effect (digoxin, beta-, or calcium channel blockers), acute inferior myocardial ischemia or infarct, intrinsic AV node disease, postcardiac surgery complications, as well as infectious processes such as myocarditis.

ED Care and Disposition

Evaluation and treatment of second-degree type I heart block depends on the patient's symptoms, stability, and likely causes of the block. The patient's medications should be reviewed to determine if one may have precipitated the block. In symptomatic patients, the evaluation typically consists of measuring serum electrolyte levels, including magnesium and calcium. Cardiac biomarkers should be obtained if there is concern for possible cardiac ischemia. If asymptomatic, the evaluation can be limited to the provider's suspicion of the underlying etiology.

In patients are hemodynamically stable, then treatment outside of withholding AV node–blocking agents may not be needed. However, if patients are suffering signs of decreased perfusion (hypotension, altered mental status, ischemic chest pain, or signs of heart failure), the use of atropine can increase conduction through the AV node (0.5 milligrams IV every 3–5 minutes to a maximum dose of 3 milligrams). If atropine is ineffective, then transcutaneous pacing is an option to

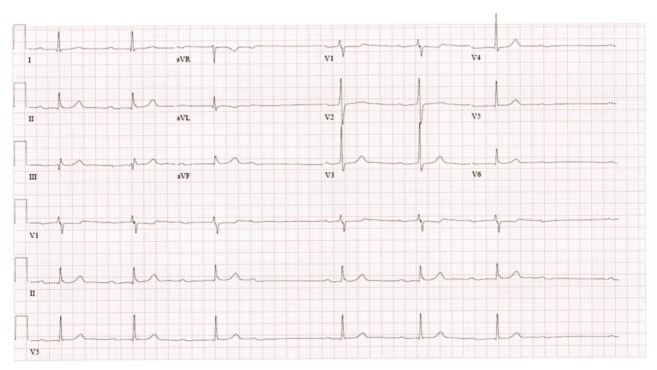

FIGURE 5.63 ■ ECG showing second-degree type I heart block. Note the progressively longer PR interval before the dropped QRS, in two sets of three conducted P waves before the nonconducted P wave.

increase cardiac output. If there is a concern for ischemia, a regimen for acute coronary syndrome should be begun.

Disposition again relates to stability and clinician suspicion of underlying etiology. For asymptomatic patients with low suspicion for underlying ischemia, then outpatient follow-up with cardiology is appropriate. However, for symptomatic patients, patients requiring treatment, or clinician concern of etiology, consultation with cardiology and hospital admission is indicated.

Pearls and Pitfalls

- Consider other types of blocks when evaluating the ECG to ensure ECG is consistent with second-degree AV block type I.
- Many patients will not require treatment, but consider for the etiology of the block.
- Review patient's medication to ensure medication or supplement is not the precipitating agent.

SECOND-DEGREE-ATRIOVENTRICULAR BLOCK, MOBITZ TYPE II

Mary A Wittler

Clinical Highlights

Second-degree atrioventricular (AV) block is a failure of conduction between the atria and ventricle where some, but not all, atrial impulses are blocked. Mobitz II blocks are infranodal and associated with degenerative and/or ischemic diseases of the His-Purkinje system. In the setting of acute anterior MI, this block often progresses to complete AV block. Clinical symptoms may be vague, including (pre)syncope, lightheadedness, dizziness, loss of exercise capacity, confusion, falls, or weakness.

The diagnosis of Mobitz II block is based on ECG criteria: the sinus rate (or P–P interval) is constant; the nonconducted atrial impulse (P wave) is preceded and followed by fixed PR intervals; at least two consecutively conducted P waves are present. The PR intervals of conducted impulses are usually normal, but can be longer than 0.2 seconds, yet are consistant in length. The QRS complex of conducted impulses can be narrow, but are usually wide secondary to infranodal conduction disturbances. A Mobitz II block can occur intermittently or in a fixed conduction ratio. A fixed 2:1 AV block can be nodal or infranodal in origin, and is difficult to classify as type I or II second-degree AV block on the basis of ECG findings (because only one PR interval is available for analysis before the block). Ultimately, because the site of the block (nodal or infranodal) carries a different prognosis regarding clinical deterioration, a 2:1 AV block should be considered to be Mobitz II until proven otherwise. Additionally, a block of two or more consecutive P waves is termed advanced or high-grade second-degree AV block.

ED Care and Disposition

Because vagal maneuvers have little effect on conduction in the His-Purkinje system, manipulation of vagal tone should not change conduction in Mobitz II block. Atropine is not indicated because it is not expected to improve infranodal conduction. Progression to third-degree AV block is common, sudden, and may result in death. All patients should have transcutaneous pacing pads applied and tested to ensure capture. Transcutaneous or transvenous pacing should be instituted for symptomatic bradycardia or clinical deterioration. Permanent or intermittent asymptomatic Mobitz II block is an indication for pacemaker placement. Urgent cardiology

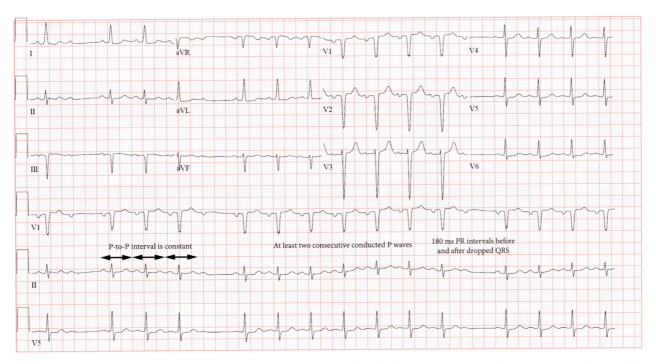

FIGURE 5.64 ■ ECG showing second-degree AV block, Mobitz type II. This ECG demonstrates the criteria for second-degree AB Block, Mobitz II: intermittently nonconducted P waves; nonconducted impulses are preceded and followed by fixed PR intervals (100 milliseconds), P-to-P intervals are constant.

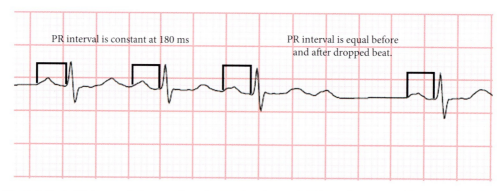

FIGURE 5.65 ■ The strip from V1 is an enlargement from the ECG in Figure 5.64. Note the uniform PR intervals before and after the nonconducted impulse, in this case, 180 milliseconds.

consultation and admission to a monitored bed is warranted for all patients.

Pearls and Pitfalls

- A salient ECG finding is the presence of a nonconducted P wave that is preceded and followed by fixed PR intervals.
- Mobitz II blocks can precipitously progress to complete heart block (CHB).
- A fixed 2:1 AV block can be nodal or infranodal in origin and carries different prognosis regarding clinical deterioration. These are best classified as advanced second-degree AV block until the location of the block is known.
- Admit all patients with type II or advanced second-degree AV block to a monitored bed, with transcutaneous and transvenous pacing capabilities, and urgent cardiology evaluation.

THIRD-DEGREE ATRIOVENTRICULAR BLOCK

Kathleen Hosmer

Clinical Highlights

Third-degree atrioventricular (AV) block, otherwise known as complete heart block CHB, occurs when there is no conduction through the AV node. The atrial pacemaker will continue to pace causing the atria to contract and P waves to occur on the ECG, but these will not correlate with the QRS complexes that are present. The block is present below the bundle of His 61% of the time. The other 39% of cases are split between a block either in the AV node or the bundle of His directly. The location of the block will correlate with the patient's heart rate on presentation. Although the atrial rate does not conduct to the ventricles, the ventricles compensate with pacemakers of their own. This rate is generally much slower than the atrial rate that often is elevated due to decreased blood pressure from the decreased ventricular rate. The most common presentation occurs with the block below the AV node, and a rate of typically <45 bpm. If the block is in the AV node the rate is generally between 45 and 60 bpm.

Patients with third-degree heart block will almost always be bradycardic, and can present with heart rates as low as in the teens. This bradycardia usually leads to hypotension and the patient's symptoms of lightheadedness, syncope, and/or generalized weakness and fatigue.

ED Care and Disposition

Treatment of third-degree heart block will vary based on the patient's hemodynamic stability and will likely directly correlate to the location of the block. If the block is at the level of the AV node, the heart rate will be higher (45–60 bpm) and patients may not need immediate intervention in the ED if they remain hemodynamically stable. These patients may also still have a response to atropine if needed. However, if the block is below the AV node, atropine is unlikely to have any effect and the patient may require pacing. Hypotensive patients can initially be temporized with external pacing, but will need a transvenous pacemaker placed quickly if cardiology is not available for permanent pacemaker placement emergently.

It is also important to consider the many potential causes of third-degree heart block, as some are reversible quickly, and therefore will not require pacemaker placement. Many drugs can cause heart block such as calcium channel blockers, beta-blockers, AV nodal–blocking agents, and digoxin. Patients may also have metabolic causes such as hyperkalemia, hypothyroidism, or hypoxia. Finally, patients may occasionally present with an acute inferior or anterior wall MI as the cause for their new-onset third-degree heart block. Prompt

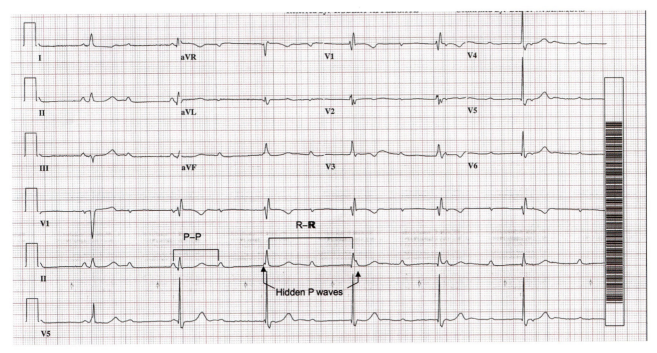

FIGURE 5.66 ■ The atrial rate on this ECG is 70 bpm, but the ventricular rate is 39 bpm, consistent with third-degree heart block. The rate tells the clinician that the block is below the AV node.

recognition of an acute STEMI on ECG and cardiac consultation for reperfusion may resolve the block without the need for a pacemaker.

Pearls and Pitfalls

- ECG analysis for third-degree heart block should demonstrate P–P intervals that are regular and likewise R–R intervals that are regular, although the rates will be different due to the different intrinsic atrial and ventricular rates. If both are not regular consider the possibility of a second-degree AV block.
- Evaluate the patient's medication list carefully for reversible causes of bradycardia, and consider treatment for possible overdoses prior to placement of transvenous pacemaker.
- If the patient has symptoms concerning for AMI, consider activating the STEMI protocol at your institution for rapid cardiology evaluation and possible reperfusion.

BIFASCICULAR BLOCK

Ahren Shubin

Clinical Highlights

Bifascicular block is a conduction abnormality below the AV node of the heart including a right bundle branch block (RBBB) with either a left anterior fascicular block (LAFB) or left posterior fascicular block (LPFB) of the left bundle branch (see Chap. 2, section on Normal Cardiac Conduction for illustration). Criteria for RBBB plus LAFB are:

(A) Prolongation of the QRS duration to 0.12 second or longer;
(B) RSR' pattern in lead V1, with a broad and slurred R' waveform;
(C) wide, slurred S waves in leads I, V5, and V6;
(D) left axis deviation in the frontal plane, from −30° to −90°; and
(E) small R wave and large S wave in II, III, and aVF.

Criteria for RBBB plus LPFB include A, B, and C above, plus the criteria for LPFB (in this setting):

(D) right axis deviation in the frontal plane of +90°, or farther to the right, usually demonstrated by a negative QRS complex in lead I, and positive QRS complexes in leads II, and III, and
(E) a small R wave and a large S wave are seen in lead I and small Q waves and large R waves are seen in leads III and aVF.

The onset of RBBB results in altered pathways for ventricular depolarization. The electrical impulse must move through muscle fibers slowing electrical movement combined with changes in the directional propagation of the impulses. As a result, there is a loss of ventricular synchrony, and there may be a drop in cardiac output. Symptoms associated with bifascicular block may include dizziness, syncope, chest pain, or shortness of breath but many patients are asymptomatic. Bifascicular block is associated with ischemic heart disease, hypertension, aortic stenosis, anterior MI, conduction system disease, congenital heart disease, neuromuscular disease, hyperkalemia, or drugs

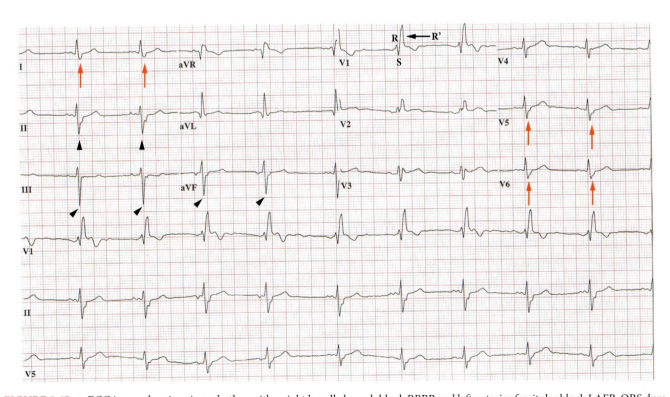

FIGURE 5.67 ■ ECG image showing sinus rhythm with a right bundle branch block RBBB and left anterior fascicular block LAFB. QRS duration is greater than 0.12 seconds, in lead V1, RSR' pattern is labeled, R' is slurred. Wide slurred S waves are seen in leads I, V5, and V6 (red arrows). Left axis deviation is noted by a positive QRS complex in lead I, with negative QRS complexes in leads II and III. Small r waves and large S waves (black arrowheads) are seen in leads II, III, and aVF.

156 ■ BIFASCICULAR BLOCK (CONTINUED)

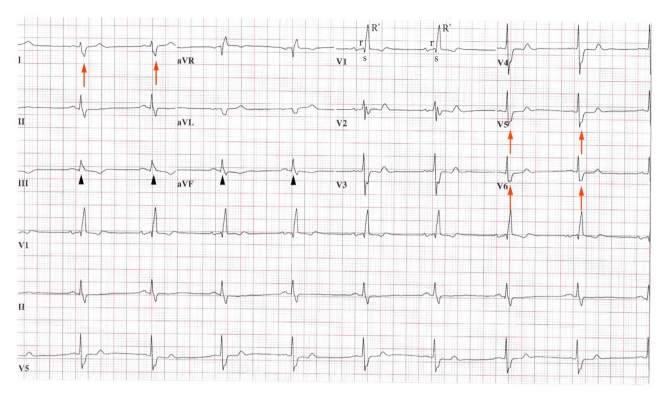

FIGURE 5.68 ■ ECG image of sinus rhythm with right bundle branch block plus LPFB. QRS duration is greater than 0.12 seconds, in lead V1, RSR' pattern is labeled, R' is slurred. Wide slurred S waves are seen in leads I, V5, and V6 (red arrows). Right axis deviation is seen in the frontal plane, demonstrated here by a negative QRS complex in lead I, and positive QRS complexes in leads II and III. A small r wave and a large S wave are seen in lead I and small q waves and large R waves (black arrowheads) are seen in leads III and aVF.

that may slow cardiac conduction and/or prolong the refractory period. Chronic bifascicular block may progress to CHB.

ED Care and Disposition

In the setting of AMI, patients with new or age-indeterminate bifascicular block with PR prolongation are at high risk for developing CHB. Temporary transvenous (preferable over transcutaneous) pacing should be considered. Treatment of chronic bifascicular block includes correcting potential etiologies of impaired cardiac conduction such as myocardial ischemia as well as stopping or avoiding drugs known to adversely affect conduction. In the absence of reversible etiologies, permanent pacemaker placement may be indicated.

Pearls and Pitfalls

- Bifascicular block signals extensive disease of the cardiac conduction system with a small percentage progressing to CHB. Risk factors for a higher rate of progression to CHB include syncope, renal failure, and a QRS duration >140 milliseconds.
- Bifascicular block in the setting of AMI is associated with higher rates of progression to CHB.
- Treatment of chronic bifascicular block includes correcting reversible causes of impaired cardiac conduction and permanent pacemaker placement in selected patients without reversible causes.

LEFT ANTERIOR FASCICULAR BLOCK

Ahren Shubin

Clinical Highlights

LAFB or left anterior hemiblock may be the result of conduction system disease in the anterior fascicle (see Chap. 2, section on Normal Cardiac Conduction) of the left bundle branch or surrounding myocardium. The left anterior fascicle is supplied by the septal branches of the left anterior descending (LAD) or AV nodal artery of the right coronary artery. Isolated LAFB without structural heart disease is usually benign and sometimes seen as a consequence of aging. There are no symptoms induced by an isolated block in the left anterior fascicle.

ECG findings characteristic of LAFB include (1) left axis deviation of greater than −45° up to −90°, yielding a positive QRS complex in lead I and negative QRS complexes in leads II, III, and aVF, (2) small q wave and tall R wave in lead aVL, (3) the beginning of the R wave to its peak is 45 milliseconds or more in aVL, and (4) a QRS duration of less than 120 milliseconds. A tall R wave in aVR and poor R wave progression in leads V1–V3 is often found. Left axis deviation, as seen in LAFB, is one of the most common abnormal ECG findings and is most commonly secondary to coronary and hypertensive heart diseases but include many others. These criteria are not applicable to patients with congenital heart disease with LAD on ECG present as an infant.

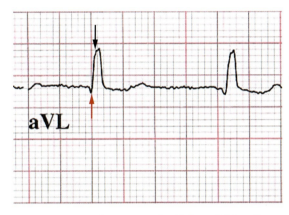

FIGURE 5.70 ■ An enlargement of AVL from ECG in Figure 5.69. The red arrow points to the small q wave and the black arrowhead point to a tall R wave in lead aVL. Note, the R wave has a slurred upstroke, measuring from onset to the peak approximately 80 milliseconds; the QRS is approximately 100 milliseconds total, meeting criteria for LAFB.

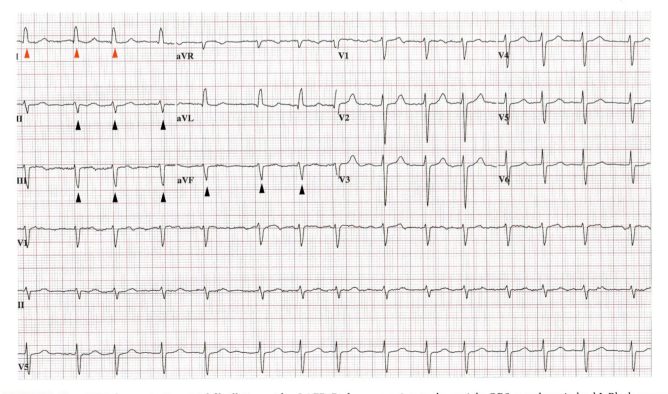

FIGURE 5.69 ■ ECG demonstrating atrial fibrillation with a LAFB. Red arrows points to the upright QRS complexes in lead I. Black arrows point to the negative QRS complexes in leads II, III, and aVF. See Figure 5.70 for discussion of aVL findings that fulfill the criteria for LAFB.

ED Care and Disposition

Isolated LAFB is not symptomatic, does not increase mortality, and does not require therapy. One exception is patients with neuromuscular disease and new fascicular block. These patients often demonstrate unpredictable and rapidly progressive conduction system disease resulting in the need for a pacemaker, and therefore need nonurgent referral to a cardiologist. Asymptomatic patients with ECG findings of LAFB on routine ECG testing should follow up with their primary care provider for regular health maintenance.

Pearls and Pitfalls

- LAFB has been associated with significant CAD in the LAD artery. LAFB presenting during an inferior wall AMI may indicate CAD of the LAD, disease of multiple coronary vessels, as well as decreased systolic function of the left ventricle.
- Isolated LAFB is asymptomatic and no treatment is indicated unless neuromuscular disease is present.

RIGHT BUNDLE BRANCH BLOCK

Erin Boyd

Clinical Highlights

RBBB occurs when conduction through the right bundle is blocked and right ventricular depolarization is delayed. Criteria for RBBB are a QRS greater than 0.12 seconds, a RSR' pattern in lead V1, and wide S waves in V5, V6, and lead I. Causes include degenerative changes in the conduction system, pulmonary embolism with overload to the right side of the heart, chronic pulmonary disease with pulmonary hypertension, pulmonary stenosis, acute anterior wall infarction, atrial septal defect, or cardiac surgery.

RBBB may also be "rate-related." This may result from a long preceding R–R interval then followed by a short cycle. After the initial aberrancy, rate-related RBBB may continue if the impulse down the left bundle reenters the right bundle branch keeping it once again refractory. This pattern may repeat itself after several cycles. This rhythm may occur in the setting of SVT such as atrial flutter.

Most commonly patients are asymptomatic, but may present with the symptoms related to an acute cause such as pulmonary embolism or myocardial ischemia. Pulmonary disease patients may present with chest pain, dyspnea, syncope, or presyncope.

ED Care and Disposition

Treatment and disposition depends on the underlying cause and symptoms of the patient. When a new RBBB is discovered and the patient is otherwise asymptomatic, then the likelihood of having another heart condition is low. In this case, follow-up with the patient's primary care physician should suffice. However, if the patient presents with symptoms including chest pain, dyspnea, or syncope in the setting of a new RBBB, then a workup to look for the underlying heart condition is important. In a case of rate-dependent RBBB, such as RBBB in the setting of atrial flutter, the patient may need pharmacologic rate control or cardioversion if unstable and referral to a cardiologist.

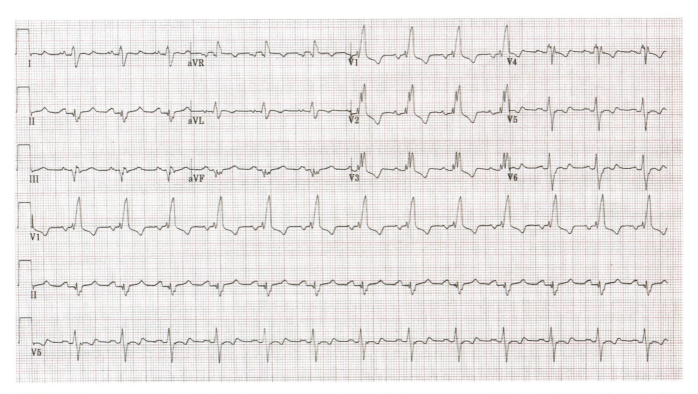

FIGURE 5.71 ■ ECG showing RBBB. QRS width is 170 milliseconds. Note tall R' wave in V1. Note RSR' pattern, best seen in here in lead V2, with large R'. Also see wide S wave in lead V6 and lead I.

RIGHT BUNDLE BRANCH BLOCK (CONTINUED)

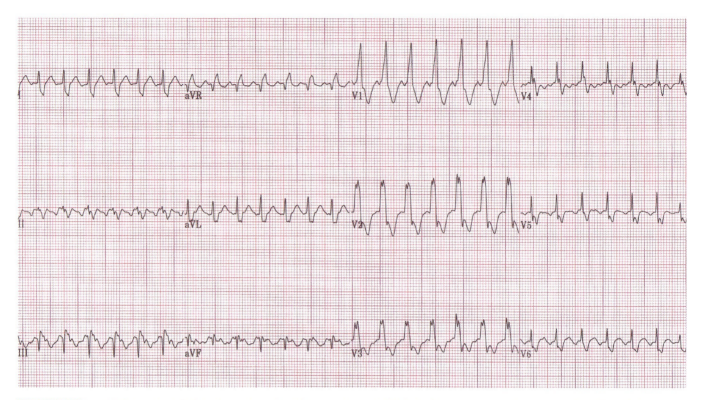

FIGURE 5.72 ■ ECG showing RBBB in the setting of atrial flutter with 2:1 AV block. Flutter waves are best seen in lead II. QRS duration is 128 milliseconds, RSR' V1 and V2, with wide S wave in V6 and lead I. The QRS pattern and width returned to normal after treatment of atrial flutter.

Pearls and Pitfalls

- Do not confuse a RBBB with a more serious condition called Brugada syndrome ("pseudo-RBBB"), which is associated with increased risk of ventricular tachyarrhythmias and sudden cardiac death.
- An RSR' pattern with a narrow QRS duration of less than 0.10 seconds and a very small terminal R' wave in V1 or V1–V2 is a common normal variant.

LEFT BUNDLE BRANCH BLOCK

Kathleen Hosmer

Clinical Highlights

LBBB is a pattern seen on an ECG when there is disruption of the conduction system after the AV node. LBBB most commonly occurs in older patients with known cardiac disease. Patients with LBBB rarely have any specific symptoms related to its occurrence; rather it is a consequence of slowly progressive disease of the conduction system. The slowed conduction through the left bundle results in a prolonged QRS duration on ECG because the electrical activation is not through the His-Purkinje system. LBBB has a characteristic appearance on an ECG, particularly when evaluating leads I, V5, and V6. The QRS duration must be ≥0.12 seconds, and in the absence of myocardial pathology, have an upright QRS in I and V6 and downward QRS in V1. There should be no q waves present in leads I, V5, and V6. The rhythm must also be a supraventricular rhythm; otherwise the widened QRS may be VT or other idioventricular rhythm. Finally, the T wave should be opposite the deflection of the QRS.

ED Care and Disposition

Because most patients will be asymptomatic, there will be no immediate care needed. It is important to determine whether the LBBB was present on prior ECGs to determine the need for further acute intervention. In patients with already diagnosed CAD, LBBB is a predictor for higher all-cause mortality. Patients who develop LBBB as a result of an acute infarction also have higher short- and long-term mortality.

If the LBBB is determined to be new and it is associated with chest pain, dyspnea, diaphoresis, or other symptoms concerning for acute myocardial ischemia, the patient needs an emergent cardiology consultation for possible AMI and reperfusion. LBBB can obscure the typical findings of ST elevation, ST depression, or T-wave inversion seen with acute ischemia.

Pearls and Pitfalls

- Inverted T waves in lateral leads do not necessarily indicate ischemia, because the T-wave deflection should be opposite to the QRS.
- T waves that are concordant with the QRS deflection should be considered concerning for ischemia, if the patient has correlating anginal symptoms.
- New onset of LBBB may indicate acute STEMI and should be treated emergently.
- If Q waves are present in I and V6 in the presence of LBBB, this likely indicates an old infarction.

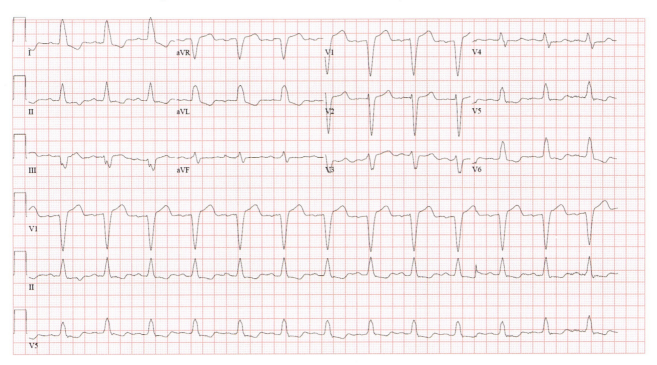

FIGURE 5.73 ■ This ECG demonstrates the typical LBBB pattern: QRS duration ≥ 0.12 seconds, upright QRS in leads I, V5, and V6, and downward QRS in V1. The T wave has an opposite deflection to the QRS.

LONG QT SYNDROME

Laura Yoder

Clinical Highlights

Long QT (or prolonged QT) syndrome is usually discovered when asymptomatic patients have ECG done for other reasons. By definition, an adult has a prolonged QTc (QT interval adjusted for heart rate) when it is longer than 0.44 seconds. These patients can present with palpitations, syncope or near syncope, seizure-like activity (usually due to syncope), or sudden cardiac death. If the patient is having symptoms, it is possible that the initial ECG may show evidence of arrhythmia. Patients suffering from other illnesses, such as acute myocardial ischemia or cerebrovascular accidents, can also be found to have long QT syndrome (LQTS) that often resolves as the patient improves.

This is an important diagnosis to consider in children who present with symptoms related to exercise or emotional stress, as there is a congenital version of LQTS. There are several gene mutations that cause congenital LQTS, one of which can also cause congenital deafness. LQTS can also be acquired due to medications (amiodarone, haloperidol, cancer drugs, and antifungals), electrolyte changes (hypomagnesemia and hypokalemia are the most common), or a combination of several factors.

Patients with long QT syndrome are at an increased risk of developing TdP. This form of PVT can lead to sudden cardiac death. Differential diagnosis includes VT not precipitated by prolonged QT syndrome and seizure disorders.

ED Care and Disposition

If a patient with a history of LQTS presents with unstable vital signs, it is possible that they have developed TdP or VT and need emergent defibrillation. If the patient has stable vital signs but has an ECG concerning for torsades, give magnesium sulfate (2 grams IV). If this does not correct the rhythm, attempt to overdrive pace of the patient with a transcutaneous pacing device. While setting up external pacing, it is possible to use isoproterenol, but there is limited data to show its benefit.

If a long QT interval is discovered in the workup for a patient with syncope or if there are other signs of ectopy on the ECG, the patient needs to be admitted to a telemetry bed for observation. Any drugs that prolong the QT interval need to be stopped (while patient is on cardiac monitoring) and all electrolyte abnormalities need to be corrected. If there is only a mild prolongation (under 0.47 seconds), it was an incidental finding, or the patient is on a drug known to prolong the QT interval, discharge can be considered if the patient is asymptomatic and without any recent syncope. The patient does need to be advised that in the future if they have a change in their offending medicine, they need to undergo cardiac monitoring during that time. If LQTS is uncovered in a young

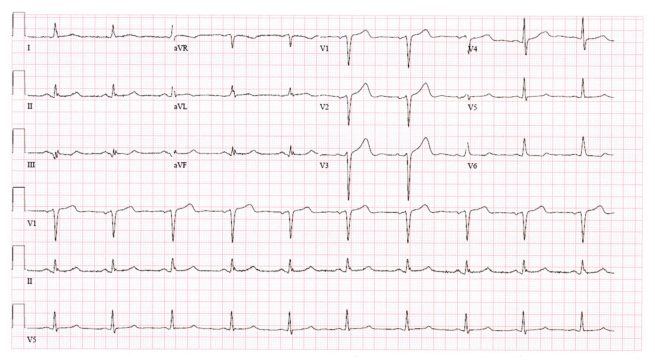

FIGURE 5.74 ■ ECG with prolonged QTc interval. QTc = 0.510 seconds.

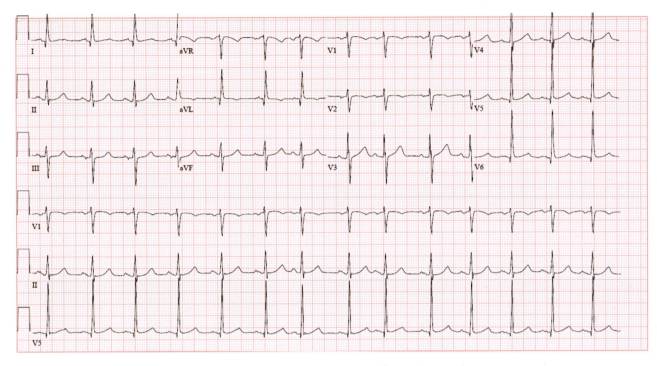

FIGURE 5.75 ■ Another example of an ECG with prolonged QTc interval. QTc = 0.550 seconds.

patient or there is concern for the congenital form of LQTS, all family members need to undergo ECG testing, as a majority of people with this syndrome are asymptomatic.

Pearls and Pitfalls

- Concern for potential arrhythmias should start when QTc exceeds 0.47 seconds.
- Admit all the patients found to have LQTS if any recent history of syncope or ectopy found on ECG—as this is concerning for an episode of arrhythmia.
- Obtain an ECG to rule out LQTS in first-time seizures or syncope, especially in children.
- Psychiatric patients getting repeat doses of haloperidol need to have their QT interval monitored.

Pacemaker Rhythms
ECG INTERPRETATION OF PACED RHYTHM

Bryon E. Rubery
Glenn M. Brammer

Clinical Highlights

The ECG pattern for a pacemaker patient depends on the pacemaker type (atrial, ventricular, dual chamber, and biventricular), location of the pacing tip (where the electrical stimulus emanates), the patient's native rhythm (without pacing), and the pacemaker mode, which determines the interaction between the patient's native rhythm and the pacemaker. This chapter attempts to present pacemaker basics succinctly. Dual-chamber pacemakers have both a right atrial pacing lead and a right ventricle lead. A biventricular pacemaker has three leads, right atrial, right ventricle, and left ventricle via the coronary sinus. Biventricular pacing facilitates cardiac resynchronization therapy for patients in advanced heart failure.

If there is a native cardiac activity faster than the programmed intervals, the pacing function is suppressed and native conduction prevails. If there is a slow cardiac activity, the pacemaker activates. Pacing spikes are recognized as vertical waveforms of short duration that precede the P wave if from an atrial lead, or precede the QRS if from a ventricular lead, provided that capture is intact. The resultant P wave in response to atrial pacing may appear abnormal or normal. The most common location for a ventricular lead is the apex of the right ventricle that produces a QRS complex resembling a left bundle branch pattern.

An atrial paced rhythm (without ventricular pacing) yields an ECG showing a pacemaker spike before the P wave (which may appear normal or abnormal) followed by a normal QRS. A ventricular demand pacing lead yields a rhythm where a pacemaker spike precedes each QRS which is wide.

A dual-chamber pacemaker (a lead in the right atrium and a lead in the right ventricle) allows for sensing and pacing of the atria as well as ventricles. Therefore, this pacemaker may yield a rhythm where the atria and ventricles are paced in sequence according to a programed set rate. Or within set

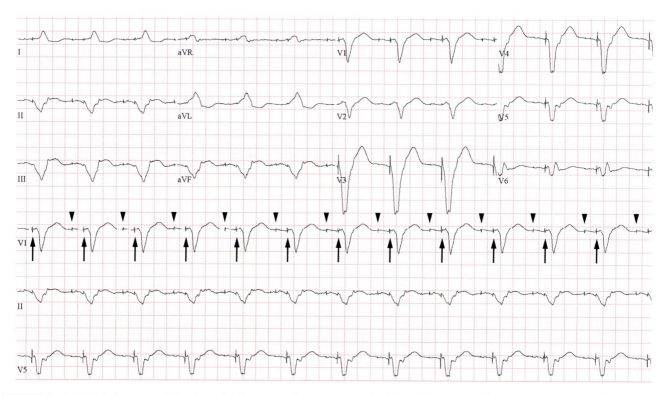

FIGURE 5.76 ■ ECG showing LBBB pattern (QRS >120 milliseconds, rS in lead V1, RsR' in lead V6) from a right ventricular apex pacemaker lead. In this example, the atrial lead is also pacing the atrium (arrowheads show atrial pacing spikes) prior to each ventricular spike (arrows) and corresponding QRS.

ECG INTERPRETATION OF PACED RHYTHM (CONTINUED)

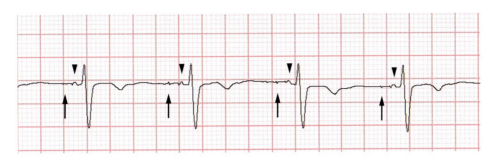

FIGURE 5.77 ■ ECG lead II strip of an atrial paced rhythm. The atrial pacing spikes are shown (arrows) followed by P waves (arrowheads) and QRS complexes that in this case are 102 milliseconds each. As shown here, pacemakers may yield pacing spikes of small amplitude, especially bipolar leads.

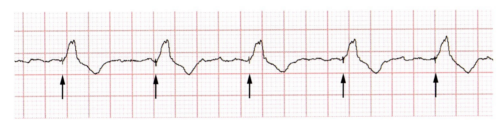

FIGURE 5.78 ■ ECG lead II strip of a ventricular paced rhythm, pacemaker spikes marked (arrowheads).

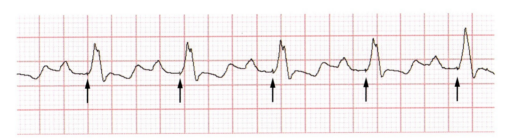

FIGURE 5.79 ■ ECG lead II strip of dual chamber pacemaker tracking sinus rhythm, ventricular pacing with pacing spikes marked (arrows).

parameters, the atrial lead can sense the native atrial impulse (sinus) and pace the ventricles in sequence at a rate determined by the native atrial rate. In contrast, in the event of a native atrial rate that rises above a set threshold, such as the onset of atrial flutter at a rate above 200, the pacemaker now switches modes and paces the ventricles at a default rate with no regard to the atrial rate until the atrial rate drops down below the set threshold.

The QRS complex with biventricular pacing will vary depending on right ventricular and left ventricular timing, but often has a tall R wave in V1 and an initial Q wave or QS complex in lead I.

Pacemaker Malfunction

There are three basic types of pacemaker failure. Loss of pacemaker capture is defined by a pacing spike with no P wave or QRS complex, when the myocardium is physiologically capable of being depolarized. Undersensing occurs when the pacemaker does not see native cardiac activity and paces inappropriately in the middle of or after a P wave or QRS complex, or has no relationship to the native cardiac signal. Oversensing occurs when the pacemaker sees nonphysiology activity and inhibits pacing. No pacing spikes are seen at the expected times.

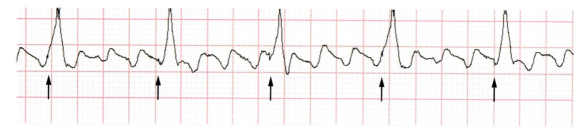

FIGURE 5.80 ■ Same patient as Figure 5.79, showing an ECG lead II strip of dual chamber pacing in the setting of new atrial flutter, pacing spikes at arrows. The ventricles are being paced at the programed rate (60 bpm); the pacemaker does not trigger the ventricular rate at this markedly elevated flutter rate (approximately 250 bpm).

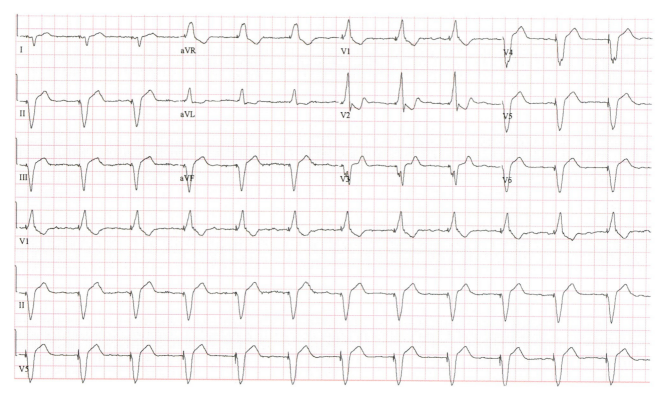

FIGURE 5.81 ■ ECG of biventricular pacemaker. Note the R wave in lead V1, and the QS complex in lead I.

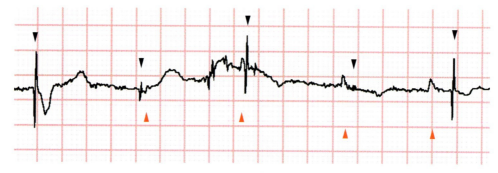

FIGURE 5.82 ■ ECG lead II strip showing ventricular undersensing. The first pacemaker spike (first black arrowhead) captures with a T wave following the induced QRS. The patient's native rhythm intervenes (red arrowheads), but the pacing spikes continue (black arrowheads). The spikes fail to pace, first on top of the first native QRS (first red arrowhead), then immediately after the remaining three native QRS complexes.

ED Care and Disposition

Patients with pacemaker malfunction and unstable vital signs should be paced transcutaneously. IV fluids and inotropic support should be given if the patient has symptomatic hypotension. In all cases of pacemaker malfunction with symptoms, a cardiologist should be consulted urgently.

Pearls and Pitfalls

- Ask the patient for his/her wallet card describing the pacemaker type and mode to help interpret the ECG.
- Both prior ECGs and prior chest x-rays will help in the assessment of pacemaker malfunction.
- Symptomatic pacemaker malfunction requires consultation with a cardiologist.

Chapter 6
VASCULAR DISEASE

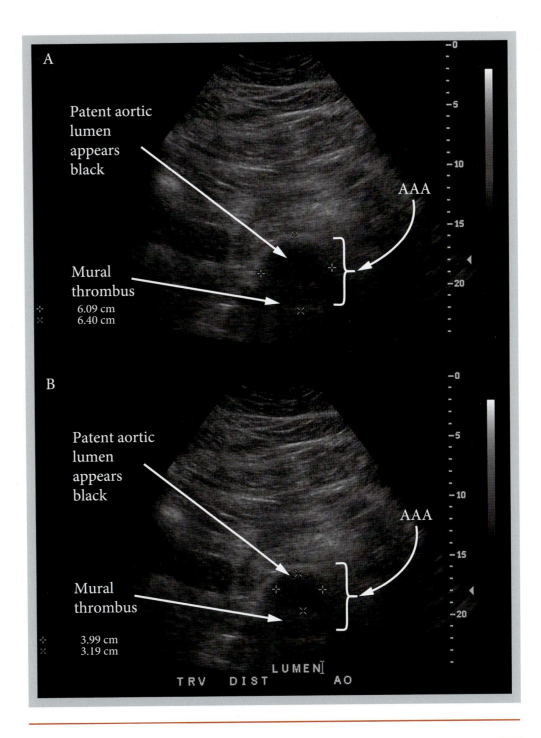

ABDOMINAL AORTIC ANEURYSM

Joshua S. Broder

Clinical Highlights

Abdominal aortic aneurysm (AAA) is defined by an abdominal aortic diameter greater than or equal to 3 cm. Aortic aneurysms occur as the elastic connective tissue of the aortic wall weakens, resulting in aortic dilatation. Risk factors include male gender, hypertension, smoking, advancing age, and family history. As the aortic diameter increases, the risk of rupture rises. Current recommendations call for elective repair of AAA ≥ 5.5 cm. Rupture of an aortic aneurysm can lead to immediate and catastrophic hemorrhagic shock. Clinical signs and symptoms of AAA rupture can include syncope or cardiac arrest, abdominal and/or back pain, lightheadedness, and hypotension. Classically, a pulsatile mass is present on exam, but the absence of this finding does not rule out the disease. More subtle presentations can include extremity or groin pain as well as neurologic symptoms related to spinal cord hypoperfusion.

In the United States, AAA rupture is among the top 15 causes of death in patients older than 60 years of age. Early mortality in AAA rupture is around 90% (including out of hospital deaths), and 20% to 30% with operative repair. Without repair, one in eight patients dies within 2 hours of arrival to the hospital.

Emergency Care and Disposition

When AAA rupture is suspected, immediate resuscitative steps should include large bore intravenous (IV) access, preoperative laboratory studies including type and cross-match for massive blood transfusion, and surgical consultation based on suspicion alone. Unstable patients should be considered for operative care before definitive diagnosis.

Bedside ultrasound can be used to assess the presence of AAA. Because ultrasound is relatively insensitive for rupture, the presence of AAA in a symptomatic patient should be considered a strong surrogate for rupture. When ultrasound is used, the entire abdominal aorta (from xiphoid process to the iliac bifurcation at the level of the umbilicus) and the proximal iliac arteries should be screened. The majority of AAAs are infrarenal. Care should be taken to identify intravascular mural thrombus, which should be included in the measurement of aortic diameter. If mural thrombus is not recognized in the lumen and the thrombus is mistaken as part of the aortic wall, aortic size may be underestimated and the diagnosis missed.

Hemodynamically stable patients can be considered for rapid computer tomographic (CT) assessment. CT without contrast media can detect the presence of AAA and AAA rupture. IV contrast can assist in delineating a subtle AAA leak and intravascular complications such as aortic dissection. Oral contrast is not needed for the diagnosis and introduces potentially fatal diagnostic delay.

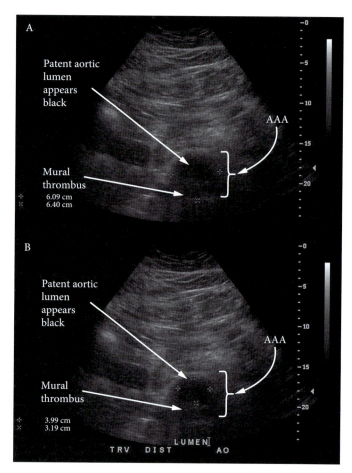

FIGURE 6.1 ■ (A) Ultrasound imaging of this acute aortic aneurysm (AAA) correctly measures the complete diameter (including mural thrombus) of the aorta at about 6 cm. (B) This ultrasound image underestimates the diameter of the aorta at about 4 cm because the patent lumen alone is measured.

ABDOMINAL AORTIC ANEURYSM (CONTINUED)

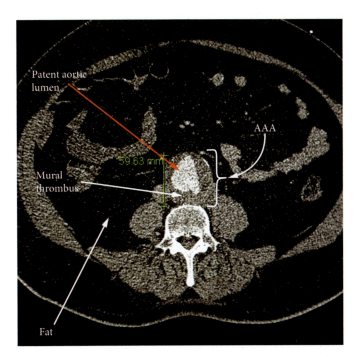

FIGURE 6.2 ■ IV contrast gives the patent aortic lumen a white appearance in this CT angiogram. Mural thrombus is also circumferentially visible at this level. The aortic diameter is about 6 cm. This aorta is not ruptured and is surrounded by fat.

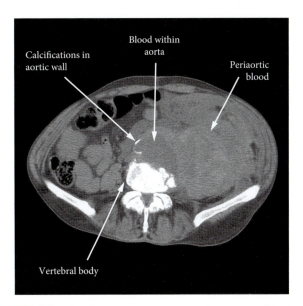

FIGURE 6.3 ■ A CT without contrast reveals a ruptured AAA. In this axial image, the aorta itself is hardly visible, but calcifications in the aortic wall (a common feature of AAA) are seen in the expected location of the aorta, anterior to a lumbar vertebral body. Blood within the aortic lumen appears dark gray in the absence of IV contrast. Blood that had already leaked from the aorta before the CT is partially clotted and appears lighter gray.

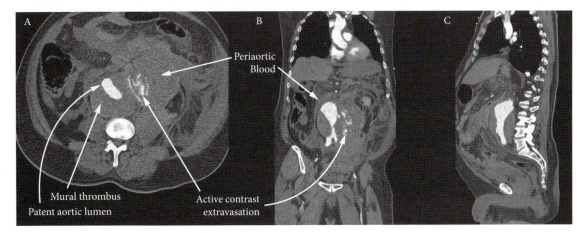

FIGURE 6.4 ■ A ruptured AAA is seen in the axial (**A**), coronal (**B**), and sagittal (**C**) reconstructions of this enhanced CT. In the axial image, blood within the aortic lumen appears bright white. Blood leaking from the aorta appears white because of active contrast extravasation. Mural thrombus within the aorta appears gray. Blood that had already leaked from the aorta before the administration of IV contrast appears gray.

Pearls and Pitfalls

- Due to similarities in the location and severity of pain, care should be taken not to mistake pain from a rupturing AAA for renal colic.
- Consult a surgeon immediately when AAA rupture is suspected, without delay for diagnostic confirmation.
- Prepare for immediate operative care with large bore IV access and massive blood transfusion.
- Assess the entire abdominal aorta with ultrasound, from xiphoid process to umbilicus, and include mural thrombus in diameter measurements to avoid underestimation of aortic size.

AORTIC DISSECTION

David James Story

Clinical Highlights

Aortic dissection is a rare disease process that carries a high rate of morbidity and mortality (27.7%). It occurs more commonly in males, African Americans, and individuals 50 to 65 years of age. Dissection occurs when an injury to the intima layer of the vessel allows for blood to tunnel into the wall of the artery, creating a false lumen.

Dissection may include the ascending aorta, aortic arch (Stanford Type A), and/or the descending aorta (Stanford Type B) with presenting complaints that vary based on the location. Typically, it is described as a sudden, severe, midsternal, tearing pain that radiates to the back and is often accompanied by nausea, vomiting, and syncope. If the injury extends into aortic tributaries or abdominal aorta, pain may be reported in the neck, jaw, arms, and/or abdomen. Neurological findings are present in up to 20% of patients and may include cerebral vascular accident, Horner syndrome, peripheral weakness or paresthesias, and altered mental status. Pericardial effusion and hypotension from tamponade can occur if the dissection originates near the aortic valve. Myocardial infarction can result concurrently if the dissection extends into the coronary arteries. Physical exam may reveal hypertension, hypotension, widened pulse pressures, asymmetric extremity blood pressures, diastolic murmurs, pulmonary crackles, muffled heart sounds, carotid bruits, and neurological abnormalities.

Emergency Care and Disposition

Diagnosis of aortic dissection is confirmed with radiographic imaging. Laboratory evaluation and electrocardiograms (ECG) typically rule out only alternative diagnoses that present similarly. Chest radiographs are abnormal in the majority of cases but consist of nondiagnostic findings, such as widening of the mediastinum. In the stable patient, CT angiography and magnetic resonance imaging (MRI) are highly sensitive and specific in identifying this vascular catastrophe. In an unstable patient, bedside transesophageal echocardiography (TEE) is the modality of choice for diagnosing aortic dissection.

Emergency care is centered on decreasing the shear stress present by controlling the blood pressure. The beta-blockers esmolol and labetalol are first-line treatments for blood

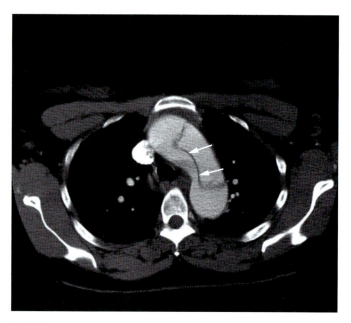

FIGURE 6.5 ■ An axial section of a chest CT through the aortic arch showing a clear intimal flap separating the true and false lumens (arrows).

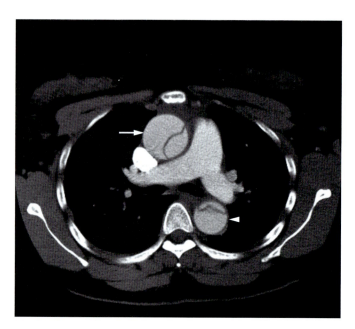

FIGURE 6.6 ■ An axial section of chest CT at the level of the right pulmonary artery showing a dissection affecting both the ascending (arrow) and descending aorta (arrowhead).

pressure control in aortic dissection. Esmolol is a pure beta antagonist administered via infusion allowing titration to effect, and often requires sequential administration of a vasodilator (ie, sodium nitroprusside) to achieve blood pressure goals. Labetalol is a mixed alpha/beta antagonist that can be

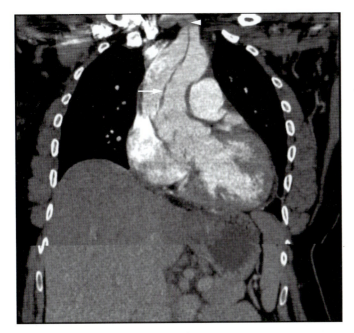

FIGURE 6.7 ■ A coronal section of chest CT scan shows the ascending aorta with a dissection flap (arrow) that extends into the brachiocephalic artery (arrowhead).

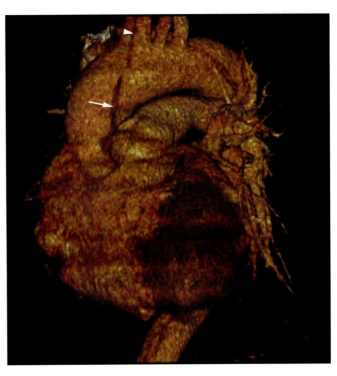

FIGURE 6.9 ■ A 3D reconstruction of a chest CT scan showing a Type A dissection. The intimal flap (arrow) can be seen in the ascending aorta and continuing into the brachiocephalic artery (arrowhead). The dissection continues in the descending aorta as well.

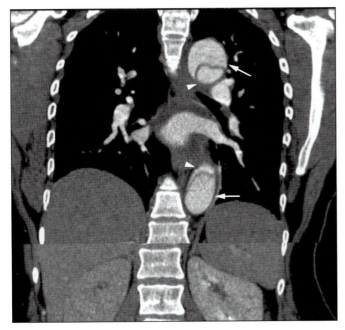

FIGURE 6.8 ■ A coronal view of a chest CT scan that catches two sections of the descending aorta with acute dissection. As is typical, the true lumen (arrowheads) is smaller than the false lumen (arrows), and as can be seen in the distal portion of the aorta, the true lumen is often crescent shaped, and the false lumen is oval or round.

used as a monotherapy, and is administered in bolus dosing or as an IV drip. The goal is the lowest systolic blood pressure that permits normal organ perfusion. Cardiothoracic surgery consultation is advised for all thoracic aortic dissections. Dissections involving the ascending aorta are treated surgically. Descending aortic dissections may be managed medically (most cases) or surgically in selected cases with aggressive blood pressure control in otherwise stable patients.

Pearls and Pitfalls

- Nifedipine, a calcium channel blocker, is not recommended for blood pressure treatment in aortic dissection because it can increase sympathetic outflow and shear stress on the vessel walls.
- Extremity exam should include evaluation of pulses and/or four extremity blood pressures to look for significant differences in arterial blood flow.
- A high index of suspicion is needed to diagnose aortic dissection as the presentation can vary greatly in location of pain and associated symptoms.

ACUTE ARTERIAL OCCLUSION

David James Story

Clinical Highlights

Acute arterial occlusion is a condition that carries high morbidity (13% amputation rate) and mortality (10%). It occurs when the blood supply to a distal part of the body (generally an extremity) is interrupted suddenly. This vascular compromise can be the result of thrombosis (50%) or an embolic event (50%). It most often affects the femoral (28%), brachial (20%), aortoiliac (18%), and popliteal artery (17%). Risk factors include peripheral arterial disease, atrial fibrillation, patent foramen ovale, hypercoagulable states, exogenous estrogen use, IV drug use, and smoking.

The diagnosis is primarily clinical. A typical patient will present with *pain*, *pallor*, and *pulselessness* (or diminished pulses) distal to the occlusion site, and may have *paresthesia*, *paralysis*, and *poikilothermia* (in this setting, cool extremity); "the 6 P's" of acute limb ischemia.

A Doppler ultrasound should be used to evaluate for any distal blood flow of an extremity where no pulse is palpated. Paresthesias and paralysis are late signs in the disease and correlate with prolonged occlusion and increased morbidity.

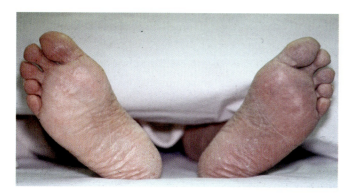

FIGURE 6.10 ■ Arterial embolus. Note the pallor of this patient's right foot, consistent with an acute arterial embolus, in this case is secondary to femoral artery occlusion. Photo contributor: Lawrence B. Stack, MD. Reproduced, with permission, from Chapter 12. Tubbs RJ, Savitt DL, Suner S. Extremity conditions. In: Knoop KJ, Stack LB, Storrow AB, Thurman R, eds. *The Atlas of Emergency Medicine*. 3rd ed. New York, NY: McGraw-Hill; 2010.

The ability to salvage the extremity decreases after 4 to 6 hours. The ankle-brachial index (ABI) is a sensitive bedside test. Using a blood pressure cuff, place a Doppler ultrasound at the brachial artery and record the pressure of occlusion. Repeat the procedure on the leg, measuring the occlusion pressure of the posterior tibial and dorsalis pedis arteries. The ABI is the highest leg occlusion pressure divided by the arm occlusion pressure; normal ABI is >0.9. A ratio lower than 0.41 is usually found in limbs with critical ischemia.

Emergency Care and Disposition

If acute limb ischemia is suspected clinically, a vascular surgeon should be consulted urgently before confirmatory imaging. Basic preoperative blood tests should be obtained. Arterial angiography is the gold standard and can be utilized to help determine etiology behind source of occlusion. CT or magnetic resonance (MR) angiography may also be utilized to confirm occlusion. Ultrasound is noninvasive but provides less information to guide the surgical approach.

Systemic anticoagulation with heparin is the mainstay of emergency department (ED) treatment. Consult vascular surgery regardless of the etiology. Thrombectomy or embolectomy needs to be performed rapidly to save the ischemic extremity. Identification of the source of an embolus is critical to preventing repeat occlusions. Treatment with intra-arterial thrombolytic therapy has shown to have potential benefits as an alternative to immediate surgery, but still requires trained interventional specialists.

Pearls and Pitfalls

- Aortic dissection can mimic an acute arterial occlusion that has extended into an extremity vessel; do not miss the correct diagnosis.
- AAAs can be the source of lower extremity emboli and should be considered.
- A history of venous thromboembolic disease does not directly predispose to acute arterial occlusion unless coagulopathy or patent foramen ovale is present.
- Inadvertent injection of drugs of abuse into the arterial system may result in acute occlusion.

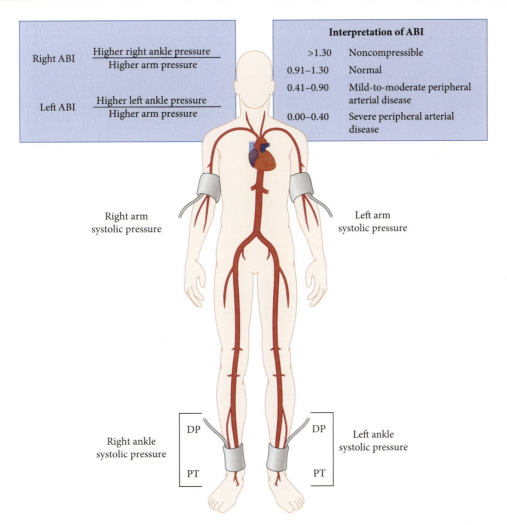

FIGURE 6.11 ■ Measurement of the ABI. Measure the systolic blood pressure using Doppler ultrasound in each arm and in the dorsalis pedis (DP) and posterior tibial (PT) arteries in each ankle. Select the higher of the two arm pressures (right vs. left) and the higher of the two pressures in the ankle (DP vs. PT). Determine the right and left ABI values by dividing the higher ankle pressure in each leg by the higher arm pressure. The ranges of the ABI and the interpretation are shown in the figure. In the case of a noncompressible calcified vessel, the true pressure at that location cannot be obtained, and alternative tests are required to diagnose peripheral arterial disease. Patients with claudication typically have ABI values ranging from 0.41 to 0.90, and those with critical leg ischemia have values <0.41. Reproduced, with permission, from Chapter 64. Chopra A, Carr D. Occlusive arterial disease. In: Tintinalli JE, Stapczynski J, Ma O, Cline DM, Cydulka RK, Meckler GD, eds. *Tintinalli's Emergency Medicine: A Comprehensive Study Guide.* 7th ed. New York, NY: McGraw-Hill; 2011.

DVT: UPPER/LOWER, PHLEGMASIA ALBA DOLENS, PHLEGMASIA CERULEA DOLENS

Derick M. Wenning

Clinical Highlights

The most common presenting complaints of a patient with deep vein thrombosis (DVT) include pain, redness, swelling, warmth, and tenderness of the affected extremity. Unfortunately, clinical symptoms are unreliable when predicting whether or not a patient has a DVT, and multiple risk factors exist for identifying who should be worked up for potential DVT. The highest risk of venous thrombosis occurs with past history of venous thrombosis, recent trauma, prolonged immobilization, recent travel, malignancy, and hereditary thrombophilia—most commonly Factor V Leiden (see Table 6.1). Physical findings vary and depend on the location degree of venous obstruction. Phlegmasia cerulea dolens is a rare presentation with massive iliofemoral thrombosis, and these patients present with an extensively swollen, painful, and cyanotic lower extremity. This amount of clot burden can compromise blood flow distally to the foot leading to bullae formation and gangrene. Phlegmasia alba dolens is also due to massive iliofemoral thrombosis. In this presentation, the extremity appears pale and white secondary to arterial vasospasm. Phlegmasia alba dolens has a common association with pregnancy.

Alternative diagnoses with similar presentation include congestive heart failure, cellulitis, myositis, fracture, superficial thrombophlebitis, lymphedema, and ruptured Baker cyst.

FIGURE 6.12 ■ Swelling and blue discoloration of the left lower extremity consistent with phlegmasia cerulea dolens in a patient with DVT. Reproduced, with permission, from Chapter 12. Tubbs RJ, Savitt DL, Suner S. Extremity conditions. In: Knoop KJ, Stack LB, Storrow AB, Thurman R, eds. *The Atlas of Emergency Medicine*. 3rd ed. New York, NY: McGraw-Hill; 2010.

Emergency Care and Disposition

The most widely accepted diagnostic test of choice for DVT is duplex ultrasonography. A quantitative D-dimer may only be used to screen select low-risk patients for DVT. Other studies for DVT include impedance plethysmography, radionuclide scintigraphy, CT venography, and MR venography. Traditional contrast venography is considered the "gold standard" for detection but is invasive and is rarely used due to diagnostic accuracy of other tests. Treatment of DVT is aimed toward prevention of thromboembolism—mainly pulmonary embolism (PE). Anticoagulation with heparin or LMWH (low-molecular-weight heparin) while bridging to oral anticoagulation with warfarin is the mainstay of treatment. LMWH has allowed outpatient management of select patients diagnosed with DVT due to its once-daily dosing. LMWH has very predictable effects and does not require routine

TABLE 6.1 ■ RISK FACTORS FOR DVT

Acquired	Inherited
Recent major surgery—especially orthopedic with immobilization	Factor V Leiden
Oral contraceptives or hormone replacement therapy	Antithrombin deficiency
Trauma	Protein C deficiency
Previous history of DVT	Protein S deficiency
Older age	Antiphospholipid antibody
Nephrotic syndrome	
Recent travel	
Smoking	

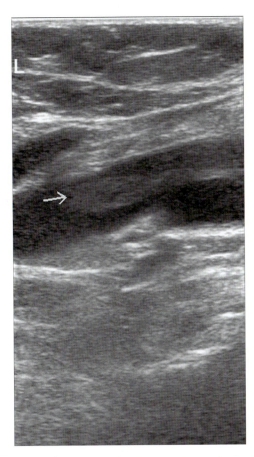

FIGURE 6.13 ■ Venous Doppler ultrasound for DVT. In this long-axis view, note the echogenic thrombus within the lumen of the popliteal vein.

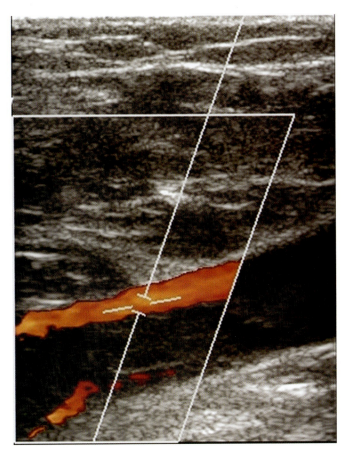

FIGURE 6.14 ■ Venous Doppler ultrasound with color flow. Here you can see the thrombus obstructing flow through the common femoral vein.

blood tests except in the setting of renal insufficiency. Patients with contraindications to anticoagulation are often admitted for inferior vena cava filter insertion.

Pearls and Pitfalls

- Occult malignancy screening as an outpatient is indicated for patients with unexplained DVT.
- Warfarin is initially a procoagulant due to inhibition of Protein C and S. Bridging therapy is required with heparin or LMWH.
- IV drug use and ipsilateral long term IV lines are risk factors for upper extremity DVT.
- The formation of a DVT is due to the presence of at least one of Virchow Triad: stasis, endothelial damage, or hypercoagulability.

PULMONARY EMBOLISM

James C. O'Neill

Clinical Highlights

PE occurs when a blood clot formed in the venous system (most commonly in the lower extremity) dislodges and travels through the heart to lodge in the pulmonary artery circulation. PE causes 250,000 hospitalizations a year, with a 3-month disease-specific mortality rate of 10%, and an initial clinical presentation of sudden death in 20% of patients. Clinical danger to the patient is dependent on the size and location of the clot as well as the patient's comorbidities and ability to compensate for the strain placed on the circulatory system. Risk factors for developing a PE include recent surgery, immobilization, use of exogenous estrogens, and familial clotting disorders. Classically, the patient presents with chest pain, dyspnea, and occasionally, hemoptysis. Syncope occurs if the clot burden causes significant strain on the cardiac circulation, sometimes as the only patient complaint. Unfortunately, presentation may be quite vague, such as chest pain or dyspnea alone.

The ECG is rarely diagnostic in patients with PE and most commonly shows sinus tachycardia. Findings of right heart strain should raise concern for PE and include T-wave inversions in anterior precordial leads, right bundle branch block, and the S1Q3T3 pattern (S wave in lead I, q wave in lead III, and a flipped t wave in lead III).

Multiple decision rules have been developed to assess for PE risk, including Wells criteria, Wicki Criteria (Geneva Rule), and pulmonary embolism rule-out criteria (PERC) scores. Patients deemed low risk could be screened with a D-dimer laboratory assay. PE is most commonly confirmed with computed tomography pulmonary angiography (CTPA) using an IV contrast bolus specifically timed for viewing pulmonary arteries. Another less preferred imaging modality is a ventilation/perfusion nuclear medicine scan.

VIDEO 6.1 ■ This CT scan of the chest is a PE protocol that shows bilateral PEs (shown by red arrows). View at http://mhprofessional.com/sites/lefebvre

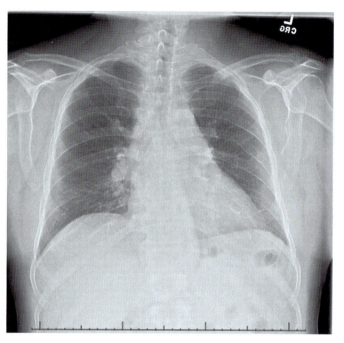

FIGURE 6.15 ■ All images in this section are from the same patient with a massive bilateral PE. Chest x-ray is usually normal in PE as shown here, but can show an area of wedge-shaped infiltrate or infarction (Hampton hump) or enlarged right descending pulmonary artery (Palla sign).

The differential diagnosis is wide, but includes acute coronary syndrome, aortic dissection, pneumonia, and pneumothorax. Having one of these other diagnoses does not exclude having a PE.

Emergency Care and Disposition

Treatment relies on stopping the generation of clot burden. IV heparin or enoxaparin intramuscular injections are the mainstays of treatment. These medications are continued until the patient can be transitioned to warfarin therapy. Consider tissue plasminogen activator (tPA) for patients having severe hemodynamic instability, severe right heart strain on echocardiogram, and elevated troponin levels due to heart strain. Patients that fail long-term anticoagulation efforts and have a second PE will often receive an inferior vena cava filter.

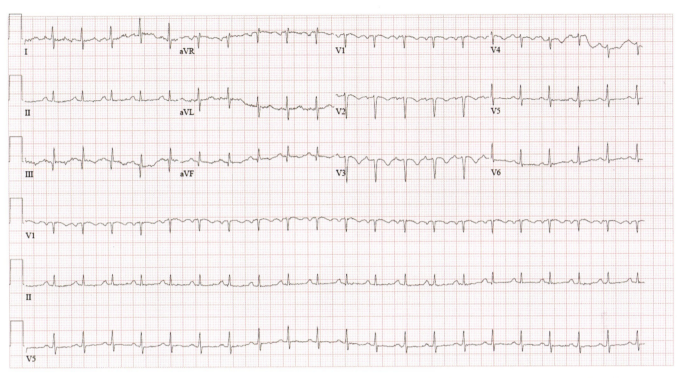

FIGURE 6.16 ■ Sinus tachycardia is commonly found on patients with PE. This ECG also shows a prominent S waves in lead I, Q waves in lead III, and a flipped T waves in lead III (S1Q3T3).

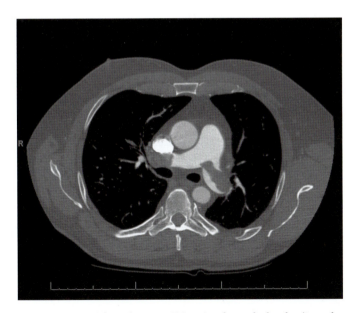

FIGURE 6.17 ■ This pulmonary CT section shows clot burden (irregular dark areas surrounded by white contrast) in bilateral pulmonary arteries.

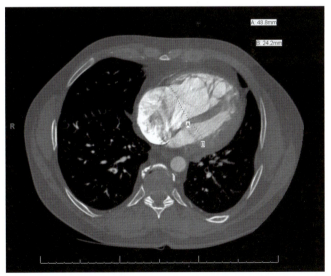

FIGURE 6.18 ■ This view of the CT angiogram is consistent with right heart strain, with dilated right ventricle at 48.8 mm, due to the massive PE.

180 ▪ PULMONARY EMBOLISM (CONTINUED)

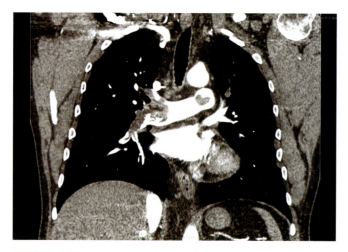

FIGURE 6.19 ▪ This coronal view of the same patient shows clot burden (irregular dark areas surrounded by white contrast) in bilateral pulmonary arteries.

Pearls and Pitfalls

- PE should be considered in all patients with chest pain, dyspnea, or syncope. Careful use of decision rules can help exclude the diagnosis or select patients for further testing.
- D-dimer tests should not be a screening tool for patients deemed moderate to high risk.
- Treatment should be started if there is high clinical suspicion of PE and imaging is delayed.

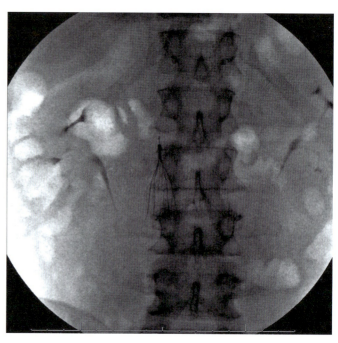

FIGURE 6.20 ▪ The patient that suffered these massive pulmonary emboli received this Greenfield filter placed in the inferior vena cava after treatment.

- If it is desired to avoid radiation or contrast bolus (pregnancy or contrast allergy), physicians can first perform lower extremity Doppler ultrasound looking for DVT because treatment for DVT and PE is the same.

SYSTEMIC AND PULMONARY HYPERTENSION

David M. Cline

Clinical Highlights

Systemic hypertension

The most common symptom of systemic hypertension is a lightheaded feeling or dizziness. Some patients report headache or blurred vision. Patients with hypertensive emergency have more specific symptoms reflecting the presence of end-organ damage (see Table 6.2).

TABLE 6.2 ■ HYPERTENSIVE EMERGENCIES

Diagnostic Category	Signs and Symptoms	Evidence of Acute End-Organ Damage
Acute aortic dissection	Chest pain, back pain Unequal blood pressures (>20 mm Hg in extremities)	Abnormal CT angiogram
Acute pulmonary edema	Shortness of breath	Interstitial edema on chest radiograph (see Chap. 3, section on Chest Radiographs)
Acute coronary syndrome	Chest pain, nausea, vomiting, diaphoresis	Changes on ECG (see Chap. 2, Acute Ischemia and Chronic Disease) or elevated biomarkers
Acute renal failure	May have systolic or diastolic abdominal bruit	Elevated serum creatinine level, proteinuria
Hypertensive retinopathy	Blurred vision	Retinal hemorrhages and cotton-wool spots hard exudates, and sausage-shaped veins
Hypertensive encephalopathy	Altered mental status, nausea, vomiting, headache, seizures	May see papilledema or retinopathy (see previous row) or changes on MRI
Subarachnoid hemorrhage	Headache, focal neurologic deficits, vomiting, syncope	Abnormal CT of the brain; red blood cells on lumbar puncture
Intracranial hemorrhage	Headache, new neurologic deficits	Abnormal CT of the brain
Acute ischemic stroke	New neurologic deficits	Abnormal MRI or CT of the brain

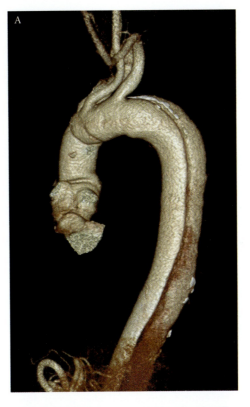

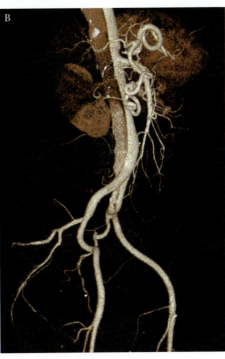

FIGURE 6.21 ■ (A) CT Angiogram, 3D volume rendering of Stanford Type B aortic dissection extending from just distal to left subclavian artery origin into the abdominal aorta. (B) Continuation of 3D CT angiogram showing dissection below the aortic bifurcation to left common iliac artery. The patient presented with severe back pain and elevated blood pressure (186/112 mm Hg).

SYSTEMIC AND PULMONARY HYPERTENSION (CONTINUED)

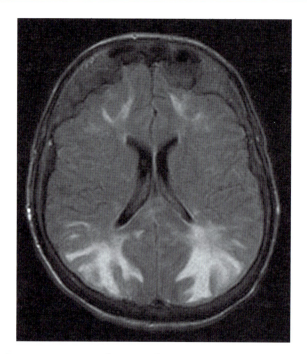

FIGURE 6.22 ■ MRI showing white matter hyperintensity in the occipital lobes bilaterally consistent with posterior reversible encephalopathy syndrome (PRES). The patient's confusion improved with blood pressure control. Repeat MRI after several days of therapy demonstrated remarkable improvement.

Pulmonary hypertension

Patients with severe pulmonary hypertension may present to the ED critically ill with signs and symptoms of right heart failure. Risks include chronic hypoxic lung disease, genetic disorders, certain toxin or drug exposures, liver disease, valvular heart disease, collagen vascular disorders, and pulmonary embolic disease. The most common symptom is dyspnea, followed by fatigue, chest pain, syncope, orthopnea, paroxysmal nocturnal dyspnea, and peripheral edema. Transthoracic echocardiography may be the best initial diagnostic test to evaluate and treat the ED patient with pulmonary hypertension. Decreased right ventricular function, right atrial hypertrophy, and right ventricular hypertrophy are indicative of more severe disease. Additional echocardiogram findings in patients with severe pulmonary hypertension include leftward deviation of the intraventricular septum and a right ventricle-to-left ventricle end-diastolic diameter ratio >1 in the four-chamber view.

ED Care and Disposition

Updated guideline decision points for the treatment of patients with systemic hypertension were published in 2014

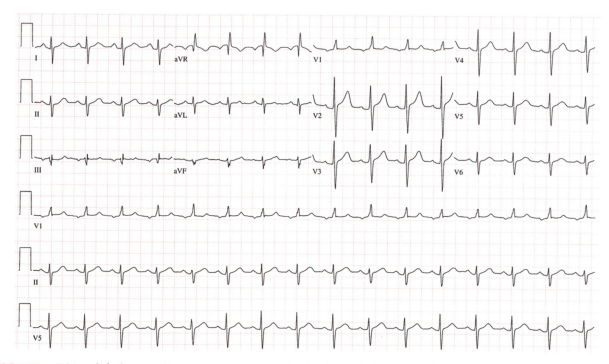

FIGURE 6.23 ■ ECG with findings predictive of pulmonary hypertension: S wave in V1 <2 mm, R/S ratio in V1 >1, R/S ratio in V6 <1, QRS axis >110°. Reproduced, with permission, from Chapter 61. Cline DM, Machado AJ. Systemic and pulmonary hypertension. In: Tintinalli JE, Stapczynski J, Ma O, Cline DM, Cydulka RK, Meckler GD, eds. *Tintinalli's Emergency Medicine: A Comprehensive Study Guide*. 7th ed. New York, NY: McGraw-Hill; 2011.

SYSTEMIC AND PULMONARY HYPERTENSION (CONTINUED)

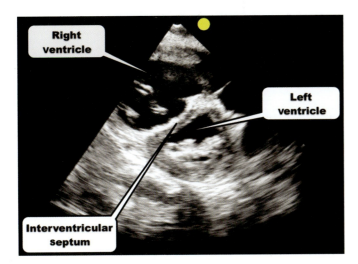

FIGURE 6.24 ■ Parasternal short-axis view of right and left ventricles of a patient with pulmonary hypertension. Notice the flattening of the interventricular septum occurring in systole, suggesting elevated right ventricular systolic pressures. This is also known as a "D"-shaped septum. Courtesy of Haney Mallemat, MD, in the Department of Emergency Medicine at the University of Maryland School of Medicine.

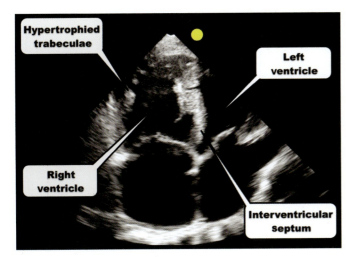

FIGURE 6.25 ■ Apical four-chamber view showing right and left ventricles of a patient with pulmonary hypertension. The right ventricle is dilated with hypertrophy of the right ventricular trabeculae, indicating chronic right ventricular overload. The interventricular septum is also shifted toward the left ventricle in systole suggesting right ventricular pressure overload. Courtesy of Haney Mallemat, MD, in the Department of Emergency Medicine at the University of Maryland School of Medicine.

and are given in Table 6.3. Recommended drugs for specific situations are given in Table 6.4.

Treatment of pulmonary hypertension is primarily treatment of the underlying condition associated with pulmonary hypertension. Therapy may include supplemental oxygen, optimizing intravascular volume, augmenting right ventricular function, maintaining coronary artery perfusion, and decreasing right ventricular afterload.

Pearls and Pitfalls

- The decision to treat a patient with hypertension in the ED should be primarily driven by the patient's symptoms and end-organ injury, rather than absolute numbers measured.
- In the patient with severe pulmonary hypertension, intubation with positive-pressure ventilation, and the effects of sedative medications on right ventricular function and systemic vascular resistance, may result in cardiovascular collapse.
- Beware of deterioration in a patient with pulmonary hypertension receiving repeated fluid boluses; recheck the patient after each 500 mL of fluid therapy.

TABLE 6.3 ■ DECISION POINTS FOR INITIATION OF TREATMENT OF CHRONIC HYPERTENSION

Population	Treatment Decision Point for Systolic Blood Pressure	Treatment Decision Point for Diastolic Blood Pressure	Strength of Evidence
General population aged ≥60 years	150 mm Hg	90 mm Hg	Grade A
General population 30–59 years old	See bottom row	90 mm Hg	Grade A
General population 18–29 years old	See bottom row	90 mm Hg	Grade E
General population 18–59 years old	140 mm Hg	See rows above	Grade E

Grade A, strong recommendation; Grade E, expert opinion.

TABLE 6.4 ■ TREATMENT RECOMMENDATIONS

Population	Recommended Agents	Therapeutic Targets
General nonblack population, including those with diabetes	A thiazide-type diuretic, CCB, ACEI, or ARB	Pressure below decision point in Table 6.3
General black population, including those with diabetes	Thiazide-type diuretic or CCB	Pressure below decision point in Table 6.3
Population aged ≥18 years with chronic kidney disease	ACEI or ARB	Pressure below decision point in Table 6.3
Aortic dissection	Esmolol labetalol, nicardipine, nitroprusside (start with beta-blocker)	SBP 100–120 mm Hg
Subarachnoid hemorrhage	Nicardipine, labetalol,	SBP <160 mm Hg to prevent rebleeding
Intracerebral hemorrhage	Nicardipine, labetalol,	SBP<200 or MAP<150 mm Hg
Acute ischemic stroke: candidate for reperfusion therapy	Labetalol, nicardipine	If fibrinolytic therapy planned, <185/110 mm Hg
Acute ischemic stroke, not a reperfusion candidate	Labetalol, nicardipine	<220/120 mm Hg
Acute hypertensive pulmonary edema	Nitroglycerin, enalaprilat, nicardipine, nitroprusside	Reduction of BP by 20%–30%.
Acute renal failure	Labetalol, nicardipine, fenoldopam,	Reduction of BP by no more than 20% acutely
Hypertensive encephalopathy	Labetalol, nicardipine, fenoldopam,	Decrease MAP by 20%–25%

ACEI, angiotensin-converting enzyme inhibitor; ARB, angiotensin receptor blocker; CCB, calcium channel blocker; DBP, diastolic blood pressure; MAP, mean arterial pressure; SBP, systolic blood pressure.

LEFT VENTRICULAR ANEUYRSM

Joshua S. Broder

Clinical Highlights

Left ventricular (LV) aneurysm results from transmural myocardial infarction of the left ventricle, with myocardial thinning, scar formation, and regional enlargement of the ventricular chamber. LV aneurysm is one of several causes of ST-segment elevation on ECG, mimicking acute myocardial infarction. Patients with LV aneurysm will typically display persistent ST-segment elevation in an ECG distribution consistent with a previous transmural myocardial infarction.

In the absence of the complications described below, LV aneurysm is usually asymptomatic. Electrocardiographic findings may be incidentally noted on an ECG obtained for unrelated reasons such as preoperative evaluation. The differential diagnosis of ST-segment elevation on ECG includes acute myocardial infarction, pericarditis, early repolarization, LV aneurysm, and LV pseudoaneurysm. The latter is similar to LV aneurysm but with complete disruption of the myocardium, such that the integrity of the ventricular wall is precariously preserved only by pericardial adhesions and hematoma. Complications of LV aneurysm include ventricular thrombus with or without systemic embolization, dysrhythmia, diminished ejection fraction, and myocardial free wall perforation resulting in pericardial tamponade. True LV aneurysms are more likely to rupture in the acute phase following acute myocardial infarction, whereas LV pseudoaneurysms may rupture at any time and should be surgically repaired.

Emergency Care and Disposition

If an ECG suggests LV aneurysm, echocardiography can be performed to confirm aneurysm, to differentiate true aneurysm from pseudoaneurysm, and to rule out complications such as ventricular thrombus, free wall rupture, and pericardial effusion or tamponade. Evaluation for acute myocardial ischemia is often indicated, even in the absence of ischemic symptoms, because of the possibility of "silent" ischemia. The current ECG should be compared with prior ECGs and with additional serial ECGs to monitor changes. In the absence of evidence for acute ischemia, dysrhythmia, symptomatically impaired ejection fraction, or other serious complications,

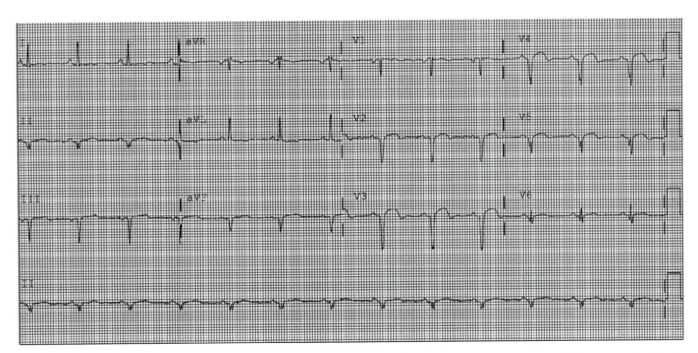

FIGURE 6.26 ■ This ECG from an asymptomatic 79-year-old male presenting for preoperative assessment reveals ST-segment elevation in leads V2–V5, suggesting acute myocardial infarction. The patient's prior ECGs did not demonstrate these findings. Serial cardiac markers were negative and an echocardiogram confirmed LV aneurysm.

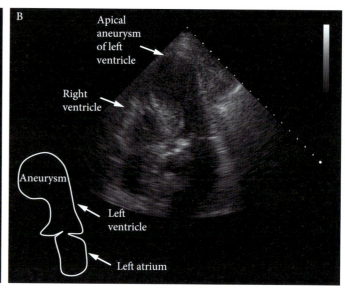

FIGURES 6.27 ■ This echocardiogram shows ventricles in diastole (**A**) and systole (**B**). The right ventricle contracts normally and thus appears smaller in systole (**B**) than in diastole (**A**). The left ventricle has an apical aneurysm, which severely impairs the LV ejection fraction. Notice that the chamber does not significantly change in size between diastole and systole, indicating a noncontractile portion of the ventricle.

chronic LV aneurysm alone is not an indication for admission or repair. When echocardiography is not diagnostic, cardiac CT or MRI can be used to evaluate for LV aneurysm.

Pearls and Pitfalls

- Suspect LV aneurysm in a patient with regional ST-segment elevation on ECG but no signs or symptoms of acute myocardial infarction.
- Consider the complications of LV aneurysm including thrombus formation, dysrhythmia, and free wall rupture with pericardial tamponade.
- Always consider acute myocardial infarction as the cause for ST-segment elevation, rather than assuming that ST-segment changes reflect LV aneurysm.

VIDEO 6.2 ■ Echocardiogram video of the same patient depicted in Figures 6.26 and 6.27. Refer to the still images in Figure 6.27 for outlines of the right ventricle, left atrium, and left ventricle expanding into LV aneurysm. Note the relative lack of movement of the wall surrounding the distal aneurysm at the top of the screen compared to the active contraction of the right ventricle and the proximal portions of the left ventricle. View at http://mhprofessional.com/sites/lefebvre

Chapter 7
CARDIOMYOPATHIES

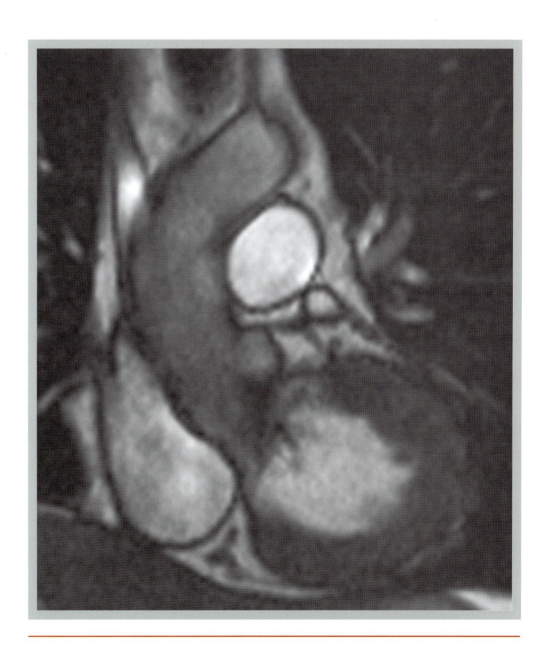

DILATED CARDIOMYOPATHY

Jieun Kim
W. Frank Peacock

Clinical Highlights

The most common ED presentation of patients with dilated cardiomyopathy is decompensated heart failure (HF). Dyspnea is the most common complaint. Other complaints suggesting HF include dyspnea on exertion, orthopnea, peripheral edema, weight gain, paroxysmal nocturnal dyspnea, cough, and fatigue. Because HF may be preceded by myocardial ischemia, risk factors for coronary artery disease should be ascertained. Conditions that worsen or precipitate HF should be considered in the differential diagnosis and include myocardial ischemia, uncontrolled hypertension, arrhythmias, dietary, and medication noncompliance. Physical examination assists in evaluating HF, with vital signs and airway stability being paramount. Pulmonary rales, peripheral edema, jugular venous distention, hepatojugular reflux, and the presence of extra heart sounds identify fluid overload. Skin mottling, indicating poor perfusion, is associated with increased acute mortality.

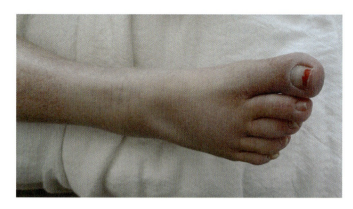

FIGURE 7.2 ■ This patient also had peripheral edema in the lower extremities demonstrated by the "pitting" that remains after gentle pressure to distal ankle and lateral proximal dorsal foot.

Appropriate testing includes an electrocardiogram (ECG) to evaluate myocardial ischemia, a chest x-ray (CXR) to assess for pulmonary edema, and lab testing for troponin, natriuretic peptide levels, renal function, electrolytes, and hemoglobin.

The salient differential diagnoses include other conditions manifesting as acute dyspnea (pulmonary embolism, chronic obstructive pulmonary disease exacerbation, or pneumonia), pathology presenting as acute volume overload or edema

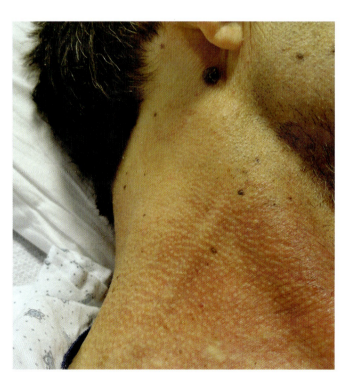

FIGURE 7.1 ■ This photograph shows a patient with jugular venous distension.

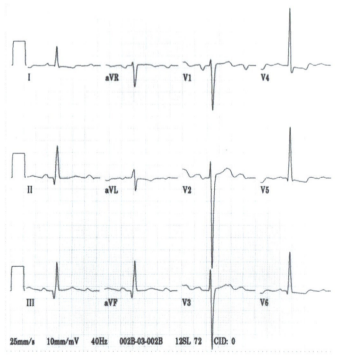

FIGURE 7.3 ■ The ECG demonstrates sinus tachycardia, without diagnostic acute ischemic changes, although there was evidence of left ventricular hypertrophy.

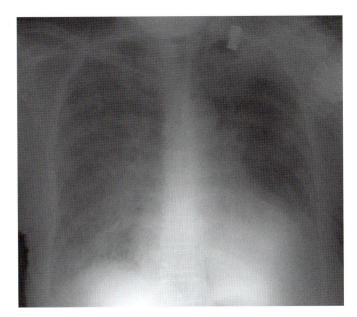

FIGURE 7.4 ■ This portable CXR demonstrates cardiomegaly, as determined by the measuring the widest width of the cardiac silhouette and dividing by the widest horizontal width of the chest from right to left pleural surface; a ratio over 0.5 meets criteria for cardiomegaly. The CXR also demonstrates pulmonary vascular congestion represented by the increased diameter of the pulmonary vessels and their hazy contours, including pulmonary vessels in the middle and upper lung fields, especially on the right side for this patient.

(eg, renal failure and liver failure), and pump failure resulting from acute myocardial infarction (AMI), acute valve dysfunction, or pericardial disease.

ED Care and Disposition

At initial presentation, the patient's airway should be evaluated and the need for noninvasive ventilation or endotracheal intubation considered. Hypertensive HF responds remarkably well to vasodilation, which may be performed via sublingual nitroglycerin until intravenous (IV) access is obtained. IV nitroglycerin is well tolerated and large doses may be required for relief of symptoms. Patients may initially be in extremis and may require rapid resuscitation. Conversely, inotropes may be indicated in the setting of symptomatic hypotension. In the volume-overloaded patient, loop diuretics may be administered after blood pressure control has been obtained, but are not necessarily critical upon initial presentation due to relatively slow onset of effect.

Disposition is dependent on the interventions required, with ICU admission indicated if airway control or vasoactive agents are necessary. Additionally, comorbidities may also prompt similar placement. The presence of coexistent renal insufficiency is particularly ominous, and identifies a cohort in whom aggressive therapy is required, as does elevated troponin, unstable vital signs, or markedly high natriuretic peptide levels. The absence of these findings, coupled with initial hypertension and symptoms that respond to therapy, identifies a cohort that is likely to be successfully managed in a 24-hour short stay unit.

Pearls and Pitfalls

- Failure to aggressively treat hypertension may result in respiratory arrest.
- Negative natriuretic peptides effectively rule out the presence of myocardial strain. However, as ventricular strain occurs in many conditions (eg, AMI and acute pulmonary embolus), elevated levels must be considered in clinical context; natriuretic peptides are falsely lowered in obesity and elevated in renal injury.

RESTRICTIVE CARDIOMYOPATHIES

Kristi Colbenson
Sean Collins

Clinical Highlights

Restrictive cardiomyopathy (RCM) is a biventricular diastolic dysfunction without ventricular dilation or hypertrophy. It is a rare form of heart failure (HF) caused by pathologic inflammation, thrombosis, infiltration, and fibrosis within the myocardium and endocardium. RCMs are classified as primary or secondary. These underlying disease processes lead to restrictive filling, reduced diastolic volume, and though systolic function is preserved, a reduced cardiac output. Patients clinically present with classic acute HF signs and symptoms (Table 7.1). Diagnostically, ECG findings include low voltage and conduction abnormalities. Unique to RCM is that the chest x-ray (CXR) lacks cardiomegaly until late in the disease when bi-atrial enlargement leads to the appearance of cardiomegaly. Bedside ultrasound will reveal a normal left ventricle with preserved systolic function. Formal echocardiogram findings include a restrictive pattern of ventricular filling (early diastolic filling velocity and decreased isovolumic relaxation time) with increased atrial contribution. Ultimate diagnosis lies in a myocardial biopsy.

The differential diagnosis includes aortic stenosis, cardiac tamponade, hypertrophic cardiomyopathy, hypertensive heart disease, and constrictive pericarditis. Nearly identical in presentation, differentiating constrictive pericarditis from RCM is difficult, but imperative, as constrictive pericarditis is curable through surgical intervention. Constrictive pericarditis will have a low natriuretic peptide level compared to elevated levels in RCM. Also, calcifications on CXR are specific for constrictive pericarditis.

ED Care and Disposition

The mainstay of treatment is supportive, as no existing treatment improves long-term outcome. The goals of therapy are to reduce symptoms of diastolic dysfunction while maintaining cardiac output and controlling for possible complications. Low to medium dose diuretics improve systemic and pulmonary congestion from diastolic dysfunction. However, cautious diuresis must be employed as RCM requires high diastolic pressures to maintain cardiac output. Small changes in filing pressures dramatically reduce cardiac index. Routine use of beta and calcium channel blockers is debatable in RCM due to deleterious effects on blood pressure and right ventricle function. However, in the setting of tachycardia, calcium channel blockers are used to improve rate control and maximize diastolic function by improving ventricular relaxation and increasing ventricular filling time.

Anatomic changes in RCM predispose patients to arrhythmias and thromboembolic events. Atrial fibrillation is the most common complication in RCM, and is disastrous due to loss of atrial contraction needed to maintain preload. First-line treatment is amiodarone, as it maintains cardiac output. Digoxin can be used, but is contraindicated in amyloidosis as it precipitates arrhythmias. Cardioversion must be used with caution as infiltrative processes damage the intrinsic

TABLE 7.1 ■ SIGNS AND SYMPTOMS OF ACUTE HEART FAILURE IN RESTRICTIVE CARDIOMYOPAHTY

LV Diastolic Dysfunction	RV Diastolic Dysfunction	Decreased Cardiac Index	General
Paroxysmal nocturnal dyspnea	Ascites and peripheral edema	Fatigue	Angina: seen primarily in amyloidosis due to coronary artery infiltration
Orthopnea	Jugular venous distention	Dyspnea on exertion	Atrial fibrillation
Dyspnea	Rapid X and Y descents of the jugular wave form	Exercise intolerance	Thromboembolic events
S3 gallop	Regurgitant v wave of tricuspid regurgitation.	Syncope	Arrhythmias and conductive disturbances
Right ventricular heave from pulmonary hypertension	Kussmaul sign	Decreased radial pulse	Clinical signs of hemachromatosis, scleroderma, sarcoidoisis, or amyloidosis
	S3 gallop		Bilateral pleural effusions: common in amlyoidosis
	Peripheral edema		

RESTRICTIVE CARDIOMYOPATHIES (CONTINUED)

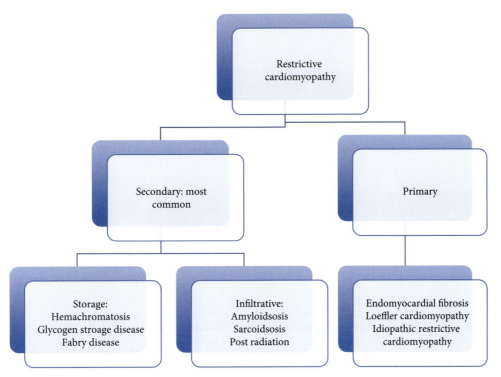

FIGURE 7.5 ■ Etiologies of restrictive cardiomyopathies.

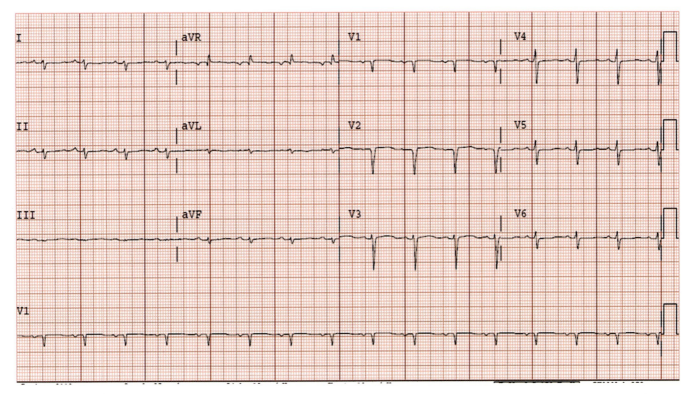

FIGURE 7.6 ■ ECG with low voltage from diffuse myocardial infiltration. Other ECG findings to look for in patients with RCM but not shown here include bundle branch blocks, atrioventricular blocks, and atrial/ventricular dysrhythmia from infiltration in the cardiac conduction pathway; pathologic Q waves caused by healing granulomas in sarcoidosis; and peaked and wide P waves due to atrial enlargement.

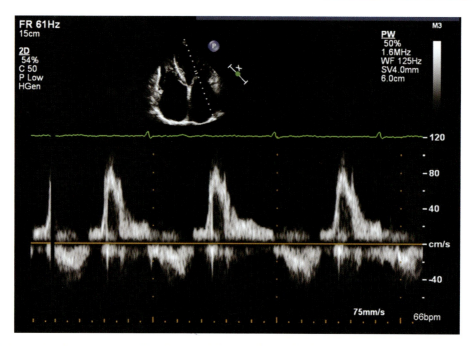

FIGURE 7.7 ■ Apical four-chamber view on cardiac ultrasound showing bi-atrial enlargement and normal ventricle size. M-mode through the mitral valve revealing restrictive filling pattern: high-peaked E (early diastolic filling), short E deceleration time (rapid filling), small a wave (reduced atrial contribution to filling), and increased E/A ratio.

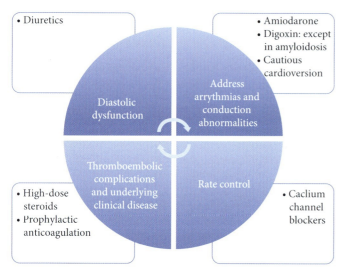

FIGURE 7.8 ■ Goals of treatment for RCM include addressing pulmonary and systemic congestion from diastolic dysfunction, maximizing diastolic function and cardiac output through rate and rhythm control, and controlling for thromboembolic complications and underlysing disease exacerbation.

pacemaker; thus, cardioversion may cause complete heart block. Patients with RCM are at increased risk for ventricular thrombus formation. Specifically, endocardial fibrosis can lead to progressive obliteration of the left ventricle from thrombus formation. Finally, treatment of the underlying disease process can be initiated in the emergency room through the use of high-dose steroids to treat underlying inflammation in Loeffler syndrome and sarcoidosis.

Pearls and Pitfalls

- RCM presents as acute diastolic HF. Its pathophysiology is unique in that systolic function is preserved and there is a lack of ventricular dilation or hypertrophy.
- Supportive care through diuresis must be performed with caution as high preloads are required to maintain cardiac output.
- Anticipate arrhythmias due to infiltrative processes in the conduction pathways; because of this, cardioversion may lead to complete heart block.

HYPERTROPHIC CARDIOMYOPATHY

Nicholas R. Phillips

Clinical Highlights

Hypertrophic cardiomyopathy (HCM) is an important diagnosis to consider in the ED. Previously known as idiopathic hypertrophic subaortic stenosis (IHSS) or hypertrophic obstructive cardiomyopathy (HOCM), this entity is the most common cause of sudden death in young athletes. It is defined by left ventricular hypertrophy that is not due to another secondary cause such as valvular disorders or hypertension. Familial HCM is inherited as an autosomal dominant trait and is a relatively common disorder affecting approximately 1 in 500 adults. There are numerous different mutations that can lead to HCM, each with differing amounts of severity and leading to varying degrees of abnormal accumulation of cardiac myocytes.

While the disease may present for the first time as sudden cardiac death, other common presenting symptoms include exertional dyspnea (most commonly), chest pain, palpitations, presyncope, and syncope.

The diagnosis is multifaceted and ultimately confirmed by echocardiography. Concern of HCM can be supported by typical history, physical exam, and ECG findings. On exam, a harsh systolic murmur is often noted at the left lower sternal border. The murmur will typically increase with valsalva and decrease with squatting and handgrip. Other possible physical exam findings are a loud S4, biphasic carotid pulse with brisk upstroke, and a prominent *a* wave in jugular vein pulsation.

The ECG changes are nonspecific but most often include left ventricular hypertrophy and prominent septal Q waves. Deep Q waves, ST segment, and T-wave changes can also be seen in the inferior or lateral leads.

Definitive diagnosis is made by echocardiography demonstrating left ventricular hypertrophy, classically affecting

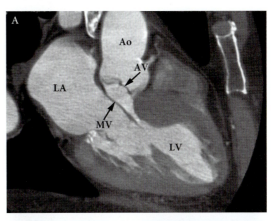

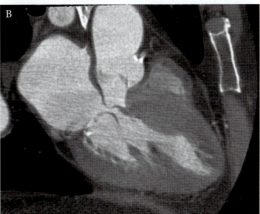

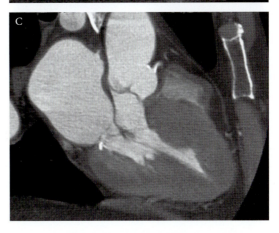

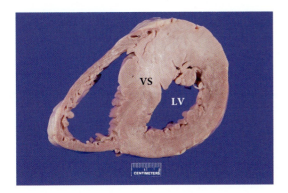

FIGURE 7.9 ■ Gross specimen of hypertrophic cardiomyopathy (HCM). This gross pathologic specimen shows the hypertrophied left ventricle wall and ventricular septum (VS) characteristic of HCM. Note that the left ventricle (LV) lumen was maintained at near normal size. Courtesy of Dr. Patrick Lantz, Department of Pathology, Wake Forest Baptist Health.

FIGURE 7.10 ■ This series of three CT images shows typical findings of the obstructive-type HCM in rotated three-chamber views. (A) Diastole; (B) mid-systole; (C) end-systole. Note that panel B clearly demonstrates systolic anterior motion of the MV leading to left ventricular outflow tract obstruction. LA, left atrium; Ao, aorta, LV, left ventricle; AV, aortic valve. Courtesy of Dr. Daniel Entrikin, Department of Radiology, Wake Forest Baptist Health.

194 ■ HYPERTROPHIC CARDIOMYOPATHY (CONTINUED)

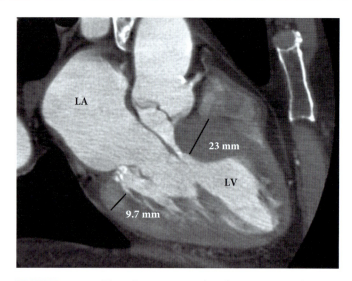

FIGURE 7.11 ■ This demonstrates the disproportionately large hypertrophy of the intraventricular septum (23 mm) as compared to the free ventricular wall (9.7 mm). LV, left ventricle; LA, left atrium. Courtesy of Dr. Daniel Entrikin, Department of Radiology, Wake Forest Baptist Health.

primarily the intraventricular septum. Cardiac CT and MRI can also be utilized in diagnostic testing.

Differential diagnosis is wide. One must rule out all other causes of secondary hypertrophy initially; then all other types of cardiomyopathies must be considered. HCM is most easily confused with other infiltrative diseases that can lead to thickened myocardium such as inherited metabolic disorders (eg, glycogen storage disease, fatty acid defects, and Fabry disease) and amyloidosis.

ED Care and Disposition

Definitive diagnosis is often not achieved in the ED; thus, care providers must maintain a high suspicion for the disorder in order to prevent subsequent complications.

When presenting in cardiac arrest, patients with HCM should be resuscitated using Advanced Cardiac Life Support (ACLS) guidelines.

Symptomatic treatment for chest pain includes beta-blockers or calcium channel blockers. Fluid status must be

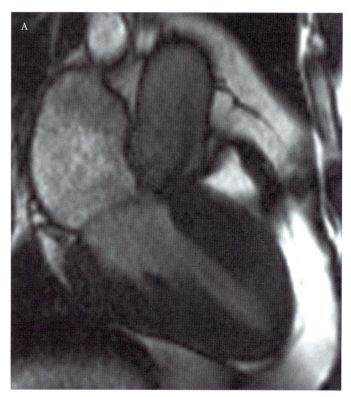
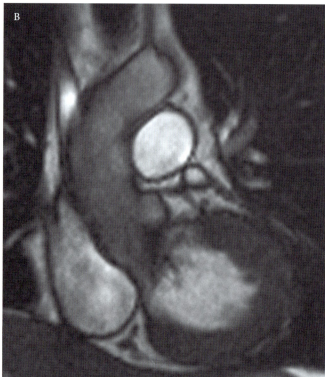

FIGURE 7.12 ■ These cardiac MRI images demonstrate another imaging modality that can be used to diagnose HCM and its potential associated obstructive variant. (A) A rotated three-chamber view; (B) a left ventricular outflow tract view. Real-time MRI in this patient also showed mitral regurgitation. Of note, MRI may potentially be useful in predicting those at risk for sudden cardiac death in patients without obstructive-type HCM by demonstrating delayed gadolinium enhancement. Courtesy of Dr. Daniel Entrikin, Department of Radiology, Wake Forest Baptist Health.

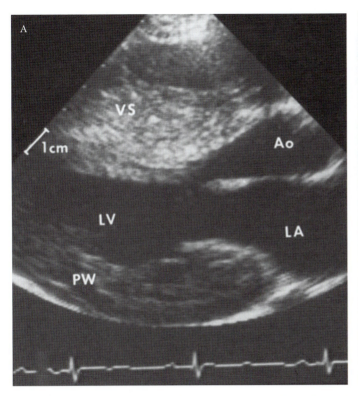 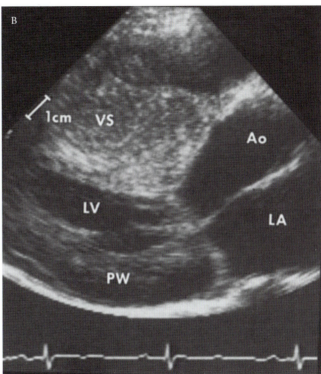

FIGURE 7.13 ■ This parasternal long-axis view on echocardiography shows the primary mode of diagnosis of hypertrophic obstructive cardiomyopathy (HOCM) by visualization of hypertrophied ventricular septum (VS). **(A)** The heart in diastole; **(B)** systolic outflow obstruction caused by anterior motion of the mitral valve. LV, left ventricle; LA, left atrium; Ao, aorta. PW, posterior wall. Reprinted, with permission, from Ommen SR, Nishimura RA, Tajik A. Chapter 33. Hypertrophic cardiomyopathy. In: Fuster V, Walsh RA, Harrington RA, eds. *Hurst's The Heart*. 13th ed. New York, NY: McGraw-Hill; 2011.

carefully monitored, as both dehydration and overhydration exacerbates symptoms. Volume depletion decreases preload and stroke volume with a subsequent increase in left ventricular outflow obstruction. Fluid overload elevates cardiac filling pressures and symptoms of HF.

Implantable cardioverter-defibrillator (ICD) placement should be considered for those at highest risk for sudden death. Strong predictive factors for sudden cardiac death (SCD) include previous cardiac arrest, exertional syncope, previous episode of ventricular tachycardia (sustained or nonsustained), left ventricle thickness greater than 30 mm, abnormal blood pressure response to exercise, and family history of SCD.

When intractable symptoms become present, other treatment options include myomectomy, either surgical or catheter-based, and ultimately cardiac transplant.

Stable patients can be safely discharged from the ED but must be referred for further cardiac evaluation on an urgent basis. All patients should be instructed to avoid strenuous activity until being seen in follow-up. A practical approach includes arranging follow-up prior to ED discharge. Consider admission for patients at high risk for SCD to expedient workup and definitive diagnosis.

Pearls and Pitfalls

- Keep HCM in the differential diagnosis for younger patients presenting with dypnea on exertion, palpitations, chest pain (typical or atypical), lightheadedness, and syncope.
- Clinical suspicion for HCM can be evaluated in the ED with a thorough history, physical exam, and ECG.
- The primary cause of symptoms in HCM is left ventricular outflow obstruction due to the displaced anterior motion of the mitral valve during systole. However, symptoms can still occur without obstruction due to diastolic dysfunction.
- Seventy-five percent of patients with hypertrophic cardiomyopathy do not have evidence of left ventricular outflow tract obstruction, but are still at risk for sudden cardiac death secondary to arrhythmias.
- The ECG may be normal in up to 25% of people with HCM.

AORTIC STENOSIS

Wiley D. Thuet
James C. O'Neill

Clinical Highlights

Aortic stenosis (AS) is a structural abnormality of the aortic valve that limits the flow of blood through the aortic valve into the systemic circulation. This loss of laminar flow and increase in turbulent flow causes reflexive concentric hypertrophy of the left ventricle that is necessary to overcome the resistance. Degenerative heart disease and valve calcifications in the elderly are the most common causes of AS. Critical AS has an estimated prevalence of 3% in patients aged 75 and older. A congenital bicuspid aortic valve (present in approximately 2% of the population) also predisposes to early onset of AS. Congenital AS, systemic lupus erythematosus (SLE), and rheumatic fever are rare causes of AS.

AS classically presents with the triad of dyspnea, chest pain, and syncope. Symptoms are secondary to inadequate blood flow from the left side of the heart with increased compensatory work of both the right and left heart. Physical exam may reveal the classic systolic crescendo decrescendo murmur that radiates to the carotids and pulmonary rales indicating pulmonary edema. Systolic blood pressures are almost never above 200 mmHg in patients with AS.

ECG findings in patients with AS, while not sensitive or specific, include left ventricular hypertrophy and occasionally a left or right bundle branch block. CXRs, also neither sensitive nor specific, may show cardiomegaly. The mainstay of diagnosis is formal echocardiography; however, this is often unnecessary in the ED and may be appropriately done in the outpatient or inpatient setting.

ED Care and Disposition

Comprehensive treatment of AS is outside the practice of emergency medicine. The emergency physician's goals in patients with AS are symptomatic control and appropriate cardiology consultation. If the patient presents with chest pain a standard cardiac workup should be initiated. The one caveat is that nitrates that are routinely given for angina symptoms may cause an unsafe drop in blood pressure as patients with AS are preload dependent.

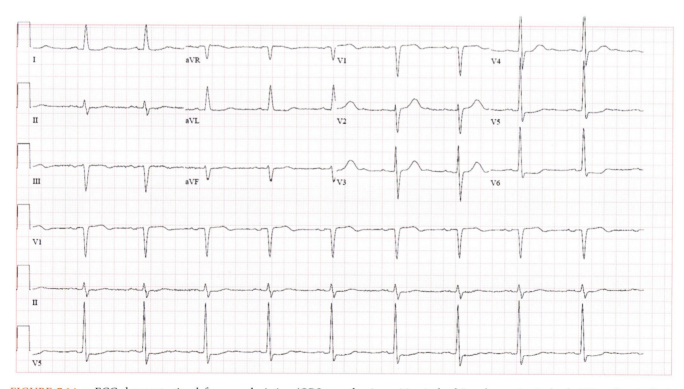

FIGURE 7.14 ■ ECG demonstrating left access deviation (QRS complex is positive in lead I and negative in lead aVF, and typically in lead II) and left ventricular hypertrophy (depth of negative S in V_1 + height of R in $V_5 \geq 35$ mm) characteristic of AS. Atrial fibrillation may also be seen.

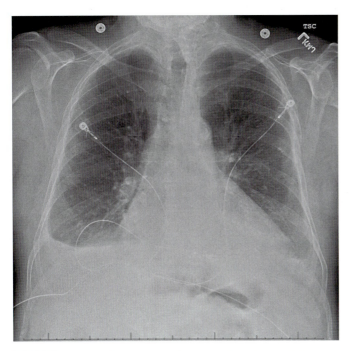

FIGURE 7.15 ■ CXR showing multiple sequelae of AS including cardiac enlargement, pulmonary vascular congestion, and pleural effusions.

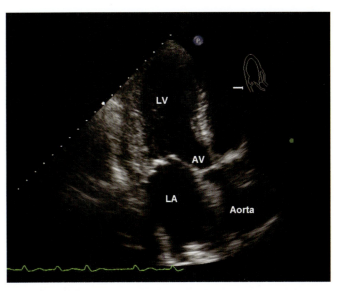

FIGURE 7.16 ■ Apical three-chamber view on echo showing thickened, calcified aortic valve and resultant dilated left atrium. Note that rhythm strip is also showing atrial fibrillation. LA, left atrium; LV, left ventricle; AV, aortic valve.

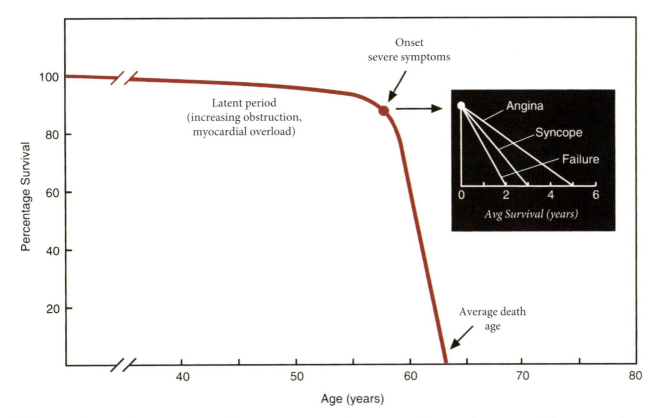

FIGURE 7.17 ■ Diagram showing the prolonged asymptomatic latent phase of AS. At the onset of AS symptoms life expectance drops significantly with a life expectancy of 2, 4, and 6 years for HF symptoms, syncope, and angina, respectively. Adapted, with permission, from Ross J Jr, et al. *Circulation*. 1968;38[suppl V]:V-61.

High-risk syncope patients will require admission to the hospital for further workup. AS presenting with pulmonary edema must be treated with appropriate respiratory support and diuretics, and will likely require admission.

New-onset atrial fibrillation in a patient with AS is an emergency requiring special care. Medications that reduce preload or afterload can precipitate profound hypotension in patient with AS. Restoration of sinus rhythm with cardioversion may be required (see the Cardioversion section of Chap. 9, Procedures).

Pearls and Pitfalls

- Patients with known AS should be advised against vigorous exercise as this may precipitate angina or syncope.
- Suspect AS if patient becomes rapidly unstable after administration of nitroglycerin.
- About 20% to 60% of patients with AS have coronary artery disease, which will complicate a definite angina diagnosis.

MITRAL STENOSIS

Wiley D. Thuet
James C. O'Neill

Clinical Highlights

Mitral stenosis restricts blood flow from the left atrium into the left ventricle. The most common cause world-wide is progressive calcification from rheumatic heart disease, however, new cases are now uncommon in developed countries. The latency period from acute rheumatic fever to valvular heart disease can last decades. As the stenosis worsens, upstream effects proliferate. Increased left atrial pressures leads to atrial dilation; as a result, atrial fibrillation will eventually occur. Further upstream, pulmonary hypertension will develop, and even further, right-sided hypertrophy, tricuspid regurgitation, and pulmonic regurgitation can all develop.

Patient presentation varies widely. In the early stages of mitral stenosis, patients are asymptomatic. As the disease progresses, patients first become symptomatic during times of increased cardiac output (eg, exercise, physical exertion, and pregnancy). Dyspnea and exercise intolerance are the most common initial complaints. As the disease progresses further, patients will start to complain of increasing pulmonary symptoms as a result of the pulmonary artery hypertension. Hemoptysis, paroxysmal nocturnal dyspnea, and increasing oxygen requirements may all be seen.

Outside of pulmonary hypertension and pulmonary venous congestion, it is important to remember that atrial fibrillation and its sequelae may also indicate mitral stenosis. Patients may present with palpitations or systemic embolic disease such as stroke, embolic MI, or splenic/renal infarcts.

Physical exam may reveal a loud S_1 and a mid-diastolic rumbling murmur with crescendo toward S_2 that will be louder with atrial fibrillation. Elements of pulmonary vascular congestion such as basilar crackles during pulmonary exam, tachypnea, and low-oxygen saturations may also be present.

Diagnosis is confirmed with echocardiography. Transesophageal echocardiography is best for measuring flow and estimating gradients; however, transthoracic echocardiography will allow for initial characterization of the valvular disease. Supporting evidence will also be noticed on ECG and CXRs. Atrial fibrillation, right atrial enlargement, and right-axis deviation can be seen on ECG, as well as pulmonary edema, Kerley B lines, and right ventricular enlargement on CXR.

ED Care and Disposition

Definitive treatment for mitral stenosis is transcutaneous balloon valvuloplasty, valve repair surgery, or valve replacement

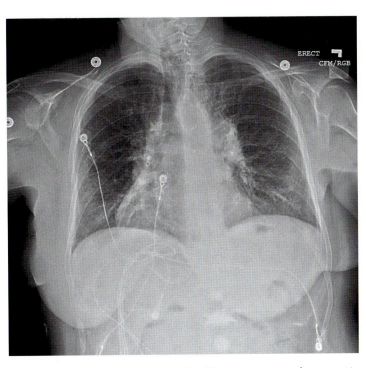

FIGURE 7.18 ■ CXR demonstrating right ventricular enlargement and mild pulmonary vascular congestion in a patient with mitral stenosis. Note that the left ventricle is mostly unchanged.

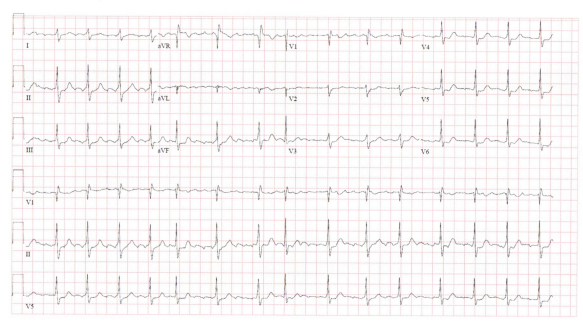

FIGURE 7.19 ■ ECG from a patient with mitral stenosis demonstrating atrial fibrillation from increased left atrial pressures and right axis deviation (net negative voltage in lead I, positive voltage in lead aVF) from increased right-sided demand.

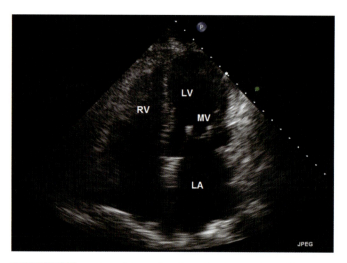

FIGURE 7.20 ■ Apical four-chamber view from echocardiography showing stenotic mitral valve (MV). Note the heavy calcifications along the valve. A dilated left atrium (LA) can also be seen, further supporting the diagnosis. LV, left ventricle; RV, right ventricle.

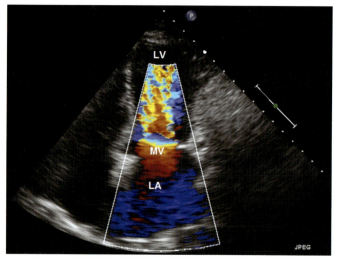

FIGURE 7.21 ■ Apical two-chamber view from echocardiography showing large turbulent jet into left ventricle (LV) during diastolic filling. LA, left atrium; MV, mitral valve.

surgery. Emergency care should be aimed at reducing pulmonary vascular congestion with diuretic therapy. Atrial fibrillation should be rate controlled with calcium channel blockers, beta-blockers, and digoxin as indicated. Anticoagulation should also be assured if the patient is in atrial fibrillation. Disposition and need for consultation is largely based on the severity of the presenting symptoms. Stable patients with mitral stenosis can follow up with cardiology on an outpatient basis.

Pearls and Pitfalls

- Mitral stenosis is becoming increasingly rare now that untreated rheumatic fever is rare.
- Massive hemoptysis from bronchial venous rupture may be seen as a result of severe mitral stenosis.
- Exertional symptoms (eg, shortness of breath and weakness) may be the only initial symptoms of mitral stenosis.

ACUTE AORTIC INSUFFICIENCY

Wiley D. Thuet
James C. O'Neill

Clinical Highlights

Acute aortic valve (AV) regurgitation (also called aortic insufficiency or aortic incompetence) is the immediate onset of diastolic regurgitation back through the aortic valve. Endocarditis and aortic dissection are the most common causes of acute aortic valve regurgitation. Other causes include rupture of congenitally malformed cusp, and occasionally blunt decelerating chest trauma.

In contrast to chronic aortic regurgitation, acute regurgitation is a surgical emergency, as the heart has not had time to slowly increase left ventricular size as a compensation mechanism.

Shortly after the commencement of acute regurgitation, patients present with sudden onset of dyspnea. Symptoms from the inciting disease may dominate the chief complaint (ie, tearing chest pain for acute dissection or fever for endocarditis). Physical exam typically reveals the manifestations of cardiogenic shock secondary to the total collapse of left ventricular outflow. Hypotension, peripheral pallor from vasoconstriction, and diaphoresis are common. Cardiac auscultation may yield a low-pitched diastolic murmur heard after S2; however, when patients are in cardiogenic shock, the gradient is reduced and the murmur may be inaudible.

Diagnosis relies on clinical suspicion for rapid stabilization with confirmation by echocardiography. CXRs will show pulmonary edema with a much smaller heart than would be expected in someone with chronic aortic regurgitation. Emergency bedside echocardiography will also help in diagnosis as a large aortic regurgitant jet will be noted. As with most valvular disorders, formal echocardiography will provide the gold standard for diagnosis. CT of the chest may be necessary as there are concerns that aortic dissection is the cause of the acute regurgitation.

ED Care and Disposition

Acute aortic valve regurgitation is a surgical emergency and mortality is very high even with treatment. Death is most often secondary to pulmonary edema, ventricular dysrhythmias, or circulatory collapse. The goal of the emergency physician is to buy time to arrange for definitive surgical management. Airway management is important given the rapidly progressing pulmonary edema. Reducing afterload

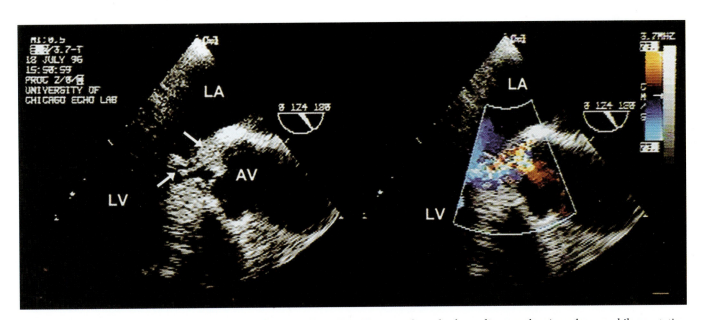

FIGURE 7.22 ■ Acute aortic regurgitation secondary to endocarditis. Transesophageal echocardiogram showing a large mobile vegetation (arrows) extending from the aortic valve (AV) into the left ventricle (LV). Doppler echocardiography reveals significant regurgitation from the aorta into the LV. LA, left atrium. Reprinted, with permission, from Sorrentino MJ. Chapter 29. Valvular heart disease. In: Hall JB, Schmidt GA, Wood LH, eds. *Principles of Critical Care*. 3rd ed. New York, NY: McGraw-Hill; 2005.

and increasing contractility are essential to promote forward flow. Nitroprusside should be used in conjunction with an ionotrope, such as dopamine or dobutamine, in those with shock too severe for nitroprusside alone. Aortic balloon pumps are absolutely contraindicated in these patients as it will increase diastolic pressure and increase regurgitant flow through the valve. Patients will need inpatient care at a facility where a cardiothoracic surgeon is available. Any delays to surgery should be weighed heavily in a hemodynamically unstable patient as very few contraindications for surgery exist in a patient with cardiogenic shock secondary to acute aortic regurgitation, including active valvular infection.

Pearls and Pitfalls

- Beware of thoracic aortic dissection in a patient who is presenting with acute aortic regurgitation.
- Classic chronic aortic regurgitation signs (wide pulse pressure, water hammer pulse, Traube sign, etc.) are most often absent with acute aortic valve regurgitation.

MITRAL REGURGITATION AND ACUTE MITRAL INSUFFICIENCY

Wiley D. Thuet
James C. O'Neill

Clinical Highlights

Mitral regurgitation (also called mitral insufficiency or mitral incompetence) includes two clinically separate entities: acute mitral regurgitation and chronic mitral regurgitation. It is important to make the distinction, as the presentation, physiology, and treatment are different.

Chronic mitral regurgitation

Up to 70% of normal healthy adults have at least trace mitral regurgitation noticeable on echocardiography. The majority of this, termed physiologic regurgitation, is not of great importance. However, if the process progresses or worsens over several years, chronic mitral regurgitation can develop. Most commonly the cause of chronic mitral regurgitation is degenerative changes of the valve itself. Another major cause of chronic mitral regurgitation is infective endocarditis.

Patient presentations of chronic mitral regurgitation vary widely. Patients may complain of exertional dyspnea, or fatigue with or without pulmonary edema, or irregular heartbeat due to atrial fibrillation. These symptoms are secondary to the regurgitant flow of blood into the left atrium and the resultant increased pressures of the pulmonary vasculature even further upstream. Physical exam in patients with chronic disease may show a holosystolic blowing murmur heard loudest at the apex.

Echocardiography will show the regurgitant jet and will be helpful in distinguishing between ischemic disease (areas of hypodynamic movement), degenerative disease, or findings of endocarditis (large valvular vegetation). CXRs may show a larger than normal left atrium and left ventricle as well as resultant pulmonary edema and congestion. ECG may show left atrial enlargement or atrial fibrillation, left ventricular enlargement, and left-axis deviation.

Acute mitral regurgitation

MI that involves the posterior descending artery yielding rupture of chordae tendineae or papillary muscles is the most common cause of acute mitral regurgitation. The resulting acute mitral regurgitation typically presents 2 to 7 days after the actual infarct. Less frequently endocarditis can cause acute rupture and few cases of traumatic rupture have also been documented.

Classically, patients with acute mitral regurgitation decompensate very rapidly. They present with acute dyspnea and tachycardia as a result of rapidly accumulating pulmonary edema. The diagnosis should be suspected in symptomatic patients with an ECG suspicious for inferior infarction or past infarction. Also, in contrast to chronic disease, the heart will be smaller than expected on CXR in the setting of pulmonary edema. With these findings, bedside echocardiography or formal echocardiography should be performed to secure the diagnosis.

Echocardiographic hallmarks of acute mitral regurgitation include a dilated right ventricle and a hyperdynamic rapidly beating left ventricle. Doppler will illustrate a large regurgitant jet through the mitral valve. Flail chordae and muscle may also be seen churning inside the ventricle.

ED Care and Disposition

Chronic mitral regurgitation

For asymptomatic chronic mitral regurgitation, no emergent treatment is necessary. Diuresis may be necessary in setting of pulmonary congestion. It is important to look for signs and symptoms of bacterial endocarditis as treatment should be initiated as soon as the organism is known or sufficient cultures have been taken. Definitive treatment in severe disease is replacement of the valve by cardiothoracic surgery.

New-onset atrial fibrillation, suspected endocarditis, or hypoxic pulmonary edema patients may need admission; however, chronic mitral regurgitation alone does not. Outpatient cardiology follow-up for those with symptomatic disease is reasonable for most patients.

Acute mitral regurgitation

Definitive care of the patient is open-heart surgery to repair or replace the valve. Medical stabilization is difficult due to complicated physiology. Reducing left ventricular afterload is key to limiting pulmonary congestion and allowing for adequate oxygenation and ventilation. Nitrates and diuretics may be used for this purpose if the patient's systemic pressures will tolerate the medications. If left ventricular aortic output is severely compromised secondary to regurgitant flow, a significant challenge is present. Bolusing fluid will likely be of little value and afterload reduction can no longer be facilitated. Dobutamine may help as an ionotrope in the severely hypotensive patient. An aortic balloon pump may

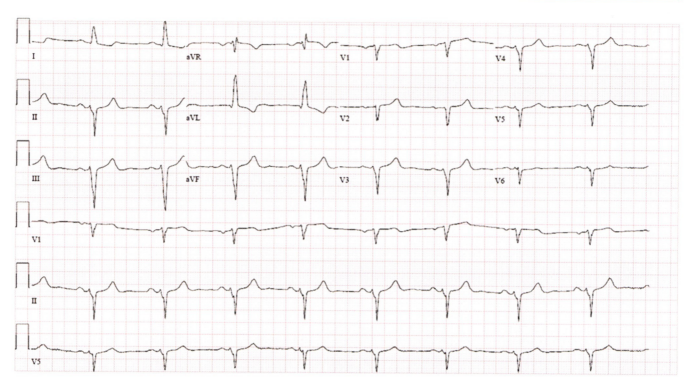

FIGURE 7.23 ■ ECG demonstrating left ventricular hypertrophy (criteria in this case is R wave in aVL ≥ 11 mm) with secondary repolarization abnormalities. Also, left atrial enlargement (bifid P wave in lead II) can be seen. Although these findings are very nonspecific, they support mitral regurgitation.

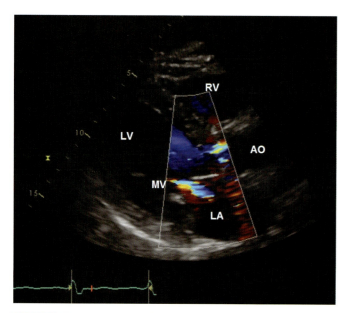

FIGURE 7.24 ■ Parasternal long view from echocardiography demonstrating regurgitant jet back into left atrium (LA). The high-velocity jet can be seen on Doppler just to the right of the mitral valve (MV) designation in the image. Note that the rhythm strip indicates that this jet is taking place in systole. LV, left ventricle; AO, aorta; RV, right ventricle.

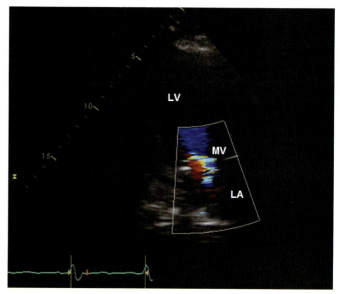

FIGURE 7.25 ■ Apical two-chamber view from echocardiography demonstrating same high-velocity regurgitant jet back into left atrium (LA) during systole. MV, mitral valve; LV, left ventricle.

MITRAL REGURGITATION AND ACUTE MITRAL INSUFFICIENCY (CONTINUED)   205

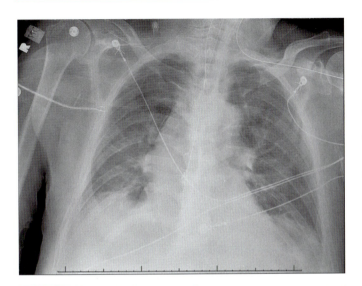

FIGURE 7.26 ■ CXR showing intubated patient from severe mitral regurgitation. Note cardiomegaly as well as increased pulmonary congestion and small pleural effusion. All are nonspecific, but certainly suggestive of mitral stenosis.

also be necessary to allow for better systemic circulation while minimizing regurgitant flow in the setting of a severely critical patient.

Pearls and Pitfalls

- Be on high alert for acute regurgitation when evaluating patients who were recently discharged for MI.
- For acute regurgitation, rapid echocardiography is crucial to establish the diagnosis.
- Nitroprusside can be useful even in normotensive patients with acute mitral regurgitation to facilitate afterload reduction if acceptable systolic pressure can be maintained with treatment.

Chapter 8
PEDIATRIC CARDIOLOGY

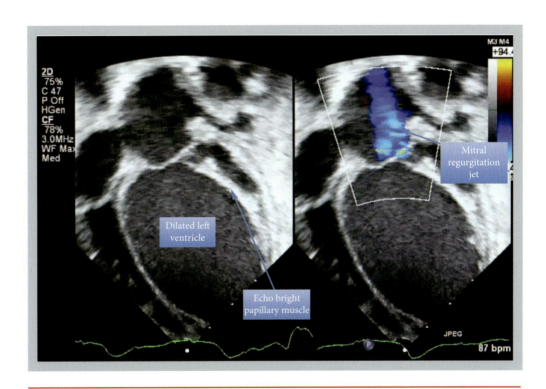

Pediatric Electrocardiogram Norms

NORMAL ECG AT AGE INTERVALS (NEWBORN, 1MO, 3MO, 12MO, 3Y, 5Y, 8Y, 13Y)

Derick M. Wenning

Clinical Highlights

Many different presentations to the pediatric emergency department (ED) warrant electrocardiogram (ECG) evaluation. These include common complaints such as chest pain, syncope, palpitations, drug exposure, and electrical burns. In young infants and neonates, an ECG may be indicated for poor feeding, cyanotic spells, or an acute life-threatening event. There are age-related changes that dramatically alter the appearance of the "normal" ECG in children (Table 8.1), and the first step in interpretation of the pediatric ECG should be noting the patient's age. The normal range for heart rate for a newborn to an infant 6 months of age is 125 to 145 beats per minute (bpm). The mean adult resting heart rate of 80 bpm is not reached until adolescence. In neonates, due to fetal circulation, the right ventricle is dominant. This leads to a normal right axis deviation in ECGs of infants. Smaller muscle mass also leads to a shorter PR interval as well as QRS duration. In younger children, the PR interval ranges between 0.08 and 0.15 seconds and in adolescents between 0.120 and 0.2 seconds. QRS duration in patients aged less than 8 years should not exceed 0.08 seconds. Adolescent QRS intervals range from 0.1 to 0.12 seconds, the latter being the normal duration for adults. The QT interval in infancy is also slightly longer. Since the QT interval varies with heart rate, calculation of the corrected QT interval is indicated. The upper limit of normal for the QT interval in infancy is 490 milliseconds, and decreases to 440 milliseconds after 6 months of age. In addition, R-wave progression does not follow the normal adult pattern until the patient is approximately 6 to 8 years of age.

T-wave changes in pediatric ECGs are nonspecific, and absolute rules for age-related changes have not been determined. The right precordial leads (V1–V3) should have upright T waves in the first week of life and inverting thereafter through early childhood. Upright T waves in leads V1 and V2 in a young child over the age of 1 week should raise suspicion for right ventricular hypertrophy (RVH) and further investigation is warranted. Inverted T waves in V1–V3 persist to 6 to 8 years of age and occasionally into adolescence.

ED Care and Disposition

Any abnormality found on ECG should be explored as a possible reason for the presenting complaint; however, a normal ECG does not rule out potential cardiac causes (see also Table 8.2). Depending on the severity of the presentation and results of other laboratory and radiographic testing, disposition may vary from inpatient hospitalization to urgent follow-up with possible cardiology consultation.

Pearls and Pitfalls

- RVH is the most common abnormality seen with congenital heart disease (CHD). Additional right precordial leads (V3R and V4R) can be used to provide more information about the right ventricle in infants.

TABLE 8.1 ■ NORMAL PEDIATRIC ECG VALUES

Age	HR (bpm)	QRS Axis (Degrees)	PR Interval (sec)	QRS Interval (s)	R in V1 (mm)	S in V1 (mm)	R in V6 (mm)	S in V6 (mm)
1st week	90–180	60–180	0.08–0.15	0.03–0.08	5–24	0–18	0–12	0–10
1–3wks	100–185	45–160	0.08–0.15	0.03–0.08	3–21	0–16	2–15	0–10
1–2 mo	120–185	30–135	0.08–0.15	0.03–0.08	3–18	0–15	5–21	0–9
3–5 mo	105–185	0–135	0.08–0.15	0.03–0.08	3–19	0–15	6–22	0–9
6–11 mo	110–170	0–135	0.07–0.16	0.03–0.08	2–20	0.5–18	6–23	0–7
1–2 yr	90–165	0–110	0.08–0.16	0.03–0.08	2–18	0.5–21	6–23	0–7
3–4 yr	70–140	0–110	0.09–0.17	0.04–0.08	1–16	0.5–23	4–26	0–5
5–7 yr	65–135	0–110	0.09–0.17	0.04–0.08	0.5–14	0.5–23	4–26	0–4
8–11 yr	60–130	−15–110	0.09–0.17	0.04–0.09	0–12	0.5–25	4–25	0–4
12–15 yr	65–120	−15–110	0.09–0.18	0.04–0.09	0–10	0.5–21	4–23	0–4

NORMAL ECG AT AGE INTERVALS (NEWBORN, 1MO, 3MO, 12MO, 3Y, 5Y, 8Y, 13Y) (CONTINUED) ■ 209

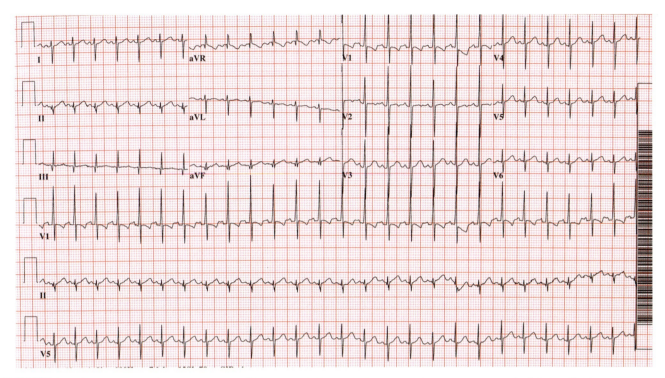

FIGURE 8.1 ■ This is a normal ECG in a 2-week old showing right axis deviation and T-wave inversion in leads V1 and V2.

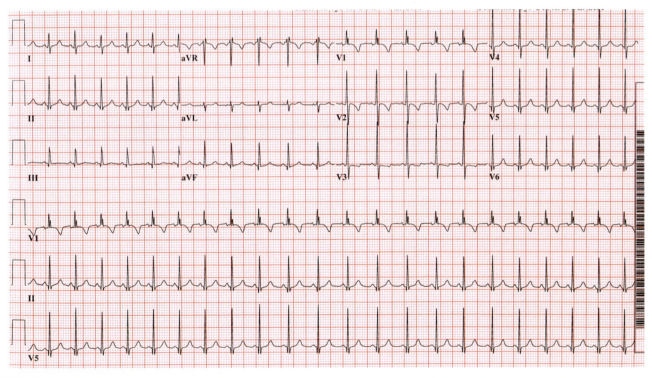

FIGURE 8.2 ■ This ECG taken in a 4-week old reveals normal axis, rate, QRS interval, and QT interval. Again normal T-wave inversions are seen in V1, V2, and V3.

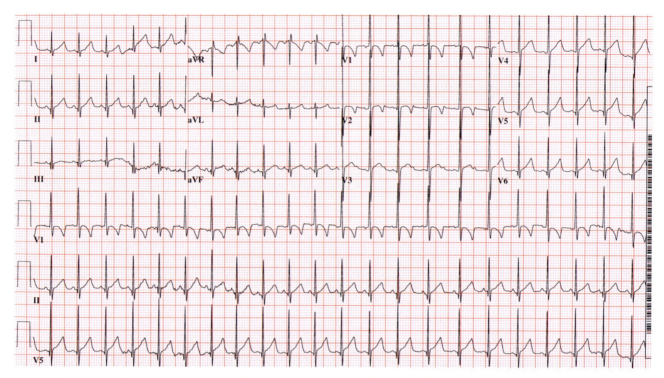

FIGURE 8.3 ■ An ECG from a normal 3-month old showing normal axis and prominent R waves with T-wave inversions in right precordial leads. Notice small Q waves in II, III, AVF, V5, and V6. These are normal and do not indicate pathology due to their small size and depth.

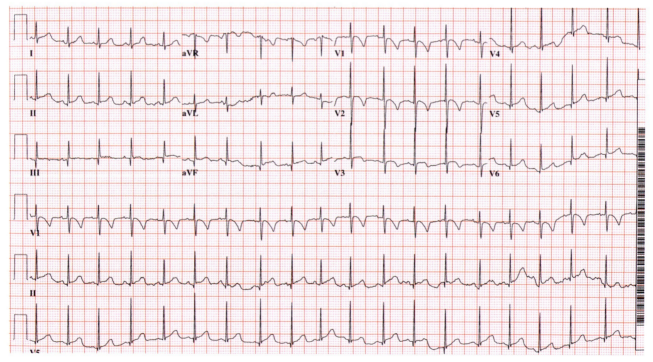

FIGURE 8.4 ■ ECG of a 1-year old. The PR interval and QRS duration are age appropriate at 0.1 and 0.06 seconds, respectively. Notice small nonpathologic Q waves in inferior (II, III, and AVF) and lateral leads (V5 and V6).

NORMAL ECG AT AGE INTERVALS (NEWBORN, 1MO, 3MO, 12MO, 3Y, 5Y, 8Y, 13Y) (CONTINUED) 211

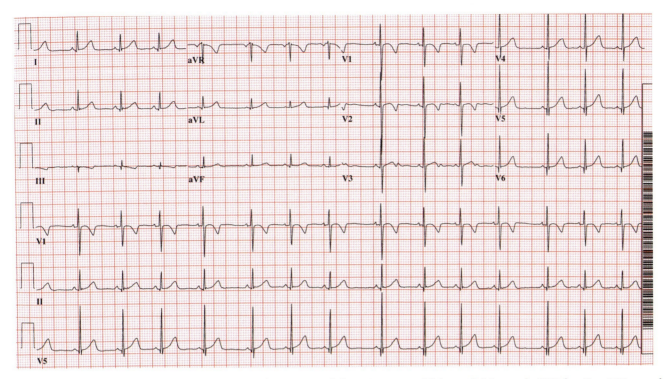

FIGURE 8.5 ■ Normal ECG in a 2-year old. This ECG shows a normal short sinus pause. PR interval, 0.1 seconds; QRS duration, 0.06 seconds; and corrected QT interval, approximately 0.4 seconds. Notice small nonpathologic Q waves in V5 and V6.

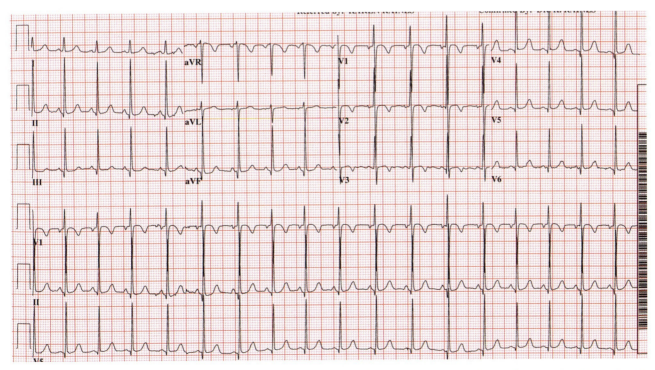

FIGURE 8.6 ■ Normal ECG in a 4-year old. Rate = 106 bpm, normal axis, PR interval = 0.1 second, QRS duration = 0.07 seconds, QTc = 0.43 seconds. Normal flipped T waves continue to persist in leads V1, V2, and V3 in this child.

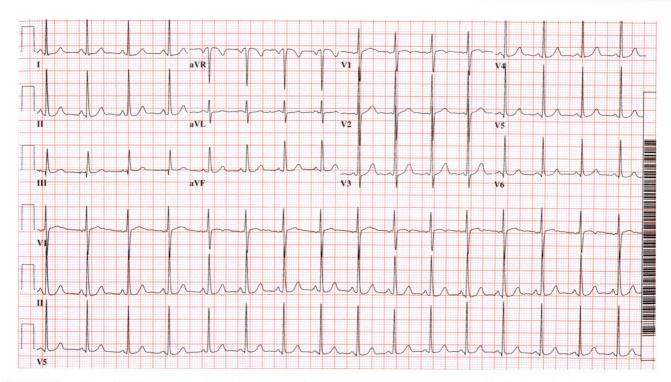

FIGURE 8.7 ■ Normal ECG in a 6-year old. The T waves have become upright in the right precordial leads (V1 and V2) in this patient.

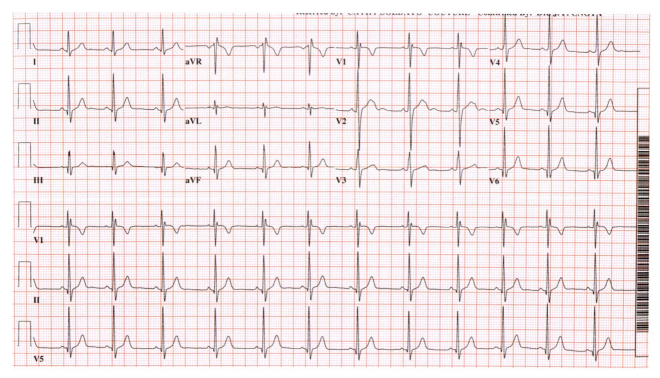

FIGURE 8.8 ■ Normal ECG in an 8-year old. Notice that this patient's ECG shows upright T waves in lead V2 but inverted in lead V1. This is a normal progression, as the T waves will turn upright in the order V3–V2–V1.

TABLE 8.2 ■ NORMAL VARIANTS OF CARDIAC RHYTHM IN PEDIATRIC PATIENTS
• Sinus arrhythmia
• Short sinus pauses < 1.8 seconds
• First-degree atrioventricular block
• Mobitz type I second-degree AV block
• Junctional rhythm
• Ventricular or supraventricular extrasystole (premature contractions)

- Correction of the QT interval can be done using the Bazett formula that divides the measured QT by the square root of the preceding R–R interval in which the QT is being measured ($QTc = QT/\sqrt{R-R}$).
- P waves should be upright in leads I, II, and aVF. Other P wave orientations in these leads suggest a nonsinus atrial rhythm.
- Q waves can be normal in the inferior and lateral leads in a child.

Congenital Heart Disease
NEONATAL CONGENITAL HEART DISEASE

Michael J. Walsh

Video in this chapter is available at http://mhprofessional.com/sites/lefebvre

Clinical Highlights

Congenital heart defects, affecting approximately 8 in 1000 live births, are the most common birth defects in newborns. With advances in fetal and postnatal echocardiography, an increasing number of diagnoses are made before newborns leave the hospital. However, in patients discharged with unrecognized cardiac disease, an accurate and timely diagnosis is essential for the reduction of morbidity and mortality.

Critical CHD commonly presents with closure of the patent ductus arteriosus (PDA) and can lead to a rapid decline in clinical status. PDA may close from the first day (most commonly) up to the 90th day (rarely) after birth in normal infants. Although echocardiography provides a definitive diagnosis, treatment often must be initiated before such a diagnosis is made. In the absence of an echocardiogram, clinicians should employ the physical examination, chest radiograph (CXR), ECG, four-extremity blood pressures, and pre- and postductal pulse oximetry in an effort to narrow the diagnosis (Table 8.3).

TABLE 8.3 ■ COMMON PRESENTATIONS OF NEONATAL CHD

Shock
    Hypoplastic left heart syndrome
    Coarctation of the aorta
    Interrupted aortic arch
    Critical aortic stenosis
Cyanosis with diminished pulmonary blood flow
    Critical pulmonary stenosis
    Tetralogy of Fallot
    Pulmonary atresia
    Ebstein anomaly of the tricuspid valve
Cyanosis with normal or increased pulmonary blood flow
    Transposition of the great arteries
    Truncus arteriosus
Respiratory distress
    Large left-to-right shunts (ventricular septal defect, patent ductus arteriosus, and AV canal)
    Truncus arteriosus
    Total anomalous pulmonary venous return

In patients with ductal-dependent systemic blood flow, ductal closure leads to a marked decrease in cardiac output, and thus, oxygen delivery—leading to metabolic acidosis and shock. Femoral pulses will be diminished or absent. Critical aortic stenosis, coarctation of the aorta (CoA), interrupted aortic arch, and hypoplastic left heart syndrome (HLHS) are the most common examples of ductal-dependent systemic blood flow.

When the pulmonary circulation is ductal dependent, PDA closure leads to profound cyanosis. This is evident in right-heart obstructive lesions, such as critical pulmonary stenosis or pulmonary atresia. Cyanosis that does not respond to oxygen therapy suggests a cardiac etiology. Cyanosis is also the most common presentation in patients with parallel circulations, as in transposition of the great arteries (TGA). Severe pulmonary edema can result from over-circulation of the lungs, as in truncus arteriosus, or from obstruction of pulmonary venous return, as seen with totally anomalous pulmonary venous return (TAPVR). Single ventricle lesions, such as double-inlet left ventricle and tricuspid atresia, can have any of the above presentations depending on the patency of the aorta and the pulmonary artery, as well as other intracardiac factors.

ED Care and Disposition

Prompt recognition and stabilization are essential for the reduction of morbidity and mortality. If cardiac disease is suspected, arrangements should be made to transfer the baby to a tertiary-care center for potential surgical or catheter-based interventions. Often, therapy must be initiated before a definitive diagnosis is made by echocardiography.

The mainstay of medical management for many of these patients is prostaglandin E1 (0.03–0.1 μg/kg/min). It is a life-saving treatment for patients with ductal-dependent lesions, and in those patients with TGA and inadequate mixing. There is a small subset of CHD patients for whom PGE makes the clinical status worse, including obstructed TAPVR. Clinicians must anticipate the side effects of apnea and hypotension. If a transfer is anticipated, consider the reliability of the airway and intravascular access before transport.

Left-sided obstructive lesions can be associated with severe heart failure after ductal closure. Catecholamines, such as dopamine and epinephrine, have an important role. Metabolic acidosis should be corrected. In patients with respiratory distress as a result of congestive heart failure, intravenous (IV) diuretics (ie, furosemide 1 mg/kg/dose IV) will be helpful.

In cases of TGA with intact ventricular septum and restrictive foramen ovale, medical management alone is often insufficient. Balloon atrial septostomy is essential to promote adequate mixing. Neurodevelopmental outcomes hinge on the speed with which this occurs. These patients underscore the need for prompt referral to a tertiary-care center. There, echocardiography can provide a definitive diagnosis and cardiothoracic surgeons can provide the lesion-specific palliation or repair.

Pearls and Pitfalls

- CHD is common and has variable presentations in the neonate. Cyanosis, a single second heart sound, diminished femoral pulses, and poor perfusion may help to distinguish CHD from other neonatal illnesses.
- If clinical suspicion for CHD is high, consultation with a pediatric cardiologist and initiation of prostaglandin E1 should be initiated without waiting for a definitive diagnosis. Neurodevelopmental outcomes can hang in the balance.

- If a transfer is anticipated, consideration must be given to the reliability of the infant's airway and intravascular access. Prostaglandin E1 must be run as a continuous infusion and can lead to apnea.

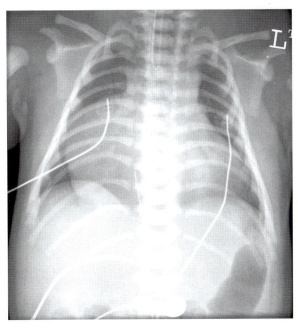

FIGURE 8.10 ■ Neonate with Ebstein anomaly of the tricuspid valve. Severe tricuspid regurgitation leads to substantial right atrial dilation—often leading to massive dilation of the cardiac silhouette on frontal radiograph.

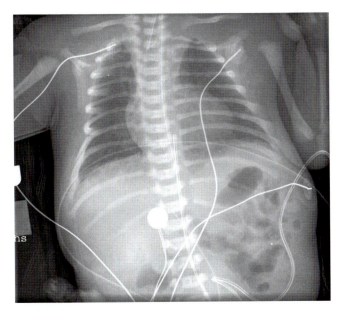

FIGURE 8.9 ■ Neonate with TGA. The orientation of the great vessels creates the appearance of a narrowed mediastinum on frontal radiograph. Along with stress-induced thymic atrophy and hyperinflated lungs, the classic "egg-on-a-string" appearance is seen.

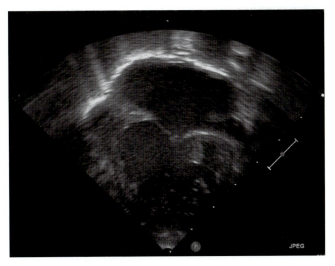

FIGURE 8.11 ■ Hypoplastic Left Heart Syndrome. From this apical view, note the appearance of the dilated right ventricle and large tricuspid valve. The left ventricle is quite small without obvious patency of the mitral valve. A muscular ventricular septal defect (VSD) is also seen.

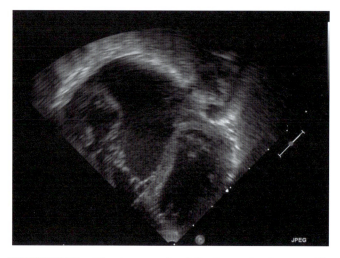

FIGURE 8.12 ■ Ebstein anomaly of the tricuspid valve. Note the inferior displacement of the tricuspid valve relative to the mitral valve. There is right atrial dilation and a large portion of "atrialized" right ventricle. The effective RV cavity is small.

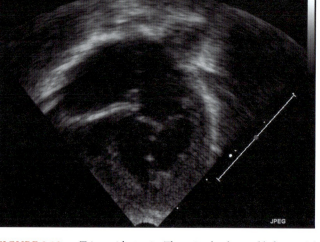

FIGURE 8.13 ■ Tricuspid atresia. The mitral valve and left ventricle have formed normally, while there is no valve connection at the right atrioventricular connection. The right ventricle is small and fed by a ventricular septal defect (VSD).

VIDEO 8.1 ■ Neonate with HLHS. Note the size discrepancy between the left and right ventricles. A VSD is also shown. On sweeping toward the outflow tracts, a hypoplastic aorta is seen arising from the left ventricle. With such a hypoplastic aorta and LV, ductal patency will be necessary for the provision of systemic blood flow.

VIDEO 8.2 ■ Ebstein anomaly of the tricuspid valve. Note the inferior displacement of the tricuspid valve relative to the mitral valve. There is right atrial dilation and a large portion of "atrialized" right ventricle. The effective right ventricular (RV) cavity is small and its ability to deliver prograde pulmonary blood flow is limited.

VIDEO 8.3 ■ Subcostal frontal view of a neonate with transposition of TGA. Sweeping from posterior to anterior, the left ventricle gives off a bifurcating great vessel posteriorly and the right ventricle gives off the aorta anteriorly.

VIDEO 8.4 ■ Tricuspid atresia. Atresias of the tricuspid valve and a small right ventricle are seen. A VSD allows blood flow into the right ventricle. Sweeping anteriorly, the great vessels (aorta from LV, then PA from RV) are seen. Without obstruction to pulmonary blood flow, this infant will present early in life with symptoms of heart failure.

INFANTILE CONGENITAL HEART DISEASE

Michael D. Quartermain

Clinical Highlights

The presentation of CHD in an infant and a child is mostly characterized by left to right shunts, left-sided outflow obstructive lesions, and cardiomyopathies (Table 8.4). The time frame of infancy and early childhood is a vulnerable period when normal decreases in the pulmonary vascular resistance (PVR) allow for the hemodynamic sequelae of CHD to become apparent. The most common defect to present to the ED in heart failure in this age range is a moderate to large ventricular septal defect (VSD). Another lesion presenting in this age group is a complete atrioventricular canal defect, which occurs in 40% of children with Trisomy 21. The defect includes a large VSD component in combination with an atrial septal defect and abnormalities of the mitral and tricuspid valves.

An isolated patent ductus arteriosis (PDA), if large, can present with similar left to right shunt symptoms of pulmonary over circulation. Coarctation of the aorta (CoA), while most common in the newborn period, can present during infancy and early childhood. Both anomalous left coronary artery from the pulmonary artery (ALCAPA) and cardiomyopathies (eg, viral, metabolic, and infectious) present with left ventricular dilation with systolic dysfunction and must be considered in this age group.

This assortment of heart defects present with overlapping features of congestive heart failure or low cardiac output. On physical examination, poor growth is evident often with height and weight less than 5th percentile and a history of feeding intolerance. Tachycardia and tachypnea with mild to moderate respiratory distress are common. Cardiac murmurs are often present along with a hyperdynamic precordium. Cool extremities with poor capillary refill and hepatomegaly are additional features often seen in these patients. Four-extremity blood pressures will identify the child with a significant CoA with gradients greater than 20 mmHg from right arm to lower extremity.

ED Care and Disposition

Pulse oximetry, accurate four-extremity blood pressure assessment, ECG, and CXRs are the initial diagnostic tools. Pulse oximetry readings are often normal or only mildly decreased secondary to pulmonary edema in these patients. ECG is valuable to rule out underlying arrhythmia, assess for prominent ventricular forces seen in large left to right shunts, and identify ischemia patterns consistent with ALCAPA. The majority of these lesions will have cardiomegaly and pulmonary edema present on CXRs. Consultation with a pediatric cardiologist is recommended for confirmatory echocardiography and development of the appropriate treatment plan for the lesion. The patient with a large left to right shunt from a VSD or PDA will benefit from diuretic therapy, usually 1 mg/kg IV furosemide. Oxygen therapy is not recommended for these patients because its vasodilatory effects may increase pulmonary blood flow and lead to worsening pulmonary edema. Admission for initiation of nasogastric feeds and digoxin therapy is often performed. Patients with a dilated cardiomyopathy often require more significant support with mechanical ventilation and IV medications such as dopamine and milrinone. If ALCAPA is suspected by echocardiography, some centers choose confirmation by cardiac catheterization prior to surgical treatment. If an arrhythmia, such as supraventricular tachycardia (SVT), is identified, then an initial treatment with adenosine (0.1 mg/kg per dose IV) to restore sinus rhythm and then hospitalization is required to begin maintenance therapy with either a beta-blocker or digoxin depending on the underlying mechanism.

Pearls and Pitfalls

- Respiratory distress in an infant or a child may not be airway disease, a cardiac etiology must always be considered.
- CXR is a simple and safe test to help identify significant CHD in this age group as most will have cardiomegaly and increased pulmonary vascular markings.
- Absent or diminished femoral pulses strongly suggest the diagnosis of a CoA and should be evaluated in any child that presents to emergency room with possible cardiac disease or right arm hypertension. In the setting of low cardiac output, a typical pressure gradient from right arm to lower extremity may not be present.

TABLE 8.4 COMMON PRESENTATIONS OF CHD IN THE INFANT AND YOUNG CHILD

Ventricular septal defect
Common AV canal
Patent ductus arteriosus
Severe aortic or mitral regurgitation
Left ventricular outflow obstruction (CoA and aortic stenosis)
Truncus arteriosus
ALCAPA
Dilated cardiomyopathies
Arrhythmia

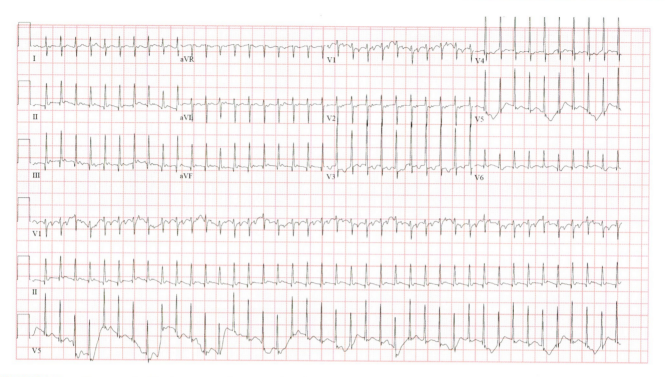

FIGURE 8.14 ■ Two-month old who presented to ER with tachycardia. The ECG demonstrates a regular, narrow complex tachycardia at 250 bpm consistent with reentry SVT. This patient returned to sinus rhythm with adenosine and demonstrated evidence of WPW syndrome.

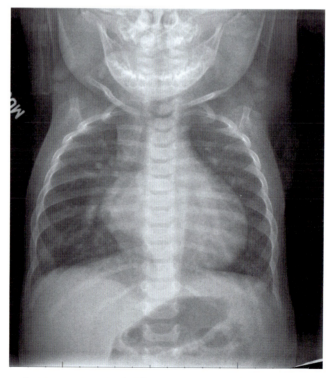

FIGURE 8.15 ■ CXR (PA) in a 3-month old with a large VSD. There is moderate cardiomegaly and increased pulmonary vascular markings consistent with a significant left to right shunt.

INFANTILE CONGENITAL HEART DISEASE (CONTINUED) ■ 219

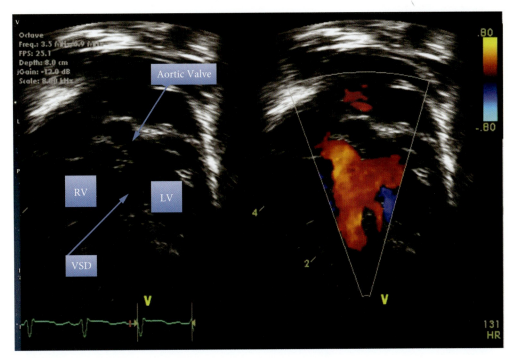

FIGURE 8.16 ■ Echo image from a standard four-chamber view in a 6-week old. The two-dimensional image on the left shows the large (1 cm) defect underneath the aortic valve. The color image highlights the left to right shunt across the VSD.

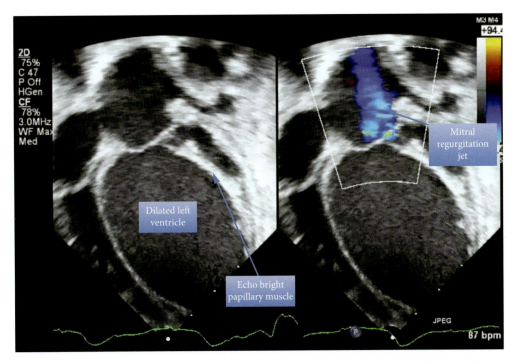

FIGURE 8.17 ■ Echo image in a 10-week-old male that presented to the ER with poor feeding and tachypnea. The image demonstrates a severely dilated left ventricle with diminished systolic function. The presence of mitral regurgitation suggests a diagnosis of ALCAPA.

FIGURE 8.18 ■ Echo image of a PDA. The classic ductal (aka "3 vessel") view demonstrates the right and left pulmonary arteries with antegrade (blue) flow and the large PDA (red) continuous flow from aorta to pulmonary artery. (RPA, right pulmonary artery; LPA, left pulmonary arter; MPA, middle pulmonary artery; DAo, descending aorta.)

PEDIATRIC CONGENITAL HEART DISEASE

Cheryl Cammock

Clinical Highlights

Older children and adolescents presenting to the emergency room with heart disease may include the following: (1) those with acquired heart disease and cardiomyopathy, (2) congenital heart defects after surgical repair, and (3) undiagnosed congenital heart defects with progressive disease. Patients in this age group may have seemingly benign complaints such as chest pain, palpitations, and dizziness. Therefore, the first major challenge for the emergency room physician is to determine whether potentially serious cardiac disease is present. Additional complaints such as anorexia, chronic cough, fatigue, and exercise-induced syncope are less common and more concerning.

The physical exam with dynamic auscultation should help determine the diagnosis and severity of the disease. Signs of heart failure may include tachypnea, tachycardia, poor perfusion, cool mottled extremities, hypotension, and sluggish capillary refill. The presence of an S4 gallop, jugular venous distention, and peripheral edema are always pathologic clinical signs. Lateral displacement of the PMI (point of maximal impulse) indicates cardiomegaly and may be seen in shunt defects or cardiomyopathy. The presence of a thrill is consistent with possible left to right shunt or a valve disease. A systolic murmur at the left lower sternal border, which increases in intensity after standing from a squat position, may indicate hypertrophic obstructive cardiomyopathy (Table 8.5).

TABLE 8.5 ■ COMMON ETIOLOGIES OF HEART FAILURE PRESENTING IN OLDER CHILDREN AND ADOLESCENTS

*Acquired Heart Disease and Cardiomypathy	*Unoperated Structural Heart Defects	*Postoperative Structural Heart Disease
KD	Mitral valve regurgitation	Left heart failure
RHD	Aortic Regurgitation	Systemic right ventricle/single ventricle/Fontan
Infective endocarditis	Progressive LVOT obstruction	Myocardial ischemia fibrosis
Marfan syndrome valvular disease	Ebstein anomaly	Residual shunts
Sickle cell anemia	Eisenmenger syndrome	Residual valve insufficiency, aortic, or truncal valve
Pulmonary hypertension		Residual outflow obstruction
Arrhythmias		
Carditis		Right heart failure
Cardiomyopathy		Residual RVOT or PA obstruction
		Pulmonary hypertenaion
		Tet repair with pulmonary insufficiency

LVOT, left ventricular outflow tract obstruction; RVOT, Right ventricular outflow tract
*Lists are not all inclusive but include the most common etiologies.

ED Care and Disposition

The second major challenge for the emergency room physician is to stabilize the patient and improve hemodynamics. Prompt reassessment of vital signs and resuscitation according to the Pediatric Advanced Life Support (PALS) guidelines is recommended including treatment of life-threatening arrhythmia. Amiodarone is useful for ventricular arrhythmias in patients with suspected left ventricle failure. Once the patient is stable, palpation of four extremities pulses, blood pressures, 12-lead ECG, and CXR may be obtained. Echocardiography is recommended for all patients with heart murmurs and signs and symptoms of heart failure. Serum B-type natriuretic peptide (BNP) may be helpful in determining the severity of heart failure. This is secreted from the ventricles in response to increased wall stress from pressure or volume load. Cardiology consultation is recommended in all patients in whom significant cardiac disease is suspected.

For ease of clinical recognition and guidance of further therapy, the pathophysiology of heart failure in older children may be divided into three categories. Category 1 includes diseases with pump dysfunction such as cardiomyopathies. Congenital heart defects rarely appear in this category. Poor cardiac output is directly related to decreased contractility. These patients may benefit from IV furosemide, fluid restriction, inotropic agents, and afterload reduction. Category 2 includes defects with normal pump function and increased preload. Previously repaired defects, such as Tetralogy of Fallot post-transannular patch with chronic pulmonary valve insufficiency or chronic aortic valve insufficiency, are the major contributors to this category.

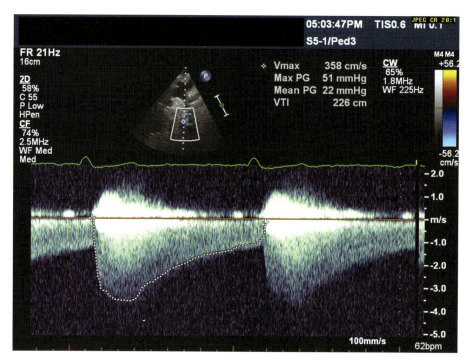

FIGURE 8.19 ▪ Aortic arch Doppler severe CoA. Twenty-two-year old with claudication and no palpable pedal pulse. Doppler of the aortic arch demonstrates forward flow across the aortic arch during systole and diastole.

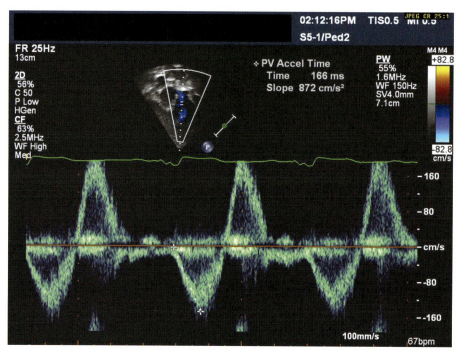

FIGURE 8.20 ▪ Doppler profile in severe pulmonary insufficiency. Eighteen-year old with early-exercise fatigue of post transannular patch repair Tetralogy of Fallot. "To and Fro" flow demonstrated during systole and diastole consistent with severe pulmonary valve insufficiency. Valve forward flow shown below the baseline, regurgitant flow shown above baseline.

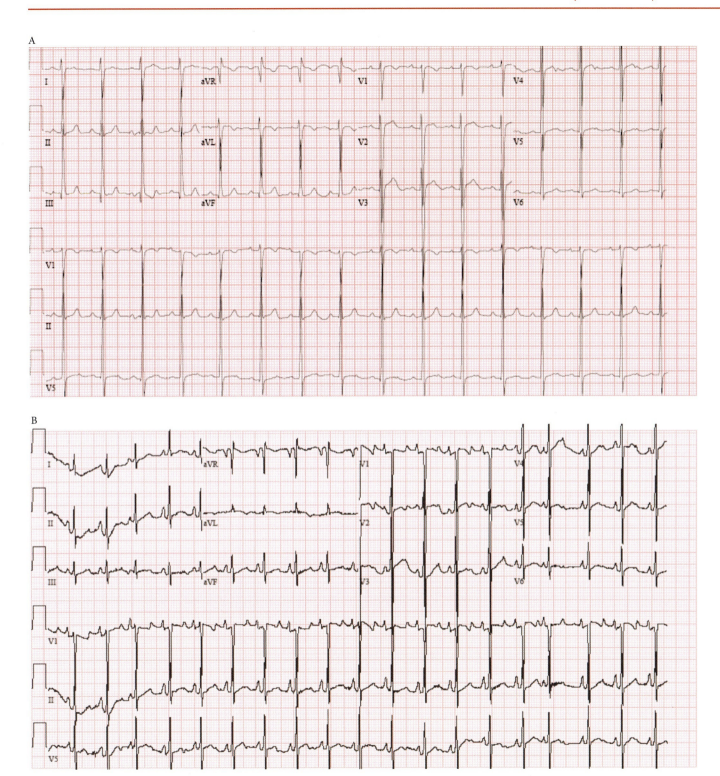

FIGURE 8.21 ■ Twelve-lead ECG hypertrophic cardiomyopathy (HCM). Two patients with HCM. **(A)** Six-year old with Hunter syndrome. Increased R-wave voltage in V5 and V6, deep S wave in V1, consistent with left ventricular hypertrophy (LVH). **(B)** Eighteen-month old with HCM and pulmonary hypertension deep S wave V1, V2 suggestive of LVH, tall P waves consistent with right atrial enlargement.

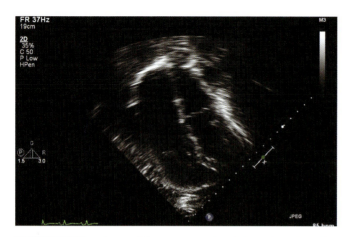

FIGURE 8.22 ■ Severe Ebstein anomaly of the tricuspid valve. Apical four-chamber view 2D echocardiography. Severe inferior displacement of the septal leaflet of the tricuspid valve. Atrialized right ventricle located between the annulus of the tricuspid valve and the septal leaflet of the tricuspid valve.

Chronic aortic valve insufficiency may be well tolerated; however, acute insufficiency can be a medical and possible surgical emergency. Afterload reduction may be helpful for this group. Category 3 consists of diseases with normal contractility and increased ventricle pressure such as aortic or subaortic stenosis. Systemic vasodilators are not recommended for this category.

Pearls and Pitfalls

- Older children with congenital heart defects usually do not present with pump dysfunction. Exceptions include patients with acute severe valve insufficiency or prior congenital heart defect surgery.
- Common adolescent complaints such as chest pain, palpitations, syncope, and fatigue accompanied by signs of volume overload should alert the physician of potential significant cardiac disease.

Inflamatory and Infectious Disorders
MYOCARDITIS AND PERICARDITIS

Sidney Larken Ware
James C. O'Neill

Clinical Highlights: Myocarditis

Myocarditis is an inflammation of the myocardium, typically involving infiltration of lymphocytes, plasma cells, and histiocytes into the myocardium. Myocarditis can range from very mild, with patients often not seeking medical attention, to severe weakness in the myocardium leading to heart failure. Fever and tachycardia out of proportion to the degree of temperature are common presenting symptoms. Patients may present with hepatomegaly, pulmonary edema, jugular venous distension, and lower extremity edema. Patients may also complain of chest pain, fever, and myalgias due to associated pericardial disease. Causative agents of myocarditis include coxsackie, echovirus, influenza, HIV, hepatitis B, and EBV. Bacterial causes include diphtheria, *Neisseria meningitidis*, *Mycoplasma*, β-hemolytic streptococcus, and Lyme disease. ECG, CXRs, cardiac enzymes, and echocardiography may be helpful in making the diagnosis.

ED Care and Disposition

Differential diagnosis for this can include any cause of heart failure and cardiomegaly: ischemic heart disease, hypertensive heart disease, valvular heart disease, CHD, and idiopathic cardiomyopathy. Treatment for myocarditis is typically supportive. Suspected bacterial causes require antibiotic therapy. Patients with myocarditis require admission and observation. If symptoms progress rapidly, extracorporeal membrane oxygenation (ECMO) may be considered.

Pearls and Pitfalls

- Consider myocarditis in someone with tachycardia out of proportion to fever.
- Although myocarditis is often caused by viral infections, there may be a bacterial cause that requires antibiotics.
- 30% to 40% of patients with pericarditis may have a myocarditis component.
- Patients who do not respond to NSAIDs or colchicine may have an underlying cause such as lupus or other autoimmune disorder.
- Patients may respond to steroids but these should not be started unless in discussion with a cardiologist and/or rheumatologist because symptoms can worsen when steroids are discontinued.

Clinical Highlights: Pericarditis

Pericarditis is inflammation of the fibrous membrane that surrounds the heart. A patient most commonly complains of either gradual or sudden-onset chest pain that radiates to the back, left shoulder, or left trapezial ridge. The chest pain often worsens with movement and inspiration. Most commonly, the pain worsens when the patient lies supine and improves with leaning forward. The patient may experience low-grade fever, shortness of breath, and difficulty in swallowing. On physical exam, patients may have a friction rub that is typically best

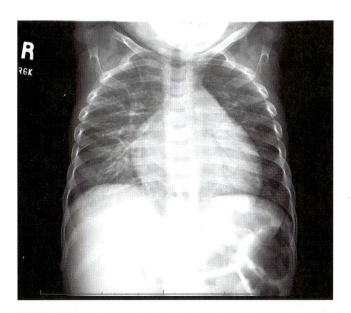

FIGURE 8.23 ■ Image taken in ED when the patient was diagnosed with myocarditis. The liver appears large. CXRs can often appear normal but this x-ray shows evidence of heart failure with cardiomegaly and pulmonary edema.

226 ■ MYOCARDITIS AND PERICARDITIS (CONTINUED)

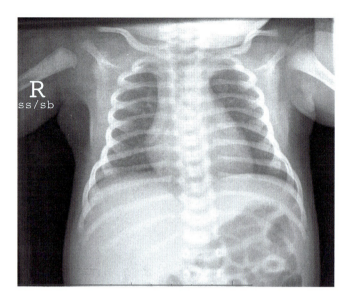

FIGURE 8.24 ■ This x-ray from the same patient from Figure 8.23 was taken 18 months prior to the diagnosis of myocarditis. The patient's cardiac silhouette was within normal limits.

heard at left sternal border or apex when patient is leaning forward.

The cause of pericarditis is often idiopathic but viral infections, such as coxsackie and HIV, bacterial infections, such as staphylococcus, β-hemolytic streptococcus, and tuberculosis, can be causative. Less common causes include malignancy, drugs such as procainamide and hydralazine, lupus, rheumatoid arthritis, and other rheumatic diseases. Pericarditis can also be seen after a myocardial infarction, with uremia, and in myxedema.

ED Care and Disposition

Diagnosis can be aided with common ECG findings. CXRs are occasionally helpful for diagnosis. An echocardiogram should be used to establish extent of effusion and to help determine hemodynamic stability. An echocardiogram can also show pericardial effusion, decreased ejection fraction,

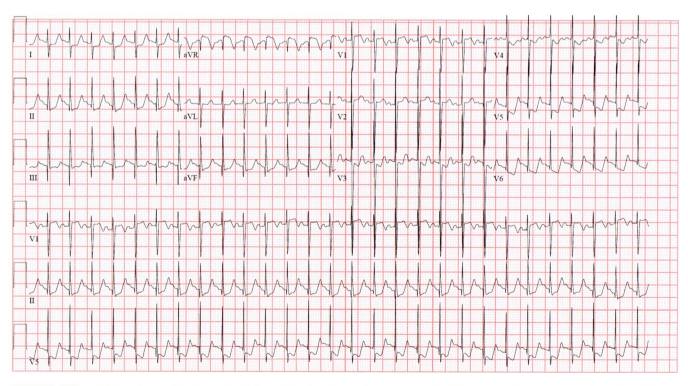

FIGURE 8.25 ■ ECG performed during patient's hospitalization shows sinus tachycardia, ST-segment depression in inferior-lateral leads, ST-segment abnormality, and T-wave inversion in lateral leads. This patient's troponin was 74 and rose to 1343.

MYOCARDITIS AND PERICARDITIS (CONTINUED)

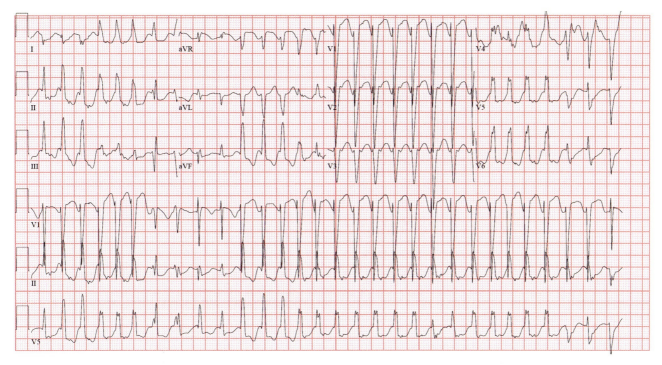

FIGURE 8.26 ■ ECG shows a wide complex tachycardia that occurred as the patient's disease progressed. This patient required ECMO after cardiac arrest.

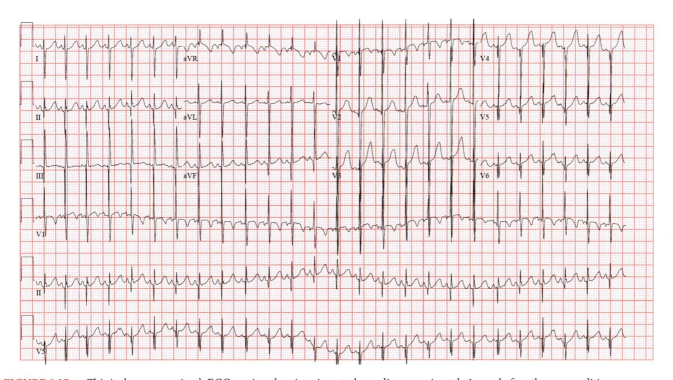

FIGURE 8.27 ■ This is the same patient's ECG tracing showing sinus tachycardia approximately 1 year before the myocarditis.

228 ■ MYOCARDITIS AND PERICARDITIS (CONTINUED)

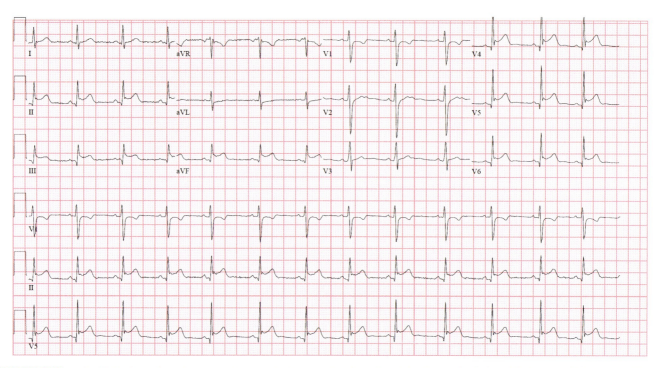

FIGURE 8.28 ■ An ECG of a patient that was subsequently diagnosed with pericarditis. Notice the diffuse ST elevation. This is typically the classic ECG for diagnosis of pericarditis.

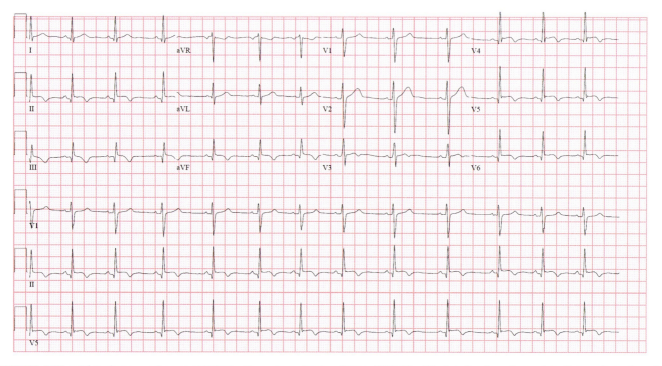

FIGURE 8.29 ■ This shows a subsequent ECG in the same patient as Figure 8.28. The ST elevation has changed to T-wave inversions in inferior-lateral leads.

MYOCARDITIS AND PERICARDITIS (CONTINUED)

or hypokinesis. Serial cardiac enzymes (most often troponin) may also point to concomitant myocarditis that is seen in between 30% and 40% of pericarditis cases. Most patients with idiopathic pericarditis respond to nonsteroidal anti-inflammatory medications in 7 to 21 days. Patients may also respond to colchicine. If a specific cause is found, then treatment should be directed toward that etiology.

Pearls and Pitfalls

- Myocarditis is concomitant in 30% to 40% of children with pericarditis.
- Bedside ultrasound looking for pericardial effusion should be considered in any profoundly symptomatic child diagnosed with pericarditis.

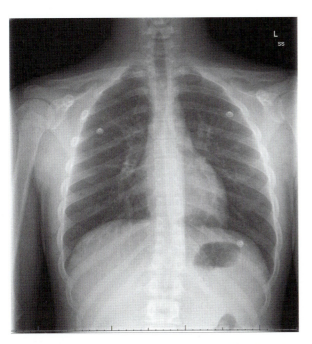

FIGURE 8.30 ■ This same patient as represented in the prior two figures with pericarditis has a normal CXR.

KAWASAKI DISEASE

Michael S. Mitchell

Clinical Highlights

Kawasaki disease (KD) is a disease that affects the pediatric population, mostly in the toddler years. The vast majority of cases are found in children under 5 years of age. While KD lacks a definitive etiology, it has distinct clinical features that aid diagnosis. A documented fever lasting for more than 5 days is the hallmark symptom, followed by a constellation of other symptoms. The diagnosis is made when at least four of the following clinical symptoms are present: (1) bilateral, bulbar, nonpurulent conjunctivitis, (2) cervical lymphadenopathy that is usually unilateral, (3) oropharyngeal mucosal changes including an injected pharynx or lips, dry lips, or strawberry tongue, (4) changes in the peripheral extremities including hand or foot edema or erythema or fingertip desquamation, and (5) polymorphous rash that is usually truncal. There is no definitive laboratory test that will diagnose KD; however, elevated inflammatory makers such as erythrocyte sedimentation rate (ESR) and C-reactive protein (CRP) can be seen as well as sterile pyuria.

KD has significant cardiac sequelae, thus, it is imperative to consider and establish the diagnosis in those children with fever for more than 5 days. KD can lead to the development of coronary artery aneurysms (can be seen in up to 20% of untreated patients), placing the patient at risk for early myocardial ischemia and infarction.

ED Care and Disposition

Confirming the diagnosis with the hallmark clinical findings is of utmost importance. To vastly reduce the risk of coronary artery aneurysms, physicians need to initiate treatment before

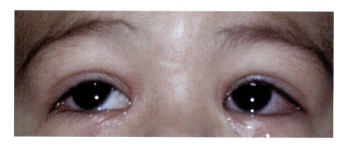

FIGURE 8.32 ■ Conjunctival injection with limbic sparing noted in KD. Reproduced, with permission, from Chapter 167. Rowley AH. Kawasaki disease. In: Goldsmith LA, Katz SI, Gilchrest BA, Paller AS, Leffell DJ, Wolff K, eds. *Fitzpatrick's Dermatology in General Medicine*. 8th ed. New York, NY: McGraw-Hill; 2012.

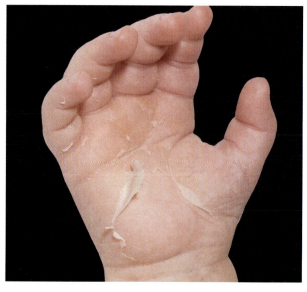

FIGURE 8.33 ■ Desquamation of the epidermis is a fairly late finding in acute KD. Note the hand swelling that is also associated with the acute process of this disease. Reproduced, with permission, from Section 14. The skin in immune, autoimmune, and rheumatic disorders. In: Wolff K, Johnson R, Saavedra AP, eds. *Fitzpatrick's Color Atlas and Synopsis of Clinical Dermatology*. 7th ed. New York, NY: McGraw-Hill; 2013.

FIGURE 8.31 ■ The toddler-aged child with dry, fissured lips and the polymorphous, erythematous exanthem noted with KD. Fissuring of the lips and an erythematous exanthem are evident in this patient with KD. Courtesy of Stephen E. Gellis, MD; with permission. Reproduced, with permission, from Harrison's Online.

the 10th day of illness. All patients in whom KD is the leading diagnosis should be admitted to an appropriate facility that can initiate treatment. Intravenous immunoglobulin (IVIG) and high-dose aspirin are the mainstays of therapy, and once given, rapidly improve the clinical syndrome. All patients with KD should have an echocardiogram to evaluate for early development of coronary artery aneurysms.

Pearls and Pitfalls

- KD should be strongly considered in all children under the age of 5 years with more than 5 days of documented fever.
- Children with KD are very irritable.
- Vast reduction in cardiac sequelae is seen if KD is treated before day 10 of illness. If a patient does not have classic disease and the diagnosis remains uncertain, it is acceptable to arrange close follow-up for the patient to see if further clinical symptoms develop as long as the patient is within the 10-day window.
- Admission and further consultation should be considered for the patient within 10 days of illness if the diagnosis remains unclear.
- The finding of sterile pyuria originates from the urethra. If attempting to check this test, it is imperative to obtain a clean catch specimen since catheterization will bypass the urethra.

RHEUMATIC HEART DISEASE

Christopher Watkins

Clinical Highlights

Rheumatic heart disease (RHD) is the most severe manifestation of rheumatic fever, a delayed autoimmune response to a pharyngeal infection due to group A β-hemolytic streptococcus, which results in valvular damage to the heart, most commonly the mitral valve. Rheumatic fever has largely become a disease of developing countries in areas of limited access to medical care or antibiotics; however, with the increasingly global nature of medicine, it is still a relevant disease to industrialized nations. Rheumatic fever typically affects children and young adults and manifests as a combination of symptoms including fever, joint pain, chorea, carditis, erythema marginatum, or subcutaneous nodules. It may begin as early as 10 days following initial pharyngeal infection. Cardiac involvement occurs in approximately 50% of rheumatic fever cases and infection may comprise myocarditis, pericarditis, and/or valvulitis. Patients may complain of chest pain, palpitations, or shortness of breath. The most common initial valvular involvement is mitral regurgitation, heard as an apical holosystolic murmur that may radiate to the axilla. Chronic RHD can progress to mitral stenosis, which is heard as a loud S1 (opening snap) followed by a diastolic rumble. A CXR may show signs of cardiomegaly or, in severe cases, pulmonary edema.

ECG findings suggestive of RHD are often nonspecific and most commonly include PR interval prolongation beyond 0.20 seconds.

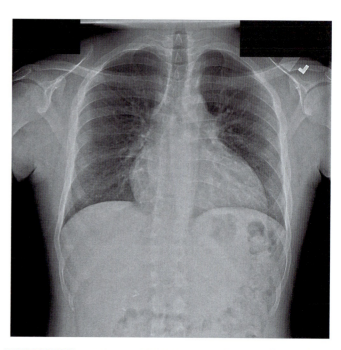

FIGURE 8.34 ■ PA view of CXR shows moderate cardiomegaly.

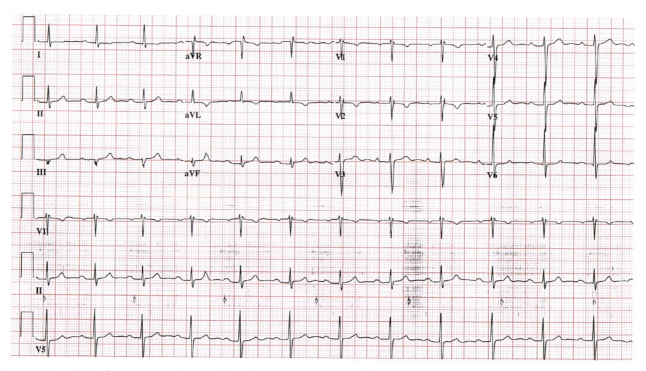

FIGURE 8.35 ■ ECG of normal sinus rhythm with moderate prolongation of PR interval.

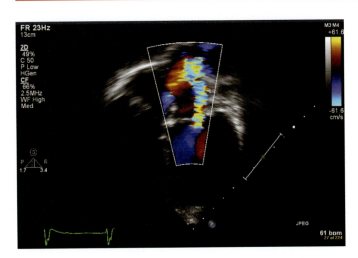

FIGURE 8.36 ■ Color-flow Doppler demonstrating mitral regurgitation.

VIDEO 8.5 ■ This apical four-chamber view shows mitral regurgitation in a patient with RHD. *View at http://mhprofessional.com/sites/lefebvre*

The most important diagnostic study is an echocardiogram to evaluate the extent of valvular damage.

ED Care and Disposition

There is no specific treatment for RHD. Therapy remains largely supportive and is directed at treatment and prevention of complicating sequelae, such as congestive heart failure and atrial fibrillation. Penicillin remains the mainstay of treatment for patients with acute rheumatic fever and as prevention of recurrent *Streptococcus pyogenes* infections that lead to reactivation of RHD. Salicylates are helpful for fever control and pain from carditis and arthralgia, but offer no protective measures. Steroids have not shown any benefit for RHD. Patients with more severe manifestations of congestive heart failure from acute valvular involvement will require admission and more urgent surgical correction of valvular damage. Patients with minor manifestations may be discharged after arranging appropriate cardiology follow-up for further evaluation and outpatient echocardiogram.

Pearls and Pitfalls

- Approximately 50% of cases of rheumatic fever and RHD have no history of preceding pharyngeal infection.
- Any new murmur in children and young adults should raise suspicion for RHD.
- Even without any cardiac signs or symptoms, all patients with rheumatic fever should have an echocardiogram for evaluation of subclinical cardiac involvement.

Obstructive Shock
CARDIAC TAMPONADE

Alan T. Chiem
Kevin Rooney
Elizabeth Turner

Clinical Highlights

Cardiac tamponade is a form of obstructive shock characterized by impedance in venous return to the right atrium due to high pressures exerted by pericardial fluid. The fluid can rapidly accumulate as in a hemopericardium from penetrating trauma to the chest or in an ascending aortic dissection. Pericardial fluid can also slowly develop over weeks to months, from effusions that slowly distend the potential space between the visceral and parietal pericardium until maximal volume is achieved and there is a resultant increase in pressure. This "last drop" phenomenon is the proposed mechanism for cardiac tamponade from slowly expanding pericardial effusions. Acute tamponade can result from as little as 100 to 200 mL of pericardial fluid, whereas subacute presentations of tamponade can result from over 1 L of pericardial fluid.

In penetrating thoracic injury, tamponade due to myocardial or great vessel injury must be considered in patients presenting with hypotension. In nontraumatic patients,

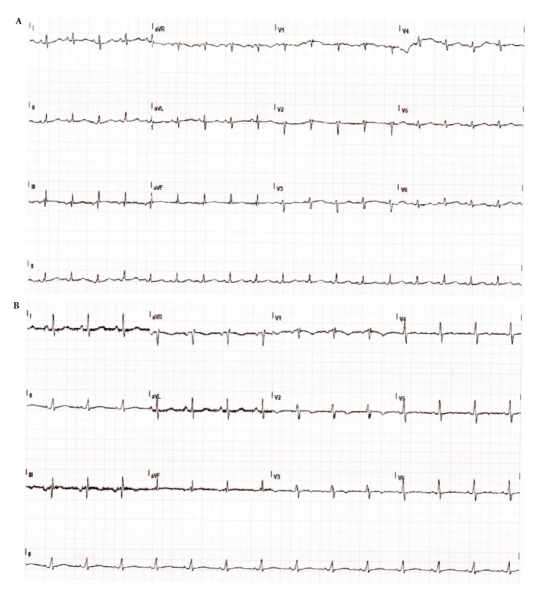

FIGURE 8.37 ■ ECG showing low voltage in precordial leads prior to pericardiocentesis (**A**) and increased voltage after pericardiocentesis (**B**).

ascending aortic dissection is an important cause of acute cardiac tamponade to consider. However, the most common causes of nontraumatic tamponade are due to malignancy (~40%), idiopathic (~20%), uremia (10%–15%), and both viral and bacterial pericarditis leading to pericardial effusion and tamponade (~10%).

Patients often present in severe discomfort, and may complain of chest pain, right upper quadrant pain due to hepatic congestion, dyspnea, and/or nausea. Physical findings include hypotension, jugular venous distension, and muffled heart sounds or a pericardial rub. Pulsus paradoxus and Kussmaul sign are classic findings, but often impractical to assess in the acute tamponade patient. ECG findings typically show low voltage or electric alternans, which can also be demonstrated via ultrasound as the swaying of the apex in the pericardial fluid. CXR may show cardiomegaly—especially a "water bottle" heart—without evidence of pulmonary congestion.

ED Care and Disposition

In trauma patients, cardiac tamponade can be assessed via the pericardial or parasternal window of the Focused Abdominal Sonography in Trauma (FAST) scan. If there is evidence of tamponade physiology, the decision must be made in concert with the trauma surgery team whether to perform ED thoracotomy or explore in the OR.

In nontraumatic patients presenting with suspected cardiac tamponade, a point-of-care (POC) ultrasound should be quickly performed to assess for pericardial effusion and RV collapse. If POC ultrasound shows evidence of cardiac tamponade, cardiology should be consulted for stat transesophageal echocardiography to evaluate for aortic dissection. In addition, cardiothoracic surgery should be consulted for possible dissection repair in the OR. Temporizing measures such as normal saline boluses may be given to

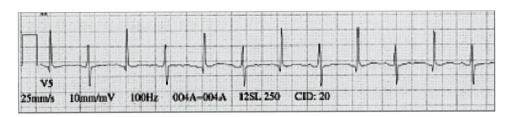

FIGURE 8.38 ■ ECG rhythm strip showing electrical alternans, which is a rhythmic alternation of the QRS axis due to swinging of the heart as it contracts in a pericardium filled with fluid. Reproduced, with permission, from Tintinalli JE, Stapczynski JS, Ma OJ, Cline DM, Cydulka RK, Meckler GD. *Tintinalli's Emergency Medicine: A Comprehensive Study Guide.* 7th ed. New York, NY: McGraw-Hill; 2011.

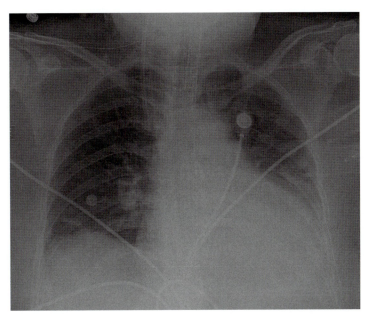

FIGURE 8.39 ■ Anterior–posterior CXR showing a "water bottle" heart. There are increased interstitial lung markings due to this patient's subacute presentation of tamponade due to cardiac neoplasm.

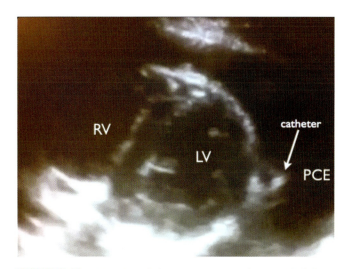

FIGURE 8.40 ■ Parasternal short-axis view on ultrasound of a large pericardial effusion after a pericardiocentesis catheter (arrow) has been placed. PCE, pericardial effusion; LV, left ventricle; RV, right ventricle.

optimize venous return and preload, and if refractory, a vasoconstrictor such as phenylephrine may be given.

Pearls and Pitfalls

- Perform a bedside ultrasound of the heart, pericardium, and pleura in any patient presenting with severe respiratory distress, chest pain, and/or hypotension.
- If ascending aortic dissection is the suspected cause of cardiac tamponade, early consultation with cardiothoracic surgery and cardiology is required.
- Inotropes should be avoided if aortic dissection is still considered as a cause of cardiac tamponade, to minimize extension of the dissection.

Cardiac Rhythm Disorders
SUPRAVENTRICULAR TACHYCARDIA IN CHILDREN

James C. O'Neill

Clinical Highlights

Although SVT is by definition any rapid heart rhythm that originates above the bundle of His, most authors use this term to refer to regular narrow-complex tachycardias. Two rhythms most commonly referred to as SVT are atrioventricular nodal reentrant tachycardia (in which the reentry circuit is located in the atrioventricular node) and atrioventricular reciprocating (reentrant) tachycardia (in which the reentry circuit involves a bypass tract). Both these rhythms create a narrow-complex regular tachycardia. SVT is the most common symptomatic arrhythmia in the pediatric population. It affects 1 in 1700 infants and can be dangerous because many younger children cannot communicate their symptoms.

ED Care and Disposition

The discomfort felt by older children with SVT often causes parents to seek medical care. In younger infants, SVT may present with lethargy, poor feeding, or a change in the child's behavior. A high index of suspicion and careful review of vital signs is important in diagnosing SVT. Infants with SVT can have tachycardia in the range of 220 to 300—much higher than what an adult or older child could tolerate without severe symptoms. Differentiating between SVT and sinus tachycardia can be difficult at high heart rates, so vagal maneuvers or adenosine use are sometimes needed to correctly diagnose SVT versus sinus tachycardia. Treatment of this rhythm requires the slowing down of atrioventricular node conduction. Once this occurs, a sinus rhythm can restart. One way to slow conduction at the AV node is to perform vagal maneuvers if a child can follow directions. These include a child trying to perform a valsalva maneuver or blowing through a straw. The most successful vagal maneuver involves placing bags of ice over the child's entire face to simulate a dive reflex. First-line therapy for SVT includes adenosine, an ultra-short acting agent that blocks at the atrioventricular node (dosed 0.1 mg/kg with additional doses of 0.2 mg/kg). Calcium channel blockers (in children older than 1 year of age), beta-blockers, procainamide, and amiodarone are considered second-line therapy, but are rarely needed. Cardioversion is immediately indicated if a child shows signs of instability, including hypotension, altered mental status, and poor perfusion. Simultaneous treatment of fever and dehydration is important in cases in which a provider has difficulty in discriminating SVT from severe sinus tachycardia.

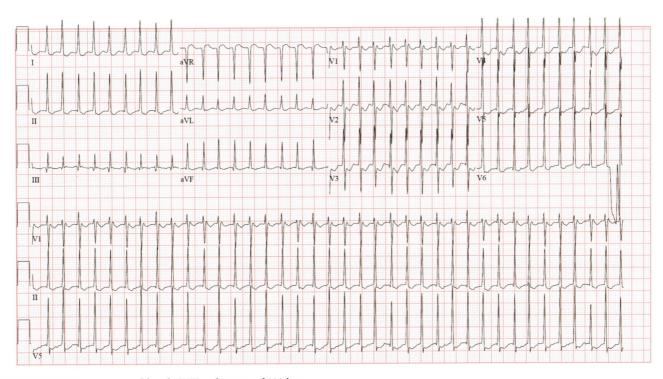

FIGURE 8.41 ■ Four-year old with SVT with a rate of 228 bpm.

Pearls and Pitfalls

- Ice applied in a vagal maneuver is more successful if the bags of ice cover the entire face, including eyes, mouth, and nose.
- Cardioversion of a child should start with 0.25 to 0.5 J/kg and may need up to 2 J/kg.

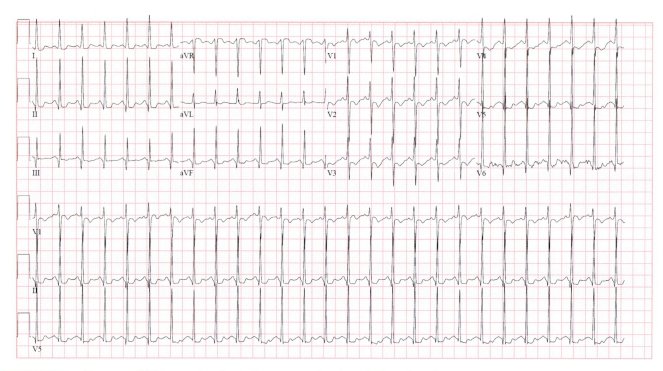

FIGURE 8.42 ■ Four-year old from previous image that converted to sinus rhythm after adenosine was given.

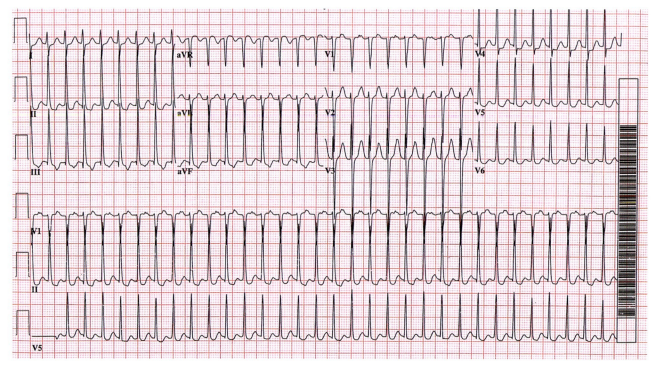

FIGURE 8.43 ■ Fourteen-year old with SVT with a rate of 198 (with inferior T-wave inversion in leads II, III, and AVF).

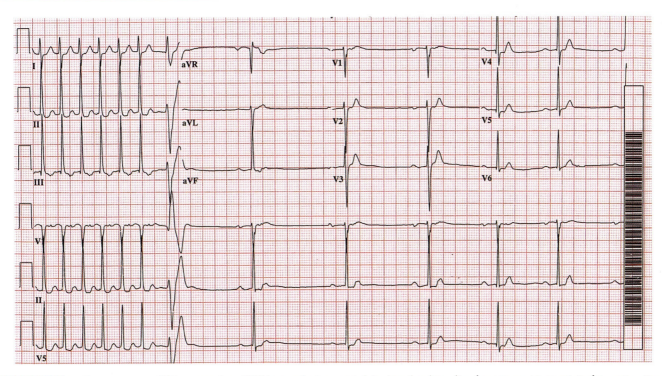

FIGURE 8.44 ■ Fourteen-year old from previous SVT image that converted to sinus bradycardia after a premature ventricular contraction.

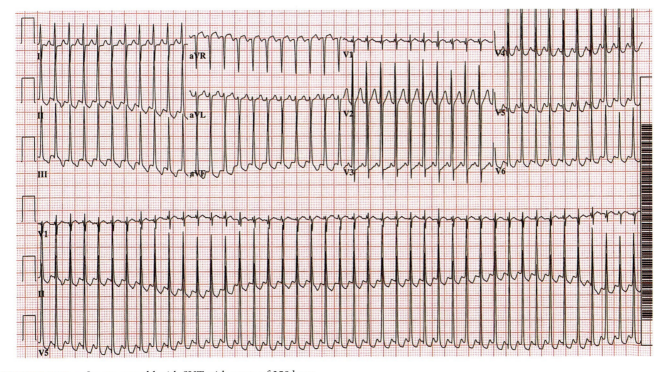

FIGURE 8.45 ■ Seven-year old with SVT with a rate of 258 bpm.

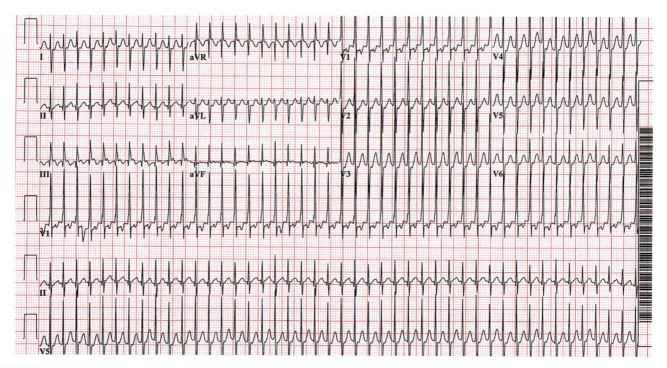

FIGURE 8.46 ■ Two-week old with SVT with a rate of 271 bpm.

HEART BLOCK IN CHILDREN

Chad McCalla

Clinical Highlights

While bradycardia is far less common in children than in adults, it can still be seen in an emergency setting and cause significant morbidity and mortality. The most common types of bradycardia in a child are sinus bradycardia and atrioventricular (AV) block. Sinus bradycardia in children is defined as a depolarization rate that is below the lowest normal heart rate values based on age. This can be a normal variant, especially in well-conditioned, athletic children. AV block causes bradycardia by either blocking or delaying impulses at the AV node. It is broken up into different degrees:

First degree: slowed conduction with no missed beats, with lengthened PR interval;

Second degree: intermittent conduction with missed beats, either with progressive prolongation of the PR interval with resultant failure of P-wave conduction (type 1/Wenckebach) or an unchanging PR interval with sudden failure of the P wave to conduct (type 2); and

Third degree/Complete: total failure of the atrial impulse to be conducted to the ventricles.

AV block can be either congenital or acquired. Common causes of congenital AV block include underlying congenital heart defects, corrective surgery of these defects that leads to injury of the conduction system, autoimmune (commonly neonatal lupus where maternal antibodies cross the placenta and damage the conduction tissue of the fetal heart), and familial AV conduction block—a rare genetically acquired condition. Causes of acquired heart block include myocarditis, acute rheumatic disease, Lyme disease, rubella, and mumps.

In older children, bradycardia presents as dizziness, syncope, fatigue, or exercise intolerance. Infants and toddlers experiencing bradycardia may demonstrate poor feeding, lethargy, or other nonspecific symptoms. The ECG will show a slow heart rate, a prolonged PR interval in the upper limits of normal based on age (first degree), progressive prolongation of the PR interval until the absence of the P-wave (Mobitz type I), P waves that suddenly fail to be conducted with no change in PR interval length (Mobitz type II), or complete dissociation of communication between atria and ventricle (third degree).

ED Care and Disposition

Acute management of bradycardia depends on the clinical presentation. Previously healthy children who are asymptomatic,

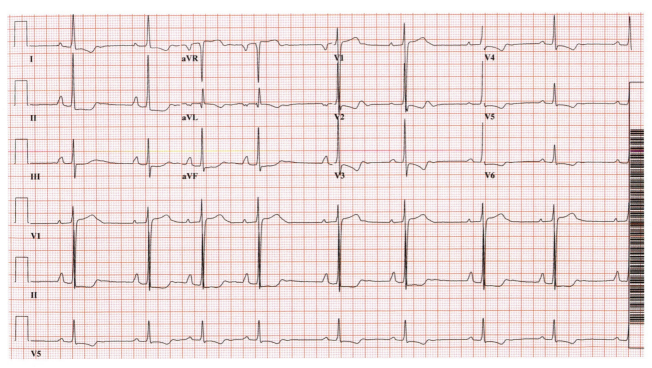

FIGURE 8.47 ■ ECG findings in a 12-year-old child with first-degree AV block. Note the slowed heart rate, prolonged PR interval, and the absence of any dropped QRS complexes.

242 ■ HEART BLOCK IN CHILDREN (CONTINUED)

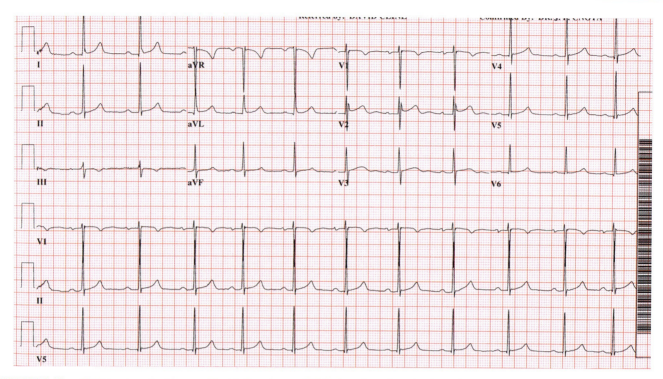

FIGURE 8.48 ■ ECG tracing of a 14-year old with first-degree AV block and resultant bradycardia.

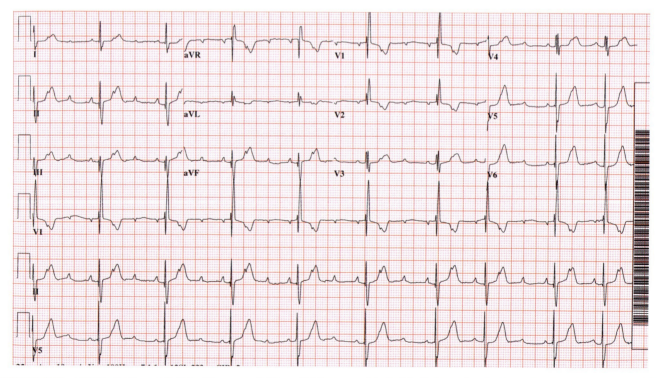

FIGURE 8.49 ■ ECG of a 3-month old with a second-degree (Mobitz type II) AV block. Note the significant bradycardia, prolonged PR interval, and intermittent failure of a QRS complex to follow a p wave.

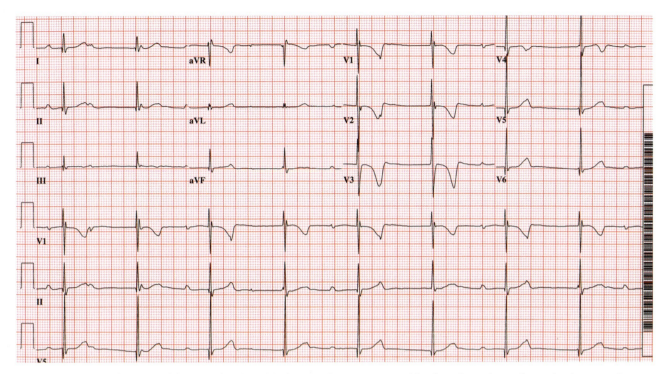

FIGURE 8.50 ■ ECG of a 3-year old in complete heart block. ECG shows a junctional bradycardia with no relationship between the P waves and QRS complexes.

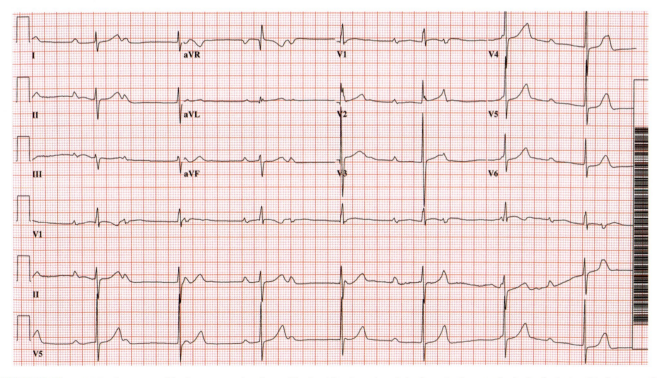

FIGURE 8.51 ■ ECG of a 9-year old, also in complete heart block with a junctional rhythm. Again note the lack of relationship between the P waves and QRS complexes.

especially patients in sinus bradycardia, can be discharged home with little to no intervention after consultation with a cardiologist. However, for children who are symptomatic—especially with poor perfusion and shock—immediate pediatric advanced life support should be initiated. The patient's airway and circulation should be assessed and treated including oxygen and intubation if indicated. Cardiopulmonary resuscitation (CPR) should be started in children with a heart rate <60 bpm despite appropriate oxygenation and ventilation. Epinephrine should be given (dose 0.01 mg/kg; 1:10,000; 0.1 mL/kg, max of 1 mg) either IV or IO, the dose can be repeated every 3 to 5 minutes as needed. If no IV/IO access has been established, epinephrine can be delivered via endotracheal tube with a higher dose concentration (0.1 mg/kg; 1:1000; 0.1 mL/kg). If still no improvement is seen, atropine at 0.02 mg/kg (minimum dose 0.1 mg) can be given and repeated once if necessary. Consider cardiac pacing for refractory bradycardia, particularly if a conduction defect is suspected.

Pearls and Pitfalls

- Normal ECG intervals are different based on the age of the patient. Standard charts can be found in multiple pediatric cardiology and emergency resources.
- Since most heart block is acquired, a thorough history, including past and recent illnesses, travel, vaccination status, should be undertaken.
- Consider neonatal lupus in a young infant with a third-degree AV block, even if the mother has not been diagnosed.
- Treatment should focus on acute reversal of the bradycardia with pharmacologic agents and/or cardiac pacing, while at the same time, the ED practitioner should be searching for a potentially reversible underlying cause.

WOLFF–PARKINSON–WHITE IN CHILDREN

Chad McCalla

Clinical Highlights

Wolff–Parkinson–White (WPW) syndrome is a congenital abnormality involving abnormal conduction tissues between the atria and the ventricles. The presence of these tissues creates an accessory conduction pathway between the atria and ventricles leading to preexcitation and premature ventricular contraction. This results in a form of SVT known as a reentrant tachycardia. This is a rare syndrome, only affecting between 0.1% and 0.3% of the general population, and the majority of children with this condition never experience symptoms. Symptomatic patients most commonly present to the ED in SVT. Infants experiencing SVT may present with irritability, poor feeding tolerance, or in more severe cases, signs of congestive heart failure. Older children may experience palpitations, chest discomfort, breathing difficulty, syncope, and rarely cardiac arrest. There are no physical exam findings diagnostic for WPW other than those features that are present in SVT. Common findings are a regular heart rhythm that is often too fast to count (200–250 bpm in infants, >180 bpm in older children), diaphoresis, and patient anxiety. There are no characteristic cardiac findings other than the tachycardia, that is, patients do not typically present with murmurs, rubs, or gallops. In severe cases, the child will show signs of cardiogenic shock, manifesting as hypotension, poor perfusion, hepatosplenomegaly, and crackles on lung exam.

Characteristic ECG findings that are associated with WPW include the following:
- Presence of a short PR interval (often <120 milliseconds).
- A widened QRS complex longer than 120 milliseconds with an abnormal sloping of the initial upstroke of the complex (delta wave). This is characteristic of WPW, however, is not universally seen.

When patients with WPW present in SVT, the rapid rhythm frequently obscures the classic ECG findings such as the delta wave making identification impossible until the SVT has been converted to sinus rhythm.

ED Care and Disposition

Patients with underlying WPW syndrome will present to the ED with SVT; therefore, initial management involves treating the SVT. In previously healthy children who are not showing signs of shock, the physician can perform maneuvers to increase vagal tone. The most common maneuvers include applying ice to the face or simulating a valsalva maneuver (having the child bear down, blow through a straw, or blow bubbles). If vagal maneuvers fail to convert the rhythm, the

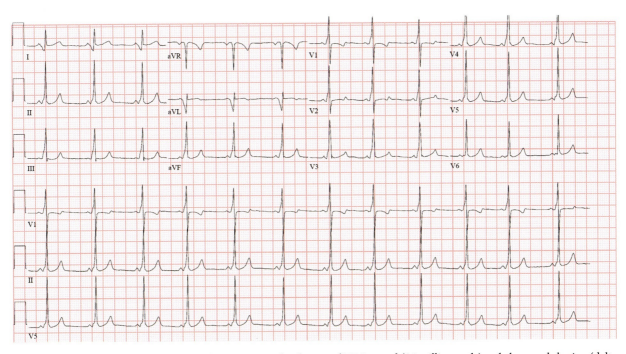

FIGURE 8.52 ■ ECG of a 13-year-old male with WPW. Note the shortened PR interval (94 milliseconds) and abnormal sloping (delta wave) on the initial upstroke of the QRS complex.

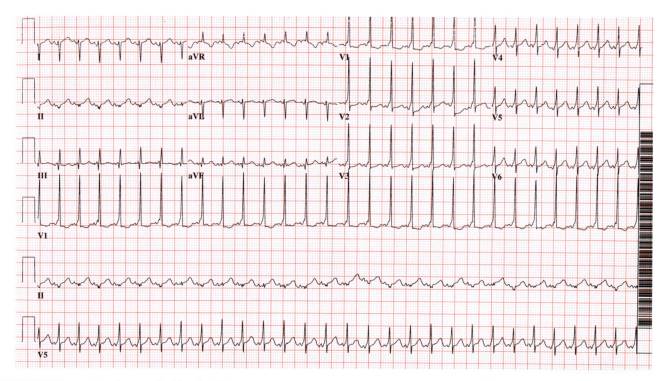

FIGURE 8.53 ■ ECG of a 3-week old with WPW, again demonstrating characteristic delta waves and PR interval changes.

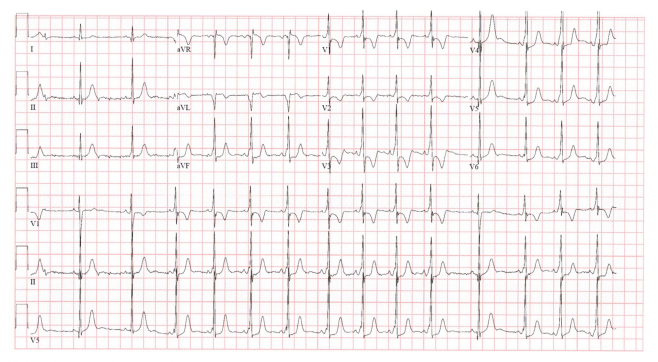

FIGURE 8.54 ■ ECG of a 6-year old with WPW.

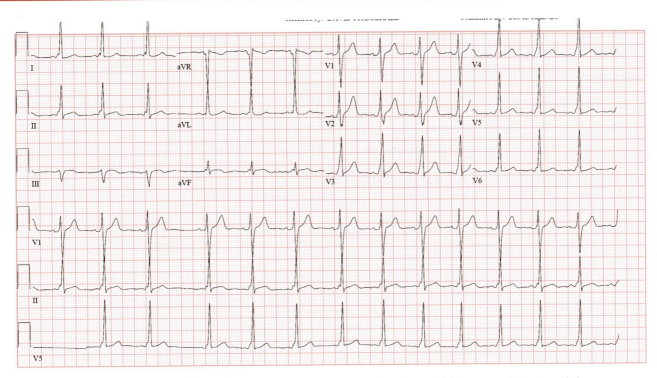

FIGURE 8.55 ■ ECG of a 17-year-old child with WPW, again demonstrating characteristic delta waves and PR interval changes.

physician should next administer adenosine. Adenosine has a very short half-life; therefore, in order to be most effective IV placement as close to the heart is needed. Initial dose is 0.1 mg/kg; double the dose to 0.2 mg/kg for the second attempt at converting the rhythm if the initial dose is unsuccessful. If adenosine is unsuccessful, try alternative medications or synchronized cardioversion in conjunction with cardiology consultation. In patients who are unstable and are showing signs of shock, proceed to cardioversion.

Long-term management often includes electrophysiological mapping and ablation of the accessory pathways or long-term pharmacologic therapies with antiarrhythmic medications.

Pearls and Pitfalls

- Children with WPW syndrome will often present in SVT; therefore, the treatment consists of stopping this arrhythmia.
- ECGs will commonly show the classic delta wave, however, many will be completely normal.
- Consider SVT on all infants with a history of poor feeding, irritability, or signs of congestive heart failure.
- Adenosine needs to be pushed rapidly and preferably through an IV in a close proximity to the heart.
- New diagnosis or suspicion of WPW warrants close cardiology follow-up or consultation in the ED to assist with management.

LONG QT SYNDROME IN CHILDREN

Shad Baab

Clinical Highlights

Long QT syndrome (LQTS) is characterized by abnormal cardiac repolarization and resultant prolongation of the QT interval on an ECG. There are both congenital and acquired forms with considerable clinical overlap.

While seven different genotypes of the congenital form have been described, three (designated LQT1, LQT2, and LQT3) are responsible for the vast majority of the clinically significant cases. The QT interval is prolonged because of mutations in the genes that encode cardiac ion channels responsible for cardiac repolarization. LQTS is usually an isolated finding, but there are also well-described phenotypes in which LQTS is commonly seen. Romano–Ward syndrome and Jervell and Lange–Nielsen syndrome are examples of syndromes that include LQTS. Acquired long QT syndrome occurs most commonly in the setting of electrolyte disturbances and in certain drug therapies, but can also occur with hypothermia, hypothyroidism, HIV infection, and intracranial lesions.

The clinical presentation of LQTS varies widely. Many patients are asymptomatic and and the disorder is discovered incidentally on an ECG. If symptomatic, patients usually present with palpitations, syncope (or presyncope), seizure (or seizure-like activity), ventricular tachyarrhythmias, or frank cardiac arrest. Frequently, these symptoms occur in with exercise or emotional stress. LQT3 symptoms occur more commonly during sleep or on awakening. Additional triggers include swimming, diving, or being startled. Even when asymptomatic, condominant ECG findings may include torsades de pointes, premature ventricular beats, monomorphic ventricular tachycardia, bradycardia, and AV block.

ED Care and Disposition

ED care depends largely on the patient's presentation. If the patient presents in cardiac arrest, ventricular tachycardia, or fibrillation, resuscitation should proceed per the current PALS or ACLS guidelines. In all cases, symptomatic or not, to the clinician should consider congenital and acquired etiologies. A careful history, paying particular attention to the patient's activity immediately prior to symptom onset, patient medications, medications in the home, as well as a family history of LQTS or sudden cardiac death, should help identify the correct etiology. If acquired LQTS is suspected, serum potassium,

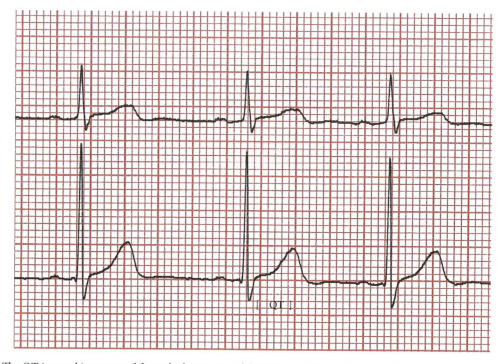

FIGURE 8.56 ■ The QT interval is measured from the beginning of the QRS complex to the end of the T wave.

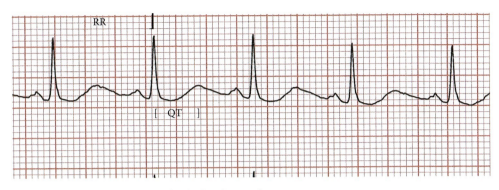

FIGURE 8.57 ■ An example of prolonged QT with a calculated QTc of 582.

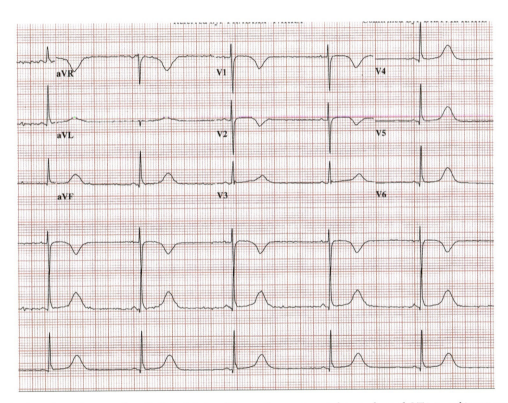

FIGURE 8.58 ■ Bradycardia and many other rhythm abnormalities can be seen even when prolonged QT interval is not apparent on an ECG.

magnesium, and calcium should be sampled and corrected. A 12-lead ECG should be performed for patients in whom LQTS is suspected. In most cases, the QT interval must be corrected (QTc) for heart rate. There are many different methods for calculating the QTc, but the most commonly used method is dividing the QT interval by the square root of the preceding RR interval. The QTc should be compared to age-based norms. For pediatric patients, 440 milliseconds and less is considered normal, 440 to 460 milliseconds is borderline, and greater than 460 milliseconds is prolonged. In addition to a prolonged QTc, the patient may have T-wave changes such as broad-based, low-amplitude, or notched T waves as well as T-wave alternans.

Except for presentations in extremis, admission is rarely indicated. Management and disposition should be performed in conjunction with a cardiologist. LQTS is only rarely formally diagnosed in the ED, and it is similarly rare to start beta-blockade (the mainstay of therapy) while in the ED. Most patients are restricted from exertion, which is thought to be protective in LQT1 and LQT2, but not helpful for patients

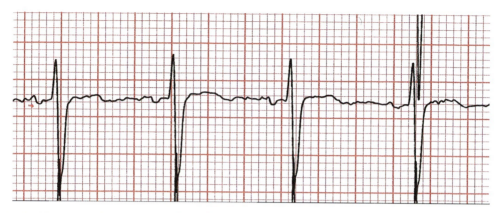

FIGURE 8.59 ■ Notched T waves in the setting of prolonged QT.

with LQT3. Patients are then referred to a cardiologist for more thorough evaluation and treatment of LQTS.

Pearls and Pitfalls

- The QT interval varies with many different factors so may not always be prolonged—a single ECG is not 100% sensitive for LQTS.
- All pediatric patients with first-time afebrile seizure should have an ECG to check for prolonged QT.
- Risk factors for sudden cardiac death include a prior episode of syncope, male gender, and QTc greater than 500 milliseconds.

Chapter 9

PROCEDURES

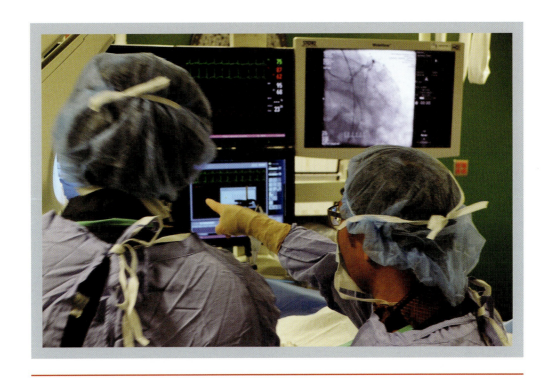

RADIOFREQUENCY ABLATION

Michael Schinlever

Indications

Cardiac radiofrequency (RF) ablation is the use of energy to damage specific cardiac tissue in an effort to inhibit pathologic conduction sources or tracts. Numerous arrhythmias can be treated with RF ablation. The success and complication rates of these ablations are highly dependent on the etiology of the arrhythmia and the targeted anatomic location. Arrhythmias that have a specific and localizable ectopic focus or conduction tract respond to RF ablation therapy with the highest rates of success. These include Wolf–Parkinson–White (WPW) syndrome, paroxysmal supraventricular tachycardias (AVNRT, unifocal atrial tachycardia, and accessory pathway–mediated tachycardia), type I atrial flutter, idiopathic ventricular tachycardia (VT; in structurally normal heart), and bundle branch reentrant tachycardia. On average, these carry success rates of 80% to 95% and have low rates of recurrence (<10%).

Ablation may be indicated for patients in whom pharmacologic management has failed, significant symptoms develop, or definitive treatment is desired. Cardiac RF ablation can be employed for atypical atrial flutter, inappropriate sinus tachycardia, and junctional tachycardia. However, RF ablation has a lower success rate in treating these rhythms; therefore, it is often reserved for cases that are refractory to drug therapy. Although controversial, asymptomatic patients who have an underlying arrhythmia prone to dangerous paroxysmal changes may benefit from ablation.

Technique

When cardiac ablation was first developed, direct current (DC) was used. With time, techniques using different forms of energy (RF, cryotherapy, laser, and acoustic) have been developed, which provide higher success rates with fewer complications. The most common energy form used for cardiac ablation is RF. RF is a low-voltage, high-frequency energy that causes resistive heating at the catheter tip and damages focused areas of cardiac tissue. The width and depth of these resultant lesions are typically 3 to 9 mm. With different approaches (eg, femoral vein, femoral artery, internal jugular vein, or subxiphoid), a variety of target sites can be reached for ablation.

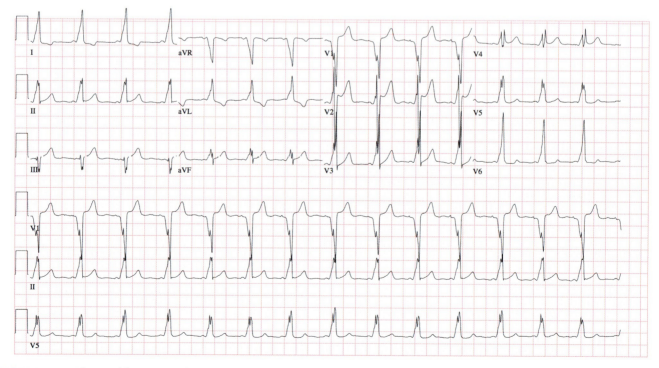

FIGURE 9.1 ■ This preablation ECG shows a short PR interval (82 milliseconds) and delta waves consistent with the preexcitation findings of the WPW syndrome.

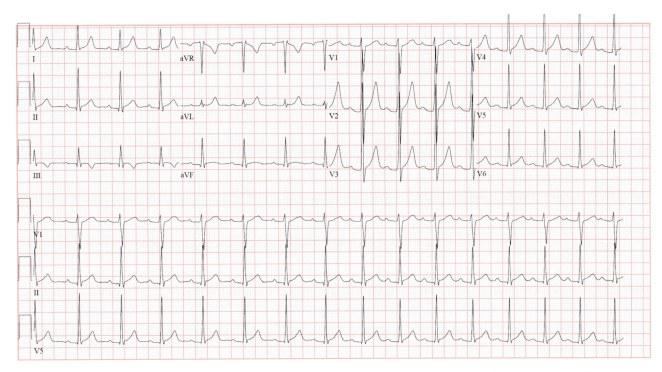

FIGURE 9.2 ■ This postablation ECG of the same patient now shows a first-degree heart block while the preexcitation findings seen earlier are absent.

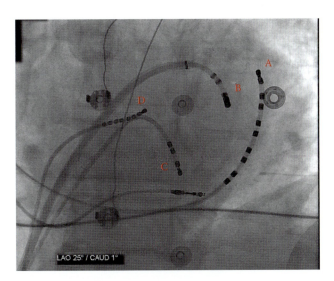

FIGURE 9.3 ■ This fluoroscopic image (left anterior oblique orientation) was obtained during cardiac RF ablation with multiple catheters at different sites; **A** is a coronary sinus electrode, **B** is an endocardial ablation catheter, lead **C** is situated at the bundle of His, and lead **D** is located in the right atrium.

The detailed mapping of cardiac conduction is a critical component of catheter ablation. Multiple catheter tips are passed through a major vessel under fluoroscopic guidance and positioned in the left or right heart. Electrophysiologists use the catheters to record internal ECG tracings, to pace different internal locations in an attempt to recreate the arrhythmia, or to locate classic areas of ectopy. Real-time fluoroscopic and ECG data can also be combined with prior CT or MR images and incorporated into mapping software. This software can create three-dimensional representations of the cardiac conduction pattern, thereby further defining ablation targets.

Complications

Cardiac ablation is relatively safe with a serious complication rate of about 1% for typical interventions. Vascular complications related to major vessel access, such as hematoma or pseudoaneurysm, can occur. Disruption of native cardiac conduction tracts may lead to heart block or new arrhythmias. Additional complications include pulmonary vein stenosis, atrial-esophageal fistulae, and cardiac perforation, resulting in tamponade.

Pearls and Pitfalls

- In patients with history of cardiac ablation, consider the possibility of recurrent/new arrhythmia, or the rare above-mentioned complications.

ANKLE BRACHIAL INDEX

Justin B. Joines
Cedric Lefebvre

Technology/Technique

Peripheral arterial disease (PAD) is the narrowing and obstruction of arteries within the peripheral vascular system. Risk factors for the development of PAD include smoking, hyperlipidemia, and diabetes mellitus. The incidence of PAD increases with age. PAD causes claudication (painful cramping of leg muscles), changes in skin color and temperature, loss of hair, and delayed healing of soft tissue wounds in the extremities.

Symptomatic patients with or without decreased peripheral pulses or bruits should be screened for PAD. The ankle brachial index (ABI) is a simple test that can detect evidence of PAD and can be performed easily in the emergency department or clinic setting. The ABI is a ratio of systolic blood pressures in the ankles/legs relative to the arms. To perform an ABI, first position a blood pressure cuff just above the ankle. Next, auscultate either the dorsalis pedis (DP) or posterior tibial (PT) artery with a Doppler device. Inflate the blood pressure cuff to just above the pressure at which the Doppler sound disappears. Allow the pressure in the cuff to release slowly until the pedal signal returns and record this systolic pressure. Repeat the measurement on the contralateral extremity using the same vessel (ie, DP or PT). Next, obtain bilateral systolic brachial artery pressures using a similar process with the blood pressure cuff located just above the elbow.

Interpretation

Calculating the ABI is achieved by dividing the higher ankle systolic pressure (DP or PT) by the higher of the two brachial artery systolic pressures (see Table 9.1 for a sample calculation). The resultant number is the ABI for the leg in question. An ABI of 0.9 to 1.3 is considered normal while an ABI of less than 0.9 is diagnostic of PAD (Table 9.2). Patients with abnormal ABI measurements should be referred to a vascular specialist for additional evaluation and treatment. Patients with an abnormal ABI should also undergo appropriate testing and treatment for other forms of atherosclerotic disease. The timing of consultation depends on the degree of ABI abnormality, the severity of symptoms, and other clinical factors.

Pearls and Pitfalls

- An abnormal ABI is associated with a higher risk of coronary artery disease (CAD), stroke, transient ischemic attack, renal disease, and all-cause mortality.

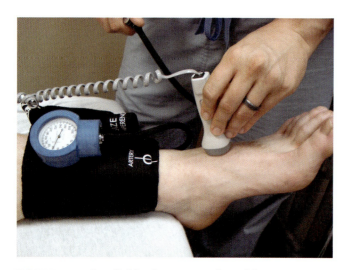

FIGURE 9.4 ■ Systolic blood pressure reading of the DP artery with a Doppler device.

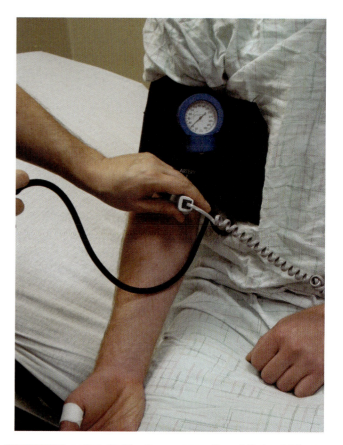

FIGURE 9.5 ■ Systolic blood pressure reading of the brachial artery with a Doppler device.

TABLE 9.1 ■ SAMPLE ABI CALCULATION FOR A LEFT LEG WITH CLAUDICATION SYMPTOMS		
	Blood Pressure	
Left brachial artery	175/99	
Right brachial artery	**178**/98	Highest brachial pressure
Left DP artery	134/87	
Left PT artery	**136**/85	Highest ankle pressure
ABI calculation	136÷178 = 0.76	Interpretation – PAD

TABLE 9.2 ■ ABI VALUE INTERPRETATIONS	
Calculated ABI	Interpretation
0.00–0.40	Severe PAD
0.41–0.90	PAD
0.91–1.30	Normal
>1.30	Noncompressible, calcified artery

- Consider obtaining ABIs in trauma patients with lower extremity injury.
- ABI of greater than 1.3 suggests calcified vasculature that is not easily compressible, leading to falsely elevated results and warrants further testing.

CARDIAC CATHETERIZATION

P. Matthew Belford
Sanjay K. Gandhi

Indications

Cardiac catheterization is an invasive procedure used to access the heart and its vessels percutaneously. It can be used to perform diagnostic coronary angiography to define anatomical and hemodynamic characteristics of the cardiac chambers, great vessels, and coronary arteries. Cardiac catheterization can also be used to perform therapeutic percutaneous coronary intervention (PCI). Indications for diagnostic cardiac catheterization include acute coronary syndromes, valvular heart disease, congestive heart failure, and pulmonary hypertension (see Table 9.3 for appropriate use criteria). The most common indication for cardiac catheterization is the evaluation, diagnosis, and treatment of CAD. Indications for *right* heart catheterization (described later) include the need for hemodynamic assessment of cardiac and pulmonary function, or for the evaluation of valvular heart disease. Contraindications for cardiac catheterization include acute renal failure, allergy to contrast media, and active severe bleeding (Table 9.4).

Cardiac catheterization with PCI has become a cornerstone in early invasive and revascularization strategies for acute coronary syndromes, particularly ST-elevation myocardial infarction (STEMI). The need for rapid recognition and management of acute coronary syndromes has prompted the development of local and regional systems of care to facilitate rapid mobilization of catheterization laboratory resources. These networks often have an established plan for immediate local catheterization, transfer to a regional facility for catheterization, or medical management with subsequent transfer to a tertiary center. PCI has evolved to include numerous therapeutic interventions such as atherectomy, as well as the

TABLE 9.3 ■ APPROPRIATE USE CRITERIA FOR DIAGNOSTIC CATHETERIZATION*

Indication	Appropriate Use Score
STEMI/suspected STEMI	A
Cardiogenic shock due to ACS	A
UA/NSTEMI	A
Symptomatic suspected CAD without stress imaging	I = if symptomatic with low pretest probability A = if symptomatic with high pretest probability
New LV systolic dysfunction (EF<40)	U = if asymptomatic A = if symptomatic
Any coronary calcium score	I = if asymptomatic Not rated if symptomatic
Known CAD with intermediate risk noninvasive study findings	U = if asymptomatic or stable A = if worsening or limiting symptoms
After VF or sustained VT without symptoms	A
After cardiac arrest with ROSC	A
After NSVT with normal LV function	U
Preoperative assessment for noncardiac surgery	I = for low risk surgery I = for >4 METS without symptoms U = prior to solid organ transplant
New LBBB	U

A, Appropriate; I, Inappropriate; U, uncertain; ACS, acute coronary syndrome; UA, unstable angina; NSTEMI, non-ST-elevation myocardial infarction; LV, left ventricular; EF, ejection fraction; ROSC, return of spontaneous circulation; NSVT, nonsustained VT; METS, metabolic equivalents; LBBB, left bundle branch block
*Patel MR, Bailey SR, Bonow RO, et al. ACCF/SCAI/AATS/AHA/ASE/ASNC/HFSA/HRS/SCCM/SCCT/SCMR/STS 2012 Appropriate Use Criteria for Diagnostic Catheterization. *J Am Coll Cardiol.* 2012; 59:1995–2027.

TABLE 9.4 ■ CONTRAINDICATIONS TO CARDIAC CATHETERIZATION*

Uncooperative patient or patient refusal
Uncontrolled severe hypertension
Decompensated congestive heart failure or pulmonary edema
Acute trauma, bleeding (including GI), or severe anemia
Acute stroke
Profound electrolyte disturbance (particularly hypokalemia)
Medication toxicity or overdose
Anticoagulation with INR > 1.8, severe coagulopathy, moderate-severe thrombocytopenia
Anaphylactic reaction to contrast medium or documented contrast allergy
Acute renal failure or severe kidney disease (in patients who are not dialysis dependent)
Active infection or unexplained fever
Limited or no peripheral venous access

GI, gastrointestinal; INR, international normalized ratio
*With the exception of patient refusal (absolute contraindication), the contraindications listed above can often be modified, controlled, or treated to enable a safe procedure.

placement of metallic stents, drug-eluting stents (DES), and most recently, bio-absorbable scaffolds with drug elution. Other methods of revascularization, such as thrombolysis and coronary artery bypass grafting (CABG), are available if PCI is not indicated or unavailable.

Technique

Cardiac catheterization is performed in a laboratory with dedicated equipment and personnel meeting regulatory and professional guidelines.

Catheterization procedures vary by indication, but can more simply be divided into right and left heart procedures. The majority of catheterization procedures are left sided, or arterial, to define left ventricular pressures, gradients, and coronary anatomy. Seldinger technique is used to enter the femoral or radial artery. After return of pulsatile, bright red blood is noted, a flexible (often 0.035-inch J tip) guide wire is advanced into the vessel through the needle. The site of entry is enlarged with a scalpel, the needle is removed, and a sheath with dilator is advanced over the wire into the vessel. The dilator is then removed, leaving the sheath in place within the vessel.

After the sheath is placed and flushed with heparinized saline, a wire is advanced in retrograde fashion to the aorta. Next, a diagnostic catheter is advanced over the wire to the aortic root. This catheter is flushed to clear any air and connected to the hemodynamic monitoring system. The guide

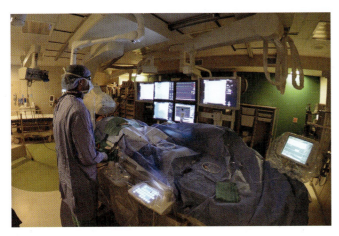

FIGURE 9.6 ■ Catheterization laboratories contain monitors, radiography equipment, sterile supplies, emergency carts, and other equipment necessary to perform the procedure. A team comprising physicians, nurses, and radiological technologists performs the procedure.

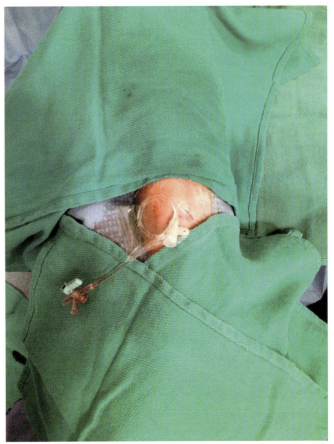

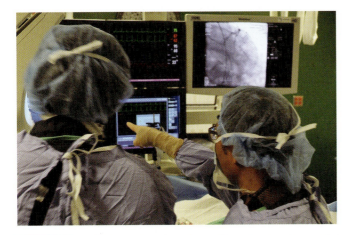

FIGURE 9.7 ■ High-resolution radiography (digital angiography) equipment, physiological monitoring systems, power injectors, and computer-based archiving and reporting systems are used by a team of providers to perform cardiac catheterization.

FIGURE 9.8 ■ A 5-French sheath has been placed in the right radial artery in preparation for cardiac catheterization. A hemostatic valve on the sheath allows catheter and wire entry.

wire is then removed. The catheter is positioned at the origin of the coronary artery (left or right) whereupon angiographic imaging begins. After contrast medium is injected into the coronary vessels, radiographic images are obtained and displayed on monitors. Operators confirm that the catheter is seated properly in the coronary artery, and then several more injections are administered to generate multiple views of each vessel. Both the left and right coronary systems are imaged independently, and then contrast is directed into the ventricle for cardiac ventriculography. Pressure tracings are obtained and monitored throughout the procedure.

If significant coronary stenosis is discovered during catheterization, such as an acute culprit lesion in a patient with STEMI, primary PCI with the intent to restore coronary blood flow is considered. Various methods are used to quantify the degree of stenosis of major epicardial vessels and ≥70% stenosis is generally considered obstructive. Factors including lesion length, vessel diameter, and lesion composition are also assessed when considering PCI. Once the decision to perform PCI has been made, implantation of a DES versus a bare-metal stent (BMS) is affected by clinical factors and vessel anatomy. Superior long-term patency and lower rates of in-stent restenosis are noted with DES. Dual antiplatelet therapy is necessary to minimize the risk of stent thrombosis, a potentially catastrophic and fatal complication. Revascularization via CABG is preferred over PCI in the setting of three-vessel obstructive disease and other clinical scenarios.

A right heart catheterization is performed to obtain diagnostic information from the right side of the heart such as pulmonary artery pressure, pulmonary capillary wedge pressure, cardiac output, and cardiac index. This information can assist in the management of pulmonary hypertension, hemodynamic instability, and valvular disease. Percutaneous access is established through a vein and the catheter can remain in place for several days to obtain serial measurements. Potential sites for access to the right side of the heart include the femoral, internal jugular, basilic, and antecubital veins. Seldinger technique is used to establish venous access, and then a pressure-sensitive, often balloon-tipped catheter is passed through the inferior or superior vena cava into the right atrium, right ventricle, and ultimately into the pulmonary artery. A Swan-Ganz catheter can be used to sample oxygen saturation, measure chamber pressures, and estimate blood flow.

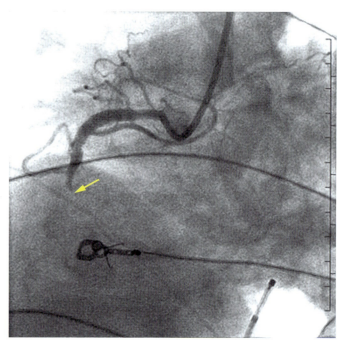

FIGURE 9.9 ■ Angiography obtained during cardiac catheterization of a patient with ST-segment elevation on ECG reveals a culprit lesion in the right coronary artery (arrow).

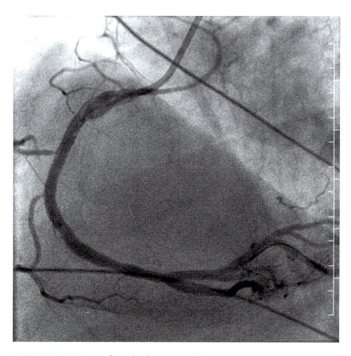

FIGURE 9.10 ■ After deployment of a coronary stent, angiography reveals restoration of flow demonstrated by radiopaque contrast material seen throughout the vessel.

Complications

Because all catheterizations are an invasive examination, the risks and complications (Table 9.5) should be understood and discussed with the patient in a process of informed consent. The procedure remains generally safe, but comorbid illnesses can increase risk. The most common complication is bleeding such as minor oozing, hematoma formation, and nonaccess site bleeding (including gastrointestinal).

Pearls and Pitfalls

- Various electrical disturbances and arrhythmias are not only associated with acute coronary syndromes, but can also result from catheterization and myocardial reperfusion after revascularization. Risks including electrolyte disturbances should be identified and corrected, and high-risk patients should be prepared for rapid defibrillation.
- The transradial approach to cardiac catheterization is gaining popularity. Benefits include a lower rate of bleeding complications and accelerated patient mobility. Confirming the presence of an intact radial arch with dual arterial supply to the hand is very important before a radial artery approach is pursued.

TABLE 9.5 ■ POTENTIAL COMPLICATIONS OF CARDIAC CATHETERIZATION

Major arrhythmia and/or death
Myocardial infarction
Local vascular injury including dissection, perforation, and pseudoaneurysm formation
Cerebrovascular accident/stroke
Need for emergent coronary artery bypass
Cardiac or major vessel perforation
Bleeding and/or need for blood transfusion
Contrast-induced nephropathy and/or renal failure
Allergic reaction including anaphylaxis
Hemodynamic complications

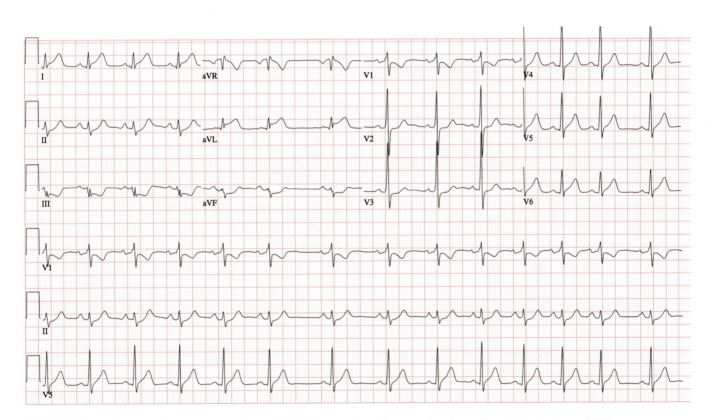

FIGURE 9.11 ■ This ECG demonstrates evidence of STEMI in a patient who was taken for cardiac catheterization and PCI.

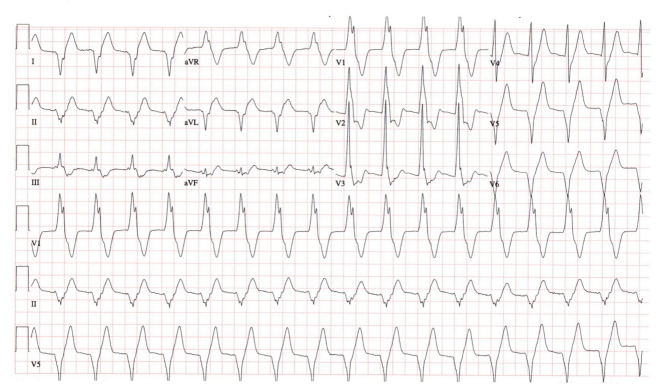

FIGURE 9.12 ■ An accelerated idioventricular rhythm, frequently associated with reperfusion, is noted in the same patient immediately after PCI has been performed.

PERICARDIOCENTESIS

Casey Jae Davis
Cedric Lefebvre

Indications

Pericardiocentesis is the removal of fluid by needle from the pericardium for diagnostic or therapeutic purposes. The pericardium normally contains 10 to 50 mL of fluid that cushions and lubricates the heart. An abnormal amount of fluid accumulation within the pericardial sac constitutes a pericardial effusion. Pericardial fluid accumulation can be caused by traumatic injury, pericarditis, infections, malignancy, myocardial infarction, congestive heart failure, renal failure, medications, and mediastinal radiation. Cardiac tamponade occurs when a pericardial effusion exerts compressive forces on the heart, reduces filling, and decreases cardiac output. Physical findings of cardiac tamponade physiology include jugular venous distention, distant heart sounds, pulsus paradoxus, and hypotension. An ECG with low-voltage QRS complexes or electrical alternans can be seen in cardiac tamponade. A chest radiograph showing an enlarged cardiac silhouette is also suggestive of a pericardial effusion. Bedside ultrasound should be used to identify a pericardial effusion and to investigate signs of cardiac tamponade such as ventricular collapse. Cardiac tamponade is a life-threatening emergency that often requires immediate pericardiocentesis to restore cardiac function.

Technique

In preparation for an emergent pericardiocentesis, resuscitation equipment should be readily available at the bedside and the patient should be placed on a cardiac monitor. After donning eye protection, sterile gloves, and gown, the physician prepares the anterior chest with antiseptic wash and a sterile drape. Emergency pericardiocentesis is usually performed on patients who have demonstrated clinical deterioration or who are being actively resuscitated. Therefore, sedation and anesthesia are seldom necessary in the emergency setting. Lidocaine infiltration can be used if the patient is conscious. An 18-gauge spinal needle is attached to a three-way stopcock and a 20- or 60-mL syringe. Several approaches for pericardiocentesis are available. The subxiphoid approach begins just below the xiphoid process and is typically used during a blind technique. The needle is advanced from a subxiphoid entry, at an angle of 45° to the skin, toward the left shoulder while aspirating continuously. Ultrasound-guided pericardiocentesis is recommended to visualize the pericardial effusion and guide the needle into correct position for aspiration. The needle is advanced under ultrasonographic guidance until entry into the pericardial sac is visualized. Potential points of entry include the left fifth or sixth intercostal space, the left or right parasternal spaces, and the left or right sternocostal margins.

Once the needle is in correct position, fluid is aspirated until vital signs normalize and no additional fluid can be removed. Obtain a chest radiograph to assess for complications such as a pneumothorax or pleural effusion after the procedure.

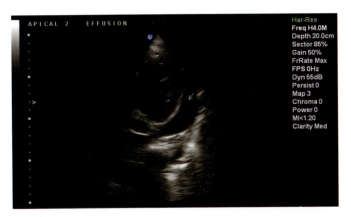

FIGURE 9.13 ■ A pericardial effusion (arrow) is seen in this cardiac ultrasound. Real-time ultrasound imaging can identify evidence of tamponade physiology such as right atrial and ventricular inversion, abnormal septal motion, and a dilated inferior vena cava diameter without variation in size with respirations.

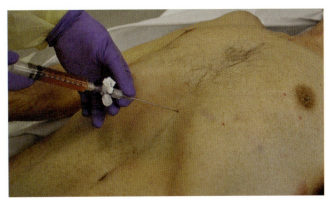

FIGURE 9.14 ■ The most common site for needle insertion during an emergent pericardiocentesis is the left sternocostal margin or the immediate subxiphoid approach. Maintain the needle in a 45° angle to the anterior abdominal wall.

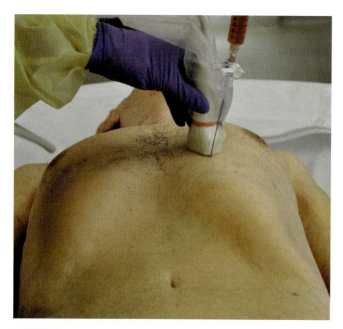

FIGURE 9.15 ■ Real-time direct ultrasonographic guidance is the most reliable method for pericardiocentesis. When bedside ultrasound imaging is available, it can be used to guide the needle into the largest collection of fluid from an entry point that is closest to the pericardial effusion while avoiding vital structures.

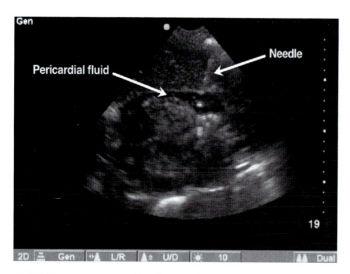

FIGURE 9.16 ■ A needle (hyperechoic structure) can be seen entering the pericardial effusion during an ultrasound-guided pericardiocentesis.

Complications

After pericardiocentesis, the patient should be monitored closely for signs of reaccumulation of fluid as well as complications from the procedure. Complications include dysrhythmias, cardiac puncture, pneumothorax, coronary and internal thoracic vessel injury, injury to the liver, stomach, or diaphragm, and death. Placement of a drain or pericardiostomy may be necessary to continue fluid drainage. In a traumatic pericardial effusion, fluid will likely rapidly reaccumulate and a temporizing pericardiocentesis should be followed by a thoracotomy.

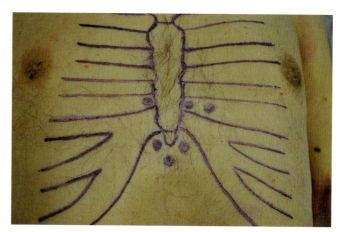

FIGURE 9.17 ■ Several anatomical points of entry are available for pericardiocentesis. Bedside ultrasound can be used to identify the entry site that provides most immediate access to the pericardial effusion.

Pearls and Pitfalls

- There are no absolute contraindications to an emergent pericardiocentesis.
- A blind approach can be performed but carries a higher risk of complications.
- Observational studies show that the parasternal or apical approaches are superior to the traditional subxyphoid approach for accessing the largest fluid collection.
- A small volume of sterile saline, stored in the syringe before the procedure, can be used to flush clotted blood that may obstruct the bore of the needle during pericardiocentesis.
- Tracings from the V_1 lead of a continuous ECG monitor, attached by an alligator clip to the base of the spinal needle, can be used to assist a blind approach. ST elevation indicates myocardial contact and should prompt needle repositioning/withdrawal.

VIDEO 9.1 ■ This ultrasound (subcostal view) demonstrates a pericardial effusion with hemodynamic compromise as evidenced by right ventricular collapse. View at http://mhprofessional.com/sites/lefebvre

PERICARDIAL WINDOW

Casey Jae Davis

Indications

A pericardial window, or pericardiostomy, is performed to treat an accumulation of fluid around the heart. By draining a compressive pericardial effusion, a pericardial window relieves cardiac tamponade and prevents cardiovascular collapse. A pericardiostomy is a surgical procedure in which an opening is created in the pericardium to allow a pericardial effusion to drain into the pleural or peritoneal cavity. A pericardial window is useful in the drainage of purulent pericardial effusions and known benign effusions that reaccumulate after pericardiocentesis. Pericardial windows are also used to mitigate hemopericardium and other pericardial collections after cardiac surgery. This procedure can be diagnostic in patients with asymptomatic pericardial effusions of unknown origin.

Technique

Echocardiography is used to assess the impact of the pericardial effusion on the heart, determine physiologic stability, and plan for the optimal surgical approach. Other imaging modalities such as CT or MRI may provide additional detailed anatomic information such as the size and location of the effusion (ie, posterior) or if any loculations are present.

A pericardial window is created via a subxiphoid incision, thoracotomy, or a thoracoscopic approach. If a patient is hemodynamically tenuous, a subxiphoid approach is employed. A 5-cm incision is made over the xiphoid and is extended into the midline of the abdomen. The retrosternal space is entered by finger dissection, the pericardium is visualized, and then incised. A drain is then secured into place. A thoracoscopic approach is preferred in patients who are hemodynamically stable as well as in patients with unilateral or posterior loculated effusions. Patients with coexisting pericardial and pulmonary pathology requiring diagnosis and therapy may also benefit from a thorascopic approach. This technique involves the introduction of trocars through two or three thoracic incisions at the level of the fourth and sixth intercostal spaces. This allows for the pericardiostomy to be performed under direct visualization. A transthoracic approach is achieved by exposure via an anterior thoracotomy in the fourth or fifth intercostal space. The pericardium is then incised and a thoracostomy tube placed in the pleural cavity.

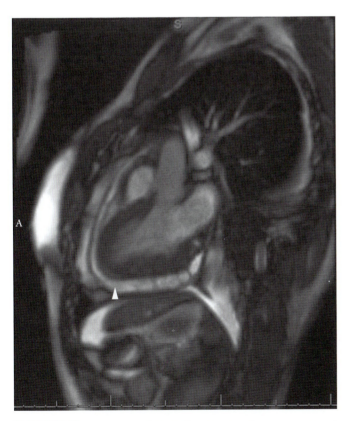

FIGURE 9.18 ■ Contrasted MRI of a patient with a recurrent pericarditis. Note the moderately sized pericardial effusion (white arrow head) is circumferential and contains multiple fibrous loculations.

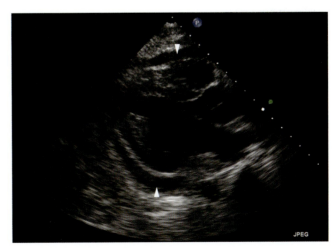

FIGURE 9.19 ■ Two-dimensional transthoracic echocardiogram with a parasternal long axis view of a heart with a moderate pericardial effusion (white arrow heads). This view is most accurate in distinguishing a pericardial effusion from a pleural effusion.

PERICARDIAL WINDOW (CONTINUED)

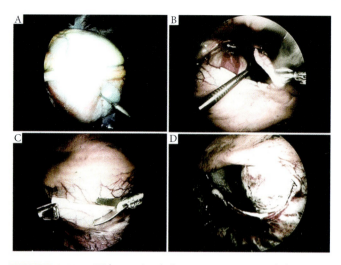

FIGURE 9.20 ■ Video-assisted thoracoscopic pericardial window. **(A)** The phrenic nerve is visualized and pericardiocentesis is performed under direct visualization. **(B)** The pericardium is incised. **(C)** Fibrinous septa and loculations are broken and the heart is freed. **(D)** A pericardial window is created. Reproduced, with permission, from Muhammad MI. The pericardial window: is a video-assisted thoracoscopy approach better than a surgical approach? *Interact Cardiovasc Thorac Surg.* 2011 Feb;12(2):174–178.

Complications

Complications from pericardiostomy are rare but include bleeding, infection, incisional hernia, pneumothorax, and cardiac injury.

Pearls and Pitfalls

- The clinical urgency of a pericardial effusion causing hemodynamic instability often favors immediate pericardiocentesis over surgical pericardiostomy to prevent cardiovascular collapse.
- A thoracoscopic approach for pericardiostomy may offer superior long-term control of effusions when compared to subxiphoid surgical drainage.
- CT-guided percutaneous drainage has drawn recent attention as a less invasive and more cost-effective management option for postsurgical pericardial effusions.

CARDIOVERSION/EXTERNAL DEFIBRILLATION

Jeffrey W. Hinshaw
Cedric Lefebvre

Indications

Defibrillation and cardioversion are electrical therapies used to treat ventricular fibrillation (VF), VT, and other abnormal cardiac rhythms. These electrical therapies are employed to terminate cardiac arrhythmias resulting in cardiac arrest or hemodynamic instability and to restore normal cardiac function. Sudden cardiac arrest is a leading cause of death in the United States, with out-of-hospital cardiac arrest affecting over 300,000 people each year. Although survival rates vary widely (from 3% to 50%) depending on several key factors, early defibrillation has been shown to improve chances of survival.

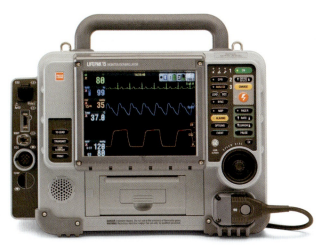

FIGURE 9.21 ■ This LifePak 15 multifunction cardiac monitor/defibrillator has several operating modes including AED and manual modes (Courtesy of PhysioControl, Inc.).

Technique

Electrical therapy with DC can be utilized in two forms during emergency treatment of tachyarrhythmias. Defibrillation (unsynchronized cardioversion) is generally used to treat VF and pulseless VT. Synchronized cardioversion is utilized to convert abnormally fast, but regular, cardiac rhythms.

Monophasic units deliver a single wave of energy through the myocardium. Biphasic units deliver a charge in one direction for the first half of the shock and in the electrically opposite direction for the second half. Less biphasic energy is required to deliver the equivalent amount of monophasic energy. Manual defibrillators require the operator to select functions on the device (eg, turn on, lead selection, energy charge, and discharge). Semiautomatic defibrillators require the operator to turn on the machine and place the electrodes onto the patient. This device analyzes the cardiac rhythm and instructs the operator to deliver the preselected energy amount. This requires less user input and decision making than with manual devices. Automated external defibrillators (AED) require only that the operator turn on the machine and place the electrodes onto the patient. The machine analyzes the rhythm and delivers shocks automatically. This device may have voice prompts to guide the user through the resuscitation. AEDs are designed for use by the layperson and are commonly found in large public areas such as airports, shopping malls, and sports complexes.

Some defibrillators employ paddles that are pressed firmly upon the patient's chest wall to deliver energy to the patient. The paddle is a metal instrument that requires the use of a gel to ensure conduction of electricity. Newer defibrillator

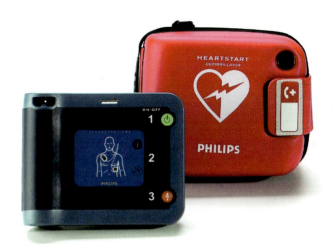

FIGURE 9.22 ■ This Philips Heartstart FRx defibrillator is a small, battery-powered AED and is one example of many types of AEDs that can be found in public areas (Courtesy of Philips, Inc.).

devices have electrodes, designed as adhesive pads, which can monitor cardiac rhythms, deliver electrical therapy, and perform transcutaneous pacing. Electrodes are also considered safer than paddles because the operator can maintain distance from the patient while delivering energy. There are several acceptable positions for the placement of defibrillator paddles and/or AED electrodes: anteroposterior, anterolateral, anterior-left infrascapular, and anterior-right infrascapular. For the anteroposterior position, electrodes are placed over the left precordium and on the back between the scapulae. When feasible, the anteroposterior configuration is preferred if long-term electrode placement and/or transcutaneous pacing is anticipated. The anterolateral approach is a reasonable configuration when the patient cannot be turned easily and when electrodes must be placed rapidly.

Delivery of electrical therapy can occur in two forms: synchronized and unsynchronized. Defibrillation is an unsynchronized delivery of electricity during any phase of the cardiac electrical cycle and is generally delivered at high energy levels. It is used for VF to briefly interrupt all electrical activity in the heart, allowing the heart's intrinsic pacemaker to resume in a more electrically coordinated fashion. Unsynchronized cardioversion is functionally similar to defibrillation. It is used for any ventricular arrhythmia without pulses (ie, pulseless VT), unstable polymorphic VT, or in cases of unstable VT in which there is uncertainty about waveform morphology. Synchronized cardioversion, on the other hand, is the delivery of a reversion shock precisely on the R wave of the QRS complex. Synchronized cardioversion in the acute setting is used for unstable supraventricular tachycardia, unstable atrial fibrillation/flutter, and unstable, regular, monomorphic, wide complex tachycardias. To deliver a synchronized electrical impulse,

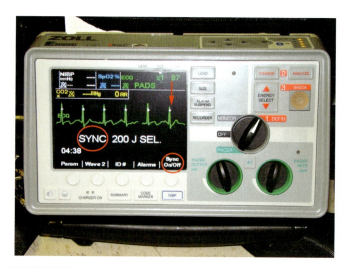

FIGURE 9.24 ■ This defibrillator device has been set to synchronized "SYNC" mode. Note the arrows pointing to each QRS complex.

the "SYNC" button is pressed on the defibrillator device. Once activated, each QRS complex will be marked by the device's internal computer. The appropriate energy level is selected and the device is charged. The discharge button is pressed and held until the energy delivers. The device senses when to deliver the electrical shock so there may be a brief delay before discharge.

Complications

The delivery of an electrical shock without proper synchronization on the R wave can result in the delivery of an impulse during cardiac repolarization that can precipitate VF. High-energy shocks can cause myocardial necrosis. Embolization of thrombi can occur when patients with atrial fibrillation are cardioverted without proper anticoagulation. Skin burns and pain may also result from electrical cardioversion.

Pearls and Pitfalls

- Defibrillation success and higher survival rates are associated with early defibrillation.
- Biphasic defibrillators allow for continuous chest compressions even during defibrillation (provided a hand barrier, such as a latex glove, is used).
- Always assure the mode of the manual device when attempting to "synchronize."
- If the R waves of a tachyarrhythmia are undifferentiated or low in amplitude, the defibrillator device may not be able to synchronize effectively and an electrical shock will not be delivered.

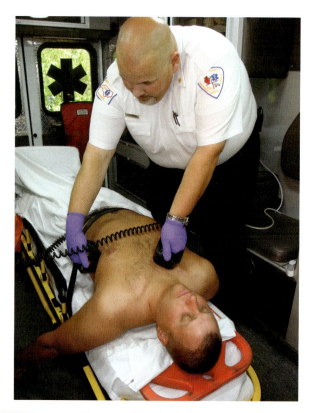

FIGURE 9.23 ■ The anterolateral configuration of paddle placement is being used here. One paddle or electrode is placed to the right of the sternum, below the clavicle, and the other is placed on the left side of the patient, below the pectoral muscle.

INDEX

Page numbers followed by "f", "t", and "v" indicate material in figures, tables, and videos respectively.

AAA. *See* Abdominal aortic aneurysm (AAA)
AAA rupture, 170, 171f
Abdominal aortic aneurysm (AAA), 170–171
Aberrant atrial conduction, 128
ABI. *See* Ankle-brachial index (ABI)
Accelerated idioventricular rhythm (AIVR), 135–136, 260f
Accelerated junctional rhythm, 130, 130f
Accessory cephalic vein, 74f
ACEIs. *See* Angiotensin-converting enzyme inhibitors (ACEIs)
Acquired long QT syndrome, 248
ACS. *See* Acute coronary syndrome (ACS)
Action potential, 14
Acute anterior wall infarction, 159
Acute aortic dissection, 181t
Acute aortic insufficiency, 201–202
Acute aortic valve regurgitation, 201
Acute arterial occlusion, 174, 175f
Acute coronary syndrome (ACS), 56, 181t
Acute ischemia, 18–22
Acute ischemic stroke, 181t
Acute LAD territory infarction, 60f
Acute limb ischemia, 174
Acute mitral regurgitation, 203
Acute myocardial infarction (AMI), 18–22
Acute myocardial ischemia, 32
Acute myocarditis, 60f
Acute pericarditis, 43
Acute pulmonary edema, 181t
Acute renal failure, 181t
Adenosine
  AVNRT, 112
  AVRT, 114
  CMR imaging, 59
  SNRT, 108
  SVT, 237
  WPW syndrome, 117, 247
Adenosine stress perfusion defect, 59f
AED. *See* Automated external defibrillator (AED)
AIVR. *See* Accelerated idioventricular rhythm (AIVR)
ALCAPA. *See* Anomalous left coronary artery from the pulmonary artery (ALCAPA)
Alcohol consumption, 124
Alcohol intoxication, 144
Ambulatory ECG, 94–95
AMI. *See* Acute myocardial infarction (AMI)
Amiodarone
  AVNRT, 112
  AVRT, 114
  LQTS, 162
  sinus bradycardia, 102
  SVT, 237
  VF, 142
  VT, 137
Amyloidosis, 191f

Anatomy, 1–12
  anomalous left coronary artery, 10–11
  cardiac valves, 6–7
  coronary arteries, 2–3
  dextrocardia, 12
  heart chambers, 4, 5f
  prosthetic valves, 8–9
Angiotensin-converting enzyme inhibitors (ACEIs), 184t
Angiotensin receptor blockers (ARBs), 184t
Ankle-brachial index (ABI), 174, 175f, 254–255
Anomalous left coronary artery, 10–11
Anomalous left coronary artery from the pulmonary artery (ALCAPA), 217, 219f
Anterolateral myocardial infarction (MI), 32f
Antiarrhythmic agents, 139
Antidepressants, 139
Antidromic AV reciprocating tachycardia, 107t, 113, 116
Antifungals, 162
Antimicrobials, 139
Antiphospholipid antibody, 176t
Antipsychotics, 139
Antithrombin deficiency, 176t
Aorta, 5f
Aortic aneurysm, 36t
Aortic balloon pump, 203
Aortic dissection, 36t, 38f, 172–173, 201
Aortic incompetence, 201
Aortic insufficiency, 201
Aortic semilunar valve, 5f
Aortic stenosis (AS), 196–198
Aortic transection, 48f
Apical ballooning, 43f
ARBs. *See* Angiotensin receptor blockers (ARBs)
Arrhythmias, 99–167
  accelerated idioventricular rhythm (AIVR), 135–136
  Ashman phenomenon, 128
  atrial fibrillation, 126–127
  atrial flutter, 124–125
  AV nodal reentrant tachycardia (AVNRT), 111–112
  AV reciprocating tachycardia (AVRT), 113–115
  bifascicular block, 155–156
  Brugada syndrome, 144–145
  ectopic atrial tachycardia (EAT), 122–123
  first-degree AV block, 146–148
  junctional escape rhythm, 129–130
  junctional tachycardia, 131–132
  left anterior fascicular block (LAFB), 157–158
  left bundle branch block (LBBB), 161
  long QT syndrome (LQTS), 162–163
  Lown–Ganong–Levine (LGL) syndrome, 119
  multifocal atrial tachycardia (MAT), 120–121
  premature atrial complex (PAC), 103–104
  premature ventricular contraction (PVC), 133–134
  right bundle branch block (RBBB), 159–160

Arrhythmias (*continued*)
   second-degree AV block, Mobitz type I, 149–150
   second-degree AV block, Mobitz type II, 151–152
   sinus arrhythmia, 102
   sinus bradycardia, 102
   sinus tachycardia, 100–101
   supraventricular tachycardia (SVT), 107–110
   third-degree atrioventricular block, 153–154
   torsades de pointes (TdP), 139–140
   ventricular fibrillation (VF), 141–143
   ventricular tachycardia (VT), 137–138
   wandering atrial pacemaker (WAP), 105–106
   WPW syndrome, 116–118
Arterial embolus, 174f
AS. *See* Aortic stenosis (AS)
Ascending aorta, 3f
Ashman phenomenon, 128
Atherectomy, 256
Atrial arrhythmia
   premature atrial complex (PAC), 103–104
   wandering atrial pacemaker (WAP), 105–106
Atrial contraction, 129
Atrial fibrillation, 108t, 116, 126–127, 190
Atrial flutter, 108t, 116, 124–125
Atrial myxoma, 44f
Atrial paced rhythm, 164, 165f
Atrial septal defect, 159
Atrial systole, 14
Atrial tachycardia
   atrial fibrillation, 126–127
   atrial flutter, 124–125
   ectopic atrial tachycardia (EAT), 122–123
   multifocal atrial tachycardia (MAT), 120–121
Atrioventricular (AV) block, 84
Atrioventricular (AV) nodal reentrant tachycardia (AVNRT), 107t, 111–112, 237
Atrioventricular (AV) node, 14, 15f
Atrioventricular (AV) reciprocating tachycardia (AVRT), 107t, 110f, 113–115, 237
Atrioventricular (AV) septum, 110f
Atrioventricular (AV) tachycardia
   AV nodal reentrant tachycardia (AVNRT), 111–112
   AV reciprocating tachycardia (AVRT), 113–115
   Lown–Ganong–Levine (LGL) syndrome, 119
   WPW syndrome, 116–118
Atropine, 130
Atypical atrial flutter, 124
Automated CPR device, 92–93
Automated external defibrillator (AED), 142, 265
AutoPulse CPR device, 93f
AV block. *See* Heart block
AV nodal-blocking agents, 153
AV nodal reentrant tachycardia. *See* Atrioventricular (AV) nodal reentrant tachycardia (AVNRT)
AV node. *See* Atrioventricular (AV) node
AV reciprocating tachycardia. *See* Atrioventricular (AV) reciprocating tachycardia (AVRT)

AVNRT. *See* Atrioventricular (AV) nodal reentrant tachycardia (AVNRT)
AVNRT reentry circuit, 111
AVRT. *See* Atrioventricular (AV) reciprocating tachycardia (AVRT)
Axial dual-energy CT angiogram, 63f

B-type natriuretic peptide (BNP), 221
Ball-valve, 8f
Basilic vein, 74f
Bazett formula, 213
Bedside echocardiogram, 39–42
Bedside ultrasound (DVT), 51–55
Beta-blockers
   aortic dissection, 172
   atrial fibrillation, 126
   AVNRT, 112
   AVRT, 114, 115
   junctional escape rhythm, 129
   Mobitz I block, 149
   restrictive cardiomyopathy, 190
   sinus bradycardia, 102
   SVT, 237
   third-degree heart block, 153
   WPW syndrome, 117
Bifascicular block, 155–156
Bigeminy, 133
Bileaflet valve, 8f, 9
Bioprosthetic valves, 9, 9f
Biphasic defibrillator, 142, 265, 266
Biventricular pacemaker, 85f, 164, 166f
BNP. *See* B-type natriuretic peptide (BNP)
Body surface mapping (BSM), 20–21
Bolusing fluid, 203
Bradycardia
   heart block (children), 241–244
   junctional rhythms, 129
   sinus, 102
   transcutaneous pacemaker, 78
   transvenous pacemaker, 81
Broad T wave, 17
Brugada syndrome, 144–145
BSM. *See* Body surface mapping (BSM)
Bundle of His, 14, 15f
Bundle of Kent, 107t, 110f, 116

CABG. *See* Coronary artery bypass grafting (CABG)
Caffeine, 134
Calcium channel blockers
   AVNRT, 112
   AVRT, 114
   hypertension, 184t
   junctional escape rhythm, 129
   Mobitz I block, 149
   restrictive cardiomyopathy, 190
   sinus bradycardia, 102
   SVT, 237

third-degree heart block, 153
WPW syndrome, 117
Cancer drugs, 162
Cardiac arrest, 92
Cardiac catheterization, 256–260
Cardiac conduction system, 15f
Cardiac CT angiography (CCTA), 56–58
Cardiac ischemia
　AIVR, 135
　catheter-induced arrhythmia, 83
　PVC, 134
　T-wave inversion, 28
Cardiac magnetic resonance (CMR) imaging, 59–61
Cardiac radiofrequency (RF) ablation, 252–253
Cardiac surgery, 159
Cardiac tamponade, 36t, 45, 234–236
Cardiac valves, 6–7
Cardiogenic shock, 49f
Cardiomegaly, 189f
Cardiomyopathy, 187–205
　acute aortic insufficiency, 201–202
　aortic stenosis (AS), 196–198
　children, 221t
　dilated, 188–189
　HOCM, 59, 61f
　hypertrophic, 193–195
　mitral regurgitation, 203–205
　mitral stenosis, 199–200
　restrictive, 190–192
　stress-induced, 43
　Takotsubo, 43, 43f
Cardiopulmonary resuscitation (CPR)
　automated CPR device, 92–93
　heart block, 244
　ventricular fibrillation, 142
Cardiothoracic surgery, 173
Cardiovascular imaging, 35–75
　bedside echocardiogram, 39–42
　bedside ultrasound (DVT), 51–55
　cardiac CT angiography (CCTA), 56–58
　chest radiograph, 36–38
　CMR imaging, 59–61
　CT angiography (pulmonary embolism), 62–63
　Doppler ultrasound (peripheral arterial system), 70–71
　Doppler ultrasound (peripheral venous system), 66–69
　transesophageal echocardiography (TEE), 46–50
　transthoracic echocardiography (TTE), 43–45
　ultrasound guided vascular access, 72–75
　V/Q scan, 64–65
Cardioversion, 265–266
　aortic stenosis, 198
　restrictive cardiomyopathy, 190
　SVT, 108, 237
　torsades de pointes, 139
　VT, 137
　WPW syndrome, 117, 118
Carditis, 221t

Carotid artery, 72f, 73f
Carotid sinus hypersensitivity, 84
Carpentier-Edwards Magna pericardial valve, 9f
Carpentier-Edwards porcine valve, 9f
Catecholamines, 214
Catheterization (subclavian vein), 72f
Catheterization laboratories, 257
Catheterization procedures, 256–260
Caval index, 39
CCTA. See Cardiac CT angiography (CCTA)
Cell-to-cell conduction, 14f
Central venous access, 72–74
Cephalic vein, 74f
CF vein. See Common femoral (CF) vein
CHB. See Complete heart block (CHB)
CHD. See Congenital heart disease (CHD)
Chest radiograph, 36–38
　3-month-old with VSD, 218f
　aortic dissection, 172
　aortic stenosis, 197f
　biventricular pacemaker, 85f
　cardiomegaly, 232f
　dilated cardiomyopathy, 189f
　dual-coil ICD, 88f
　LVAD and implantable defibrillator, 91f
　mitral regurgitation, 205
　mitral stenosis, 199f
　myocarditis, 226f
　pacemaker wire fracture, 86f
　RV pacemaker lead tip, 84f
　transvenous pacemaker wire, 82f
　water bottle heart, 235f
Children. See Pediatric cardiology
Chordae tendineae, 5f, 6
Chronic aortic valve insufficiency, 224
Chronic mitral regurgitation, 203
Chronic obstructive pulmonary disease (COPD), 43
Circumflex artery, 2f, 3f
Circumflex artery occlusion, 24, 25f
Classic atrial flutter, 124
Clonidine, 102
CMR imaging. See Cardiac magnetic resonance (CMR) imaging
Coarctation of the aorta (CoA), 217, 222f
Cocaine, 144
Codominant system, 26
Colchicine, 229
Combination ICD-pacemaker, 88
Common femoral artery, 71f
Common femoral (CF) vein, 52f, 66f, 67f, 68f
Complete heart block (CHB), 153
Computed tomography pulmonary angiography (CTPA), 178
Concealed WPW syndrome, 107t
Conduction disorders
　bifascicular block, 155–156
　first-degree AV block, 146–148
　left anterior fascicular block (LAFB), 157–158
　left bundle branch block (LBBB), 161

Conduction disorders (*continued*)
   long QT syndrome (LQTS), 162–163
   right bundle branch block (RBBB), 159–160
   second-degree AV block, Mobitz type I, 149–150
   second-degree AV block, Mobitz type II, 151–152
   third-degree AV block, 153–154
Congenital bicuspid aortic valve, 196
Congenital heart disease (CHD), 214–224
   infants/toddlers, 217–220
   neonates, 214–216
   older children/adolescents, 221–224
Congestive heart failure, 43
Conjunctival injection with limbic sparing, 230f
Continuous monitor, 94
Contrast-induced nephropathy, 63
Conus arteriosus, 5f
COPD. *See* Chronic obstructive pulmonary disease (COPD)
CoreValve transcatheter pericardial valve, 9f
Coronary arteries, 2–3
Coronary artery bypass grafting (CABG), 257–258
Coronary artery stenosis, 59
Coronary calcium scoring, 56
Coronary veins, 3
Corrected QT interval (QTc)
   Bazett formula, 213
   LQTS, 163, 163f, 249
   prolonged QTc interval, 17
   sudden cardiac death, 250
CPR. *See* Cardiopulmonary resuscitation (CPR)
Cribier-Edwards transcatheter pericardial valve, 9f
Crista terminalis, 5f
CT angiography (pulmonary embolism), 62–63
CT coronary angiography (CTCA), 11
CT-guided percutaneous drainage, 264
CT venography (CTV), 62
CTCA. *See* CT coronary angiography (CTCA)
CTPA. *See* Computed tomography pulmonary angiography (CTPA)
CTV. *See* CT venography (CTV)
Cusps, 6
CXR. *See* Chest radiograph
Cyanosis, 214

D-dimer laboratory dimer, 178
D-shaped septum, 183f
D-shaped ventricle, 40
Deep femoral artery, 53f
Deep femoral vein, 53f
Deep vein thrombosis (DVT), 176–177
   bedside ultrasound, 51–55
   Doppler ultrasound, 66–69
Defibrillation, 265–266
   torsades de pointes, 139
   VF, 142
Defibrillation pads, 142f
Delta waves, 116, 116f, 117f, 247f
Depolarization-repolarization cycle, 14
DES. *See* Drug-eluting stent (DES)

Descending aorta, 3f
Descending aortic dissection, 173
Desquamation of the epidermis, 230f
Devices, 77–98
   ambulatory ECG, 94–95
   automated CPR device, 92–93
   external rhythm recorder, 94–95
   extracorporeal membrane oxygenation (ECMO), 96–98
   implanted cardioverter-defibrillator (ICD), 88–89
   left ventricular assist device (LVAD), 90–91
   pacemaker dysfunction, 84–87
   transcutaneous pacemaker, 78–80
   transvenous pacemaker, 81–83
Dextrocardia, 12
Dextrocardia without situs inversus, 12
Diagnostic catheterization, 256t
Diastolic dysfunction, 39
Digitalis, 129
Digoxin
   atrial fibrillation, 126
   Mobitz I block, 149
   restrictive cardiomyopathy, 190
   sinus bradycardia, 102
   third-degree heart block, 153
   VT, 138
Dilated cardiomyopathy, 188–189
Diltiazem
   atrial fibrillation, 126
   WPW syndrome, 117
Diuretics, 184t
   dilated cardiomyopathy, 189
   mitral regurgitation, 203
Dobutamine
   CMR imaging, 59
   mitral regurgitation, 203
Doppler ultrasound
   peripheral arterial system, 70–71
   peripheral venous system, 66–69
Drug-eluting stent (DES), 257–258
DTPA aerosol, 64
Dual antiplatelet therapy, 258
Dual AV nodal conduction, 109f
Dual-chamber pacemaker, 164–165, 165f, 166f
Dual chamber pacemaker tracking sinus rhythm, 165f
Dual chamber pacing, 166f
Dual-coil ICD, 88f
Dual-energy CT angiogram, 63f
Ductal-dependent systemic blood flow, 214
Duplex ultrasonography
   DVT, 51
   peripheral arterial system, 70–71
DVT. *See* Deep vein thrombosis (DVT)
Dyspnea, 199

E-point septal separation, 41f
EAT. *See* Ectopic atrial tachycardia (EAT)
Ebstein anomaly, 215f, 216f, 216v, 224f

ECG. *See* Electrocardiogram (ECG)
ECMO. *See* Extracorporeal membrane oxygenation (ECMO)
ECMO machine, 96f
ECMO oxygenator, 97f
ECMO sweep monitor, 97f
ECMO ventilation monitor, 97f
Ectopic atrial tachycardia (EAT), 108t, 122–123
Ejection fraction, 39, 40v, 42f
Electrical alternans, 235f
Electrical cardiac cycle, 14
Electrocardiogram (ECG), 13–34
    acute ischemia, 18–22
    arrhythmias. *See* Arrhythmias
    BSM, 20–21
    children, 208–213
    hyperacute T-waves, 29
    interpretation, 16–17
    interval measurements, 17t
    LVAD, 91f
    normal ECG waveform, 17t
    normal resting ECG, 16f
    pacemaker rhythms, 164–167
    PE, 178
    posterior leads, 19
    Q waves, 32
    right-sided leads, 20
    ST-segment depression, 30–31
    ST-segment elevation. *See* ST-segment elevation
    STEMI, 23–27
    T-wave inversion, 28
    third-degree heart block, 78f
    Wellens syndrome, 33–34
Electrolyte abnormalities, 144
Empty space, 73f
Enalaprilat, 184t
Endocarditis
    acute aortic insufficiency, 201
    mitral regurgitation, 203
Endomyocardial fibrosis, 191f
Enoxaparin, 178
Esmolol, 172, 184t
Esophageal rupture, 36t
Event type recorder, 94
Excitation-contraction coupling, 14
Exercise intolerance, 199
External jugular vein, 72f
External rhythm recorder, 94–95
Extracorporeal membrane oxygenation (ECMO), 96–98

Fabry disease, 191f
Factor V Leiden, 176, 176t
Familial AV conduction block, 241
FAST scan. *See* Focused abdominal sonography in trauma (FAST) scan
Fast-slow AVNRT, 107t, 111
Femoral artery, 53f, 73f
Femoral nerve, 73f

Femoral vein, 53f, 73f
Fibrinolytic therapy, 26
First-degree AV block, 146–148, 241f, 242f
Fixed 2:1 AV block, 151
Fluid overload, 188, 195
Focal atrial tachycardia, 108t, 122–123
Focused abdominal sonography in trauma (FAST) scan, 235
Fossa ovalis, 5f

Gadolinium, 59
Gap junction, 14f
Geneva rule, 178
Glycogen storage disease, 191f
Greater saphenous vein, 52f

Haloperidol, 162
Hampton's hump, 36t, 62f, 178f
Hancock Modified Orifice II porcine valve, 9f
HCM. *See* Hypertrophic cardiomyopathy (HCM)
Heart, 4
Heart block, 146–154
    children, 241–244
    first-degree AV block, 146–148
    second-degree AV block, Mobitz type I, 149–150
    second degree AV block, Mobitz type II, 151–152
    third-degree atrioventricular block, 153–154
Heart chambers, 4, 5f
Heart "dominance," 2–3, 25–26
Heart failure
    dilated cardiomyopathy, 188
    restrictive cardiomyopathy, 190
Heart rate, 100
Heart rhythm abnormalities. *See* Arrhythmias
Hemachromatosis, 191f
Hemodynamically unstable LVAD patient, 90
Hemopericardium, 263
Hemoptysis, 200
Heparin, 90, 176, 178
Hepatojugular reflux, 188
Hereditary thrombophilia, 176
His bundle, 14, 15f
HLHS. *See* Hypoplastic left heart syndrome (HLHS)
HOCM. *See* Hypertrophic obstructive cardiomyopathy (HOCM)
Holiday heart syndrome, 124
Holter monitor, 94–95
Holter monitor lead placement, 95f
Hyperacute T-waves, 29
Hyperkalemia, 29, 153
Hypertension, 181–184
Hypertensive emergencies, 181t
Hypertensive encephalopathy, 181t
Hypertensive retinopathy, 181t
Hyperthyroidism, 134
Hypertrophic cardiomyopathy (HCM), 193–195, 221, 223f
Hypertrophic obstructive cardiomyopathy (HOCM), 59, 61f, 193, 195f

Hypokalemia
    LQTS, 162
    PVC, 134
    ST-segment depression, 31
Hypomagnesemia, 134, 162
Hypoplastic left heart syndrome (HLHS), 214, 215f, 216v
Hypotension, 172
Hypothermia-induced bradycardia, 78
Hypothyroidism, 153
Hypoxia
    atrial flutter, 124
    multifocal atrial tachycardia, 120
    third-degree heart block, 153

ICD. *See* Implanted cardioverter-defibrillator (ICD)
ICD shocks, 88
Idiopathic hypertrophic subaortic stenosis (IHSS), 193
Idiopathic pericarditis, 229
Idiopathic restrictive cardiomyopathy, 191f
IHSS. *See* Idiopathic hypertrophic subaortic stenosis (IHSS)
Imaging studies. *See* Cardiovascular imaging
Implanted cardioverter-defibrillator (ICD), 88–89, 195
Inducible ischemia, 59
Infective endocarditis, 221t
Inferior myocardial infarction (MI), 20
Inferior vena cava (IVC), 5f, 39, 40f, 40v
Infiltrative cardiomyopathy, 59
Inflammatory and infectious disorders, 225–233
    Kawasaki disease (KD), 230–231
    myocarditis, 225–229
    pericarditis, 225–229
    rheumatic heart disease (RHD), 232–233
Inotropes, 189, 236
Intermittent monitor, 94
Internal jugular vein, 72f, 73f
Interstitial prominence, 38f
Intracranial hemorrhage, 181t
Inverted T wave, 17
Ischemic chest pain, 126
Ischemic heart disease, 59
Isoelectric line, 17f
Isoelectric signals, 22f
Isolated LAFB, 158
Isoproterenol, 139
IVC. *See* Inferior vena cava (IVC)

James fibers, 110f, 119
Jervell and Lange–Nielsen syndrome, 248
JET. *See* Junctional ectopic tachycardia (JET)
Jugular venous distention, 188
Junctional bradycardia, 243f
Junctional ectopic tachycardia (JET), 108t, 131, 132, 132f
Junctional escape rhythm, 129–130
Junctional rhythm
    junctional escape rhythm, 129–130
    junctional tachycardia, 131–132
Junctional tachycardia, 129, 131–132

Kawasaki disease (KD), 221t, 230–231
Kent bundle, 107t, 110f, 116
King of Hearts monitor, 94–95
King of Hearts monitor lead placement, 94f
Kussmaul sign, 235

LA. *See* Left atrium (LA)
Labetalol, 172, 184t
LAD. *See* Left anterior descending artery (LAD)
LAD occlusion. *See* Left anterior descending
    artery (LAD) occlusion
LAFB. *See* Left anterior fascicular block (LAFB)
Last drop phenomenon, 234
Lateral antebrachial cutaneous nerve, 74f
LBBB. *See* Left bundle branch block (LBBB)
LCA. *See* Left coronary artery (LCA)
Leaflets, 6
Left anterior descending artery (LAD), 2f, 3f, 23, 23f
Left anterior descending artery (LAD)
    occlusion, 31f
Left anterior fascicle, 15f, 157
Left anterior fascicular block (LAFB), 157–158
Left atrium (LA), 3f, 4, 5f
Left axis deviation, 157
Left bundle branch, 14
Left bundle branch block (LBBB), 26, 27f, 161
Left coronary artery (LCA), 2, 2f, 3f, 10, 23
Left coronary artery occlusion, 23
Left dominant heart, 2–3, 25–26
Left lateral decubitus position, 42
Left posterior fascicle, 15f
Left pulmonary artery, 3f
Left pulmonary vein, 3f
Left-sided obstructive lesions, 214
Left-sided pneumothorax, 85f
Left ventricle (LV), 3, 4, 5f
Left ventricular (LV) aneurysm, 185–186
Left ventricular assist device (LVAD), 90–91
Left ventricular (LV) hypertrophy, 193
Left ventricular thrombus, 45f
LGL syndrome. *See* Lown–Ganong–Levine (LGL) syndrome
Lidocaine, 261
    AIVR, 135
    torsades de pointes, 139
    VF, 142
    VT, 138
LifePak 15 multifunction cardiac monitor/defibrillator, 265
LifeStat system, 92f
Lithium, 129
LMCA. *See* Left main coronary artery (LMCA)
LMWH. *See* Low-molecular-weight heparin (LMWH)
Loeffler cardiomyopathy, 191f
Long QT syndrome (LQTS), 139
    adults, 162–163
    children, 248–250
Long-short rule, 128
Loop recorder, 94

Loss of pacemaker capture, 165
Low cardiac output states, 83
Low-molecular-weight heparin (LMWH), 176
Lower extremity arterial disease, 70t
Lown–Ganong–Levine (LGL) syndrome, 108t, 110f, 119
LQTS. See Long QT syndrome (LQTS)
LUCAS chest compression system, 92f
LV. See Left ventricle (LV)
LV aneurysm. See Left ventricular (LV) aneurysm
LVAD. See Left ventricular assist device (LVAD)

Magnesium sulfate
   torsades de pointes, 139
   VT, 138
Mahaim fiber tachycardia, 108t, 110f
Main pulmonary artery, 3f
Manual defibrillator, 265
Marfan syndrome valvular disease, 221t
Marginal artery, 2f
MAT. See Multifocal atrial tachycardia (MAT)
McCullen's sign, 44f
Mechanical CPR device, 92–93
Mechanical valves, 8–9
Median antebrachial cutaneous nerve, 74f
Median antebrachial vein, 74f
Medical procedures. See Procedures
Medtronic Freestyle stentless valve, 9f
Metabolic acidosis, 214
Methadone, 139
Metoprolol, 121
MI. See Myocardial infarction (MI)
Mitral incompetence, 203
Mitral insufficiency, 203
Mitral regurgitation, 44f, 50f, 203–205, 219f, 233f, 233v
Mitral stenosis, 199–200
Mitral valve, 5f, 6, 6f
Mitroflow pericardial valve, 9f
Mobitz type I block, 149–150
Mobitz type II block, 151–152, 242f
Moderator band, 5f
Monomorphic ventricular tachycardia (VT), 137
Monophasic defibrillator, 265
Monophasic waveform (Doppler ultrasound), 70v
Mosaic stented porcine valve, 9f
Multifocal atrial tachycardia (MAT), 105, 108t, 120–121
Multiform premature ventricular contraction (PVC), 134
Mural thrombus, 169, 171f
Musculi pectinati, 5f
Myocardial bridging, 10, 11f
Myocardial infarction (MI). See also Acute myocardial infarction (AMI)
   aortic dissection, 172
   ventricular tachycardia, 138
Myocardial ischemia, 43, 138
Myocardial necrosis, 266

Myocarditis, 225–229
Myocardium, 5f

Neck, 72f
Neonatal lupus, 241
Nicardipine, 184t
Nifedipine, 173
Nitrates, 203
Nitroglycerin, 184t, 189
Nitroprusside
   acute aortic insufficiency, 202
   aortic dissection, 172
   hypertension, 184t
   mitral regurgitation, 205
Noncontrast cardiac CT exam, 56
Nonsteroidal anti-inflammatory medications, 229
Normal cardiac conduction, 14–15

Obstructive shock, 234–236
Obtuse marginal, 23f, 24f
Open heart surgery, 124
Opiate analgesics, 139
Orthodromic AV reciprocating tachycardia, 107t, 113, 116
Overdrive pacing, 78, 80
Oversensing, 165

P wave, 16, 17f
PAC. See Premature atrial complex (PAC)
Pacemaker
   complications, 84–87
   ECG interpretation, 164–167
   hematoma, 87
   infection, 87
   lead dislodgement, 85
   lead fracture, 86
   lead perforation, 86–87
   loss of pacemaker capture, 165
   oversensing, 165
   pneumothorax, 85
   skin erosion, 87
   transcutaneous, 78–80
   transvenous, 81–83
   undersensing, 165, 166f
Pacemaker dysfunction, 84–87
Pacemaker wire fracture, 86f
Pacing spikes, 164
PAD. See Peripheral arterial disease (PAD)
Palla sign, 178f
Papillary muscle rupture, 44f, 49f
Papillary muscles, 5f
Patent aortic lumen, 169, 171f
Patent ductus arteriosus (PDA), 214, 217, 220f
Pathological Q wave, 17
PCI. See Percutaneous coronary intervention (PCI)
PDA. See Patent ductus arteriosus (PDA)
PE. See Pulmonary embolus (PE)
Peak systolic velocity (PSV), 70t

Peaked T wave, 17, 29
Pediatric cardiology, 207–250
   cardiac rhythm disorders, 237–250
   cardiac tamponade, 234–236
   congenital heart disease, 214–224
   heart block, 241–244
   infantile congenital heart disease, 217–220
   inflammatory and infectious disorders, 225–233
   Kawasaki disease (KD), 230–231
   long QT syndrome (LQTS), 248–250
   myocarditis, 225–229
   neonatal congenital heart disease, 214–216
   normal ECG values, 208–213
   normal variants of cardiac rhythm, 213t
   obstructive shock, 234–236
   pediatric congenital heart disease, 221–224
   pericarditis, 225–229
   rheumatic heart disease (RHD), 232–233
   SVT, 237–240, 247
   WPW syndrome, 245–247
Penetrating thoracic injury, 234
PERC. See Pulmonary embolism rule-out criteria (PERC)
Percutaneous coronary intervention (PCI), 256, 258
Pericardial effusion, 39, 39f, 42, 45, 45f, 172, 236f, 261, 261f, 262v, 263f
Pericardial fluid accumulation, 261
Pericardial window, 263–264
Pericardiocentesis, 261–262
Pericardiostomy, 263–264
Pericarditis, 225–229
Peripheral arterial disease (PAD), 254
Peripheral arterial system, 70–71
Peripheral edema, 188
Peripheral venous access, 72, 74–75
Peripheral venous system, 66–69
Permanent junctional reciprocating tachycardia (PJRT), 131, 131f
Phenylephrine, 236
Phenytoin, 139
Philips Heartstart FRx defibrillator, 265
Phlegmasia alba dolens, 176
Phlegmasia cerulea dolens, 176, 176f
Piston chest compression device, 92, 92f
PJRT. See Permanent junctional reciprocating tachycardia (PJRT)
Pleural effusion, 38f, 263f
Pneumonia, 36t
Pneumothorax
   chest radiograph, 36t
   ICD, 85, 88
   pacemaker, 85
Point-of-care (POC) ultrasound, 235
Polymorphic ventricular tachycardia (VT), 137
Popliteal artery, 53f
Popliteal vein, 53f, 54f
Popliteal vein trifurcation, 54f
Positive pressure ventilation, 42
Posterior descending artery, 2f, 25
Posterior descending artery occlusion, 25–26, 26f

Posterior myocardial infarction, 18
Posterior myocardial infarction (MI), 19, 19f, 24
Posterior reversible encephalopathy syndrome (PRES), 181f
Posterior STEMI, 19f
Potassium, 138
P–P interval, 151
PR interval, 16, 17f
PR segment, 17f
Preexcitation, 116, 245
Preexcitation syndrome, 118
Premature atrial complex (PAC), 103–104
Premature ventricular con-traction (PVC), 133–134, 245
PRES. See Posterior reversible encephalopathy syndrome (PRES)
Principles of cardiovascular imaging. See Cardiovascular imaging
Procainamide
   SVT (children), 237
   VT, 137
Procedures, 251–266
   ankle brachial index (ABI), 254–255
   cardiac catheterization, 256–260
   cardioversion/external defibrillation, 265–266
   pericardial window, 263–264
   pericardiocentesis, 261–262
   radiofrequency ablation, 252–253
Prolonged QT interval, 249f
Prolonged QT syndrome, 162
Prolonged QTc interval, 17
Prostaglandin E1, 214
Prosthetic valves, 8–9
Protein C deficiency, 176t
Protein S deficiency, 176t
Pseudo-RBBB, 160
PSV. See Peak systolic velocity (PSV)
Pulmonary artery, 2f
Pulmonary CT angiogram, 62–63
Pulmonary edema, 36t, 38f, 49f
Pulmonary embolism (PE), 178–180
   atrial flutter, 124
   chest radiograph, 36t
   CT angiogram, 62–63
   DVT, 176
   RBBB, 159
   TTE, 43
   V/Q scan, 64
Pulmonary embolism rule-out criteria (PERC), 178
Pulmonary hypertension, 182, 182f, 183f, 221t
Pulmonary insufficiency, 222f
Pulmonary rales, 188
Pulmonary stenosis, 159
Pulmonary trunk, 5f
Pulmonary valve, 5f, 6f
Pulmonary vascular congestion, 189f
Pulsed Doppler imaging (superficial femoral vein), 68f
Pulseless ventricular tachycardia (VT), 137
Pulsus paradoxus, 235

Purkinje fibers, 15f
PVC. *See* Premature ventricular contraction (PVC)

Q wave, 17, 17f, 32
QRS complex, 16
QRS duration, 17f
QT interval, 17, 17f, 248f, 250
QT-prolonging drugs, 139
QTc interval. *See* Corrected QT interval (QTc)

R wave, 17
R-wave progression, 17
RA. *See* Right atrium (RA)
Radiofrequency (RF) ablation, 252–253
Rate-related RBBB, 159
RBBB. *See* Right bundle branch block (RBBB)
RCA. *See* Right coronary artery (RCA)
RCM. *See* Restrictive cardiomyopathy (RCM)
Recalcitrant tachyarrhythmia, 78
Reentrant tachycardia, 245
Regadenoson, 59
Respiratory variation of vena cava, 40v
Restrictive cardiomyopathy (RCM), 190–192
Return of spontaneous circulation (ROSC), 143
Revascularization, 257–258
RF ablation. *See* Radiofrequency (RF) ablation
RHD. *See* Rheumatic heart disease (RHD)
Rheumatic fever, 196, 232
Rheumatic heart disease (RHD), 221t, 232–233
Right atrium (RA), 3f, 4
Right auricle, 5f
Right bundle branch, 14, 15f
Right bundle branch block (RBBB), 159–160
Right coronary artery (RCA), 2, 2f, 3f, 24
Right coronary artery occlusion, 24–25, 25f
Right dominant heart, 2, 2f, 3, 25
Right heart catheterization, 258
Right marginal artery, 24
Right pulmonary artery, 3f
Right pulmonary vein, 3f
Right ventricle (RV), 4, 5f
Right ventricular hypertrophy (RVH), 208
Right ventricular (RV) infarction, 18, 20f
Romano–Ward syndrome, 248
ROSC. *See* Return of spontaneous circulation (ROSC)
R-to-R interval
    Ashman phenomenon, 128
    Mobitz I block, 149
    PVC, 133f, 134f
    RBBB, 159
R-on-T phenomenon, 134
Ruptured AAA, 170, 171f
RV. *See* Right ventricle (RV)
RV infarction. *See* Right ventricular (RV) infarction
RV lead perforation, 86f
RVH. *See* Right ventricular hypertrophy (RVH)

S wave, 17, 17f
SA node. *See* Sinoatrial (SA) node
Salicylates, 233
Sarcoidosis, 191f
SCD. *See* Sudden cardiac death (SCD)
Second-degree AV block, Mobitz type I, 149–150
Second-degree AV block, Mobitz type II, 151–152, 242f
Seldinger technique, 257–258
Semiautomatic defibrillator, 265
Semilunar valves, 6, 7f
Septal Q wave, 193
Serial cardiac enzymes, 229
Sgarbossa criteria, 26
Sick sinus syndrome, 84
Sickle cell anemia, 221t
Simpson's method of disks, 42f
Sinoatrial (SA) node, 14, 15f
Sinus arrhythmia, 102
Sinus bradycardia, 102, 241
Sinus node reentry tachycardia (SNRT), 108, 108t
Sinus tachycardia, 100–101, 179f
Situs inversus totalis, 12, 12f
Situs inversus with dextrocardia, 12
Situs inversus with levocardia, 12
SLE. *See* Systemic lupus erythematosus (SLE)
Slow-fast AVNRT, 107t, 111
Slow-slow AVNRT, 111–112
SNRT. *See* Sinus node reentry tachycardia (SNRT)
Sodium nitroprusside, 172. *See* Nitroprusside
S1Q3T3 pattern, 178
ST-elevation myocardial infarction (STEMI), 23–27
    cardiac catheterization, 256
    circumflex artery occlusion, 24
    ED care and disposition, 26–27
    left coronary artery occlusion, 23
    posterior descending artery occlusion, 25–26
    right coronary artery occlusion, 24–25
    Sgarbossa criteria, 26
ST segment, 17, 17f
ST-segment depression, 30–31
    BSM torso color display, 22f
    posterior AMI, 19f
    subendocardial ischemia, 31
ST-segment elevation
    BSM torso color display, 22f
    circumflex artery occlusion, 25f
    inferior leads, 18f
    left anterior descending artery occlusion, 31f
    PDA occlusion, 26f
    posterior AMI, 19f
    RCA occlusion, 25f
    transmural infarction, 31
    V1R-V6R, 20f
Stanford Type A aortic dissection, 172, 173f
Stanford Type B aortic dissection, 172, 181f
STEMI. *See* ST-elevation myocardial infarction (STEMI)
Stress, 134

Stress-induced cardiomyopathy, 43
Stress test, 34
Subarachnoid hemorrhage, 181t
Subendocardial ischemia, 31
Sudden cardiac death (SCD), 195, 265
Superficial femoral artery, 53f
Superficial femoral vein, 53f, 68f
Superficial veins, 69f
Superficial venous thrombosis, 69f
Superior vena cava, 3f, 5f
Supraventricular tachycardia (SVT)
  adults, 107–127. See also Arrhythmias
  children, 237–240, 247
Surgical procedures. See Procedures
SVT. See Supraventricular tachycardia (SVT)
Swan-Ganz catheter, 258
Sympathomimetic drugs, 134
Synchronized cardioversion, 265, 266. See also Cardioversion
Systemic hypertension, 181
Systemic lupus erythematosus (SLE), 196
Systolic blood pressure reading, 254f
Systolic dysfunction, 42f

T wave, 17, 17f
T-wave inversion, 28, 31f
Takotsubo cardiomyopathy, 43, 43f
Tall T waves, 29
TAPVR. See Totally anomalous pulmonary venous return (TAPVR)
Tc99m. See Technetium-99m (Tc99m)
TdP. See Torsades de pointes (TdP)
Technegas, 64
Technetium-99m (Tc99m), 64
TEE. See Transesophageal echocardiography (TEE)
Temporary transvenous pacing generator, 82f
TGA. See Transposition of the great arteries (TGA)
Third-degree atrioventricular block, 78f, 153–154
Thoracic aortic dissection, 43
Thoracoscopic approach for pericardiostomy, 263–264
Thrombosed veins, 67
Thyroid stimulating hormone, 127
Tilting disc valve, 8f, 9
Tissue plasminogen activator (tPA), 178
Toronto Stentless porcine valve, 9f
Torsades de pointes (TdP), 137, 138f, 139–140
Totally anomalous pulmonary venous return (TAPVR), 214
tPA. See Tissue plasminogen activator (tPA)
Trabeculae carneae, 5f
Transcutaneous pacemaker, 78–80
Transesophageal echocardiography (TEE), 46–50
Transmural infarction, 31
Transposition of the great arteries (TGA), 214, 215f, 216v
Transradial approach to cardiac catheterization, 259
Transthoracic echocardiography (TTE), 43–45
Transvenous pacemaker, 81–83
Tricuspid atresia, 216f, 216v
Tricuspid valve, 5f, 6

Trigeminy, 133
Triphasic femoral artery spectral waveform, 71f
Triphasic waveform (Doppler ultrasound), 70, 70v
TTE. See Transthoracic echocardiography (TTE)
Twisting of the points, 139
2:1 AV block, 151
Type A dissection, 48f
Type I atrial flutter, 124
Type I Brugada tachycardia, 144, 144f
Type II Brugada tachycardia, 144, 144f
Type III Brugada tachycardia, 144, 145f
Typical atrial flutter, 124

U wave, 17, 17f
Ultrasound guided pericardiocentesis, 261
Ultrasound guided vascular access, 72–75
Undersensing, 165, 166f
Upper extremity, 74f
Upper extremity arterial duplex, 70t

VA ECMO. See Venoarterial extracorporeal membrane oxygenation (ECMO)
Vagal maneuvers
  AVNRT, 112
  AVRT, 114
  SNRT, 108
  SVT, 237
  WPW syndrome, 117
Vagal tone, 144
Vascular disease, 169–186
  abdominal aortic aneurysm (AAA), 170–171
  acute arterial occlusion, 174, 175f
  aortic dissection, 172–173
  deep vein thrombosis (DVT), 176–177
  hypertension, 181–184
  left ventricular (LV) aneurysm, 185–186
  pulmonary embolism (PE), 178–180
Vasodilation, 189
Vena cava, 2f
Vena cava size, 40f
Vena mediana cubiti, 74f
Venoarterial extracorporeal membrane oxygenation (ECMO), 96–97
Venous thrombosis, 176
Venovenous extracorporeal membrane oxygenation (ECMO), 96–97
Ventilation/perfusion scan (V/Q scan), 64–65, 178
Ventricular arrhythmia
  accelerated idioventricular rhythm (AIVR), 135–136
  Brugada syndrome, 144–145
  premature ventricular contraction (PVC), 133–134
  torsades de pointes (TdP), 139–140
  ventricular fibrillation (VF), 141–143
  ventricular tachycardia (VT), 137–138
Ventricular fibrillation (VF), 78, 80, 141–143
Ventricular preexcitation physiology, 114
Ventricular septal defect (VSD), 215f, 216f, 216v, 217, 218f

Ventricular systole, 14
Ventricular tachycardia (VT), 80, 137–138
Ventricular undersensing, 166f
Verapamil
    MAT, 120
    WPW syndrome, 117
VF. *See* Ventricular fibrillation (VF)
Video-assisted thoracoscopic pericardial window, 264f
Virchow triad, 177
Volume depletion, 195
V/Q scan. *See* Ventilation/perfusion scan (V/Q scan)
VSD. *See* Ventricular septal defect (VSD)
VT. *See* Ventricular tachycardia (VT)
VV ECMO. *See* Venovenous extracorporeal membrane oxygenation (ECMO)

Wall motion abnormalities, 41v
Wandering atrial pacemaker (WAP), 105–106

WAP. *See* Wandering atrial pacemaker (WAP)
Warfarin, 177
Water bottle heart, 235, 235f
Wellens syndrome, 33–34
Wells criteria, 178
Wenckebach block, 149
Westermark sign, 36t
Wicki criteria, 178
Widow maker lesion, 33
Wolff–Parkinson–White (WPW) syndrome
    adults, 110f, 116–118
    children, 245–247
    WPW syndrome with narrow complex SVT, 107t
    WPW syndrome with wide complex SVT, 108t
WPW syndrome. *See* Wolff–Parkinson–White (WPW) syndrome

X-ray. *See* Chest radiograph
Xenon-133, 64